Practical Urology
for the General Surgeon

Editors

LISA T. BEAULE
MORITZ H. HANSEN

SURGICAL CLINICS
OF NORTH AMERICA

www.surgical.theclinics.com

Consulting Editor
RONALD F. MARTIN

June 2016 • Volume 96 • Number 3

ELSEVIER

1600 John F. Kennedy Boulevard • Suite 1800 • Philadelphia, Pennsylvania, 19103-2899

http://www.surgical.theclinics.com

SURGICAL CLINICS OF NORTH AMERICA Volume 96, Number 3
June 2016 ISSN 0039–6109, ISBN-13: 978-0-323-44636-5

Editor: John Vassallo, j.vassallo@elsevier.com
Developmental Editor: Colleen Viola

Photocopying

Single photocopies of single articles may be made for personal use as allowed by national copyright laws. Permission of the Publisher and payment of a fee is required for all other photocopying, including multiple or systematic copying, copying for advertising or promotional purposes, resale, and all forms of document delivery. Special rates are available for educational institutions that wish to make photocopies for non-profit educational classroom use. For information on how to seek permission visit www.elsevier.com/permissions or call: (+44) 1865 843830 (UK)/(+1) 215 239 3804 (USA).

Derivative Works

Subscribers may reproduce tables of contents or prepare lists of articles including abstracts for internal circulation within their institutions. Permission of the Publisher is required for resale or distribution outside the institution. Permission of the Publisher is required for all other derivative works, including compilations and translations (please consult www.elsevier.com/permissions).

Electronic Storage or Usage

Permission of the Publisher is required to store or use electronically any material contained in this periodical, including any article or part of an article (please consult www.elsevier.com/permissions). Except as outlined above, no part of this publication may be reproduced, stored in a retrieval system or transmitted in any form or by any means, electronic, mechanical, photocopying, recording or otherwise, without prior written permission of the Publisher.

Notice

No responsibility is assumed by the Publisher for any injury and/or damage to persons or property as a matter of products liability, negligence or otherwise, or from any use or operation of any methods, products, instructions or ideas contained in the material herein. Because of rapid advances in the medical sciences, in particular, independent verification of diagnoses and drug dosages should be made.

Although all advertising material is expected to conform to ethical (medical) standards, inclusion in this publication does not constitute a guarantee or endorsement of the quality or value of such product or of the claims made of it by its manufacturer.

Surgical Clinics of North America (ISSN 0039–6109) is published bimonthly by Elsevier Inc., 360 Park Avenue South, New York, NY 10010-1710. Months of publication are February, April, June, August, October, and December. Business and Editorial Offices: 1600 John F. Kennedy Blvd., Suite 1800, Philadelphia, PA 19103-2899. Periodicals postage paid at New York, NY and additional mailing offices. Subscription prices are $375.00 per year for US individuals, $707.00 per year for US institutions, $100.00 per year for US students and residents, $455.00 per year for Canadian individuals, $895.00 per year for Canadian institutions, $510.00 for international individuals, $895.00 per year for international institutions and $250.00 per year for Canadian and foreign students/residents. To receive student/resident rate, orders must be accompanied by name of affiliated institution, date of term, and the signature of program/residency coordinator on institution letterhead. Orders will be billed at individual rate until proof of status is received. Foreign air speed delivery is included in all Clinics subscription prices. All prices are subject to change without notice. POSTMASTER: Send address changes to Surgical Clinics, Elsevier Health Sciences Division, Subscription Customer Service, 3251 Riverport Lane, Maryland Heights, MO 63043. **Customer Service (orders, claims, online, change of address): Telephone: 1-800-654-2452 (U.S. and Canada); 314-447-8871 (outside U.S. and Canada). Fax: 314-447-8029. E-mail: journalscustomerservice-usa@elsevier.com (for print support); journalsonline support-usa@elsevier.com (for online support).**

Reprints. For copies of 100 or more, of articles in this publication, please contact the Commercial Reprints Department, Elsevier Inc., 360 Park Avenue South, New York, New York 10010-1710. Tel. 212-633-3874, Fax: 212-633-3820, E-mail: reprints@elsevier.com.

The Surgical Clinics of North America is also published in Spanish by McGraw-Hill Interamericana Editores S.A., P.O. Box 5-237 06500 Mexico D.F. Mexico; and in Portuguese by Interlivros Edicoes Ltda., Rua Comandante Coelho 1085, CEP 21250, Rio de Janeiro, Brazil; and in Greek by Paschalidis Medical Publications, Athens Greece.

The Surgical Clinics of North America is covered in MEDLINE/PubMed (Index Medicus), EMBASE/Excerpta Medica, Current Contents/Clinical Medicine, Current Contents/Life Sciences, Science Citation Index, and ISI/BIOMED.

Contributors

CONSULTING EDITOR

RONALD F. MARTIN, MD, FACS
Lead Surgeon, York Hospital System, York, Maine; Colonel (ret.), United States Army Reserve

EDITORS

LISA T. BEAULE, MD
Co-Chief and Medical Director, Division of Urology, Maine Medical Center, Assistant Clinical Professor, Tufts University School of Medicine, Portland, Maine

MORITZ H. HANSEN, MD
Division of Urology, Maine Medical Center, Assistant Clinical Professor, Tufts University School of Medicine, Portland, Maine

AUTHORS

ILIJA ALEKSIC, MD
Resident, Division of Urology, Albany Medical College, Albany, New York

GABRIELLA J. AVELLINO, MD
Urology Resident, Department of Urology, Boston Medical Center, Boston University School of Medicine, Boston, Massachusetts

LISA T. BEAULE, MD
Co-Chief and Medical Director, Division of Urology, Maine Medical Center, Assistant Clinical Professor, Tufts University School of Medicine, Portland, Maine

GABRIEL V. BELANGER, MD
Chief Resident, Division of Urology, Maine Medical Center, Portland, Maine

SANCHITA BOSE, MD
Urology Resident, Department of Urology, Boston Medical Center, Boston University School of Medicine, Boston, Massachusetts

DAVID J. CHALMERS, MD
Division of Urology, Maine Medical Center, Assistant Clinical Professor, Tufts University School of Medicine, Portland, Maine

ELISE J.B. DE, MD
Associate Professor of Surgery, Division of Urology, Albany Medical College, Albany, New York

HARCHARAN S. GILL, MD, FRCS, FACS
Professor of Urology, Department of Urology, Stanford University Hospital, Stanford, California

MORITZ H. HANSEN, MD
Division of Urology, Maine Medical Center, Assistant Clinical Professor, Tufts University School of Medicine, Portland, Maine

MATTHEW HAYN, MD
Division of Urology, Maine Medical Center, Assistant Clinical Professor, Tufts University School of Medicine, Portland, Maine

JOHANN P. INGIMARSSON, MD
Fellow in Endourology, Department of Urology, Mayo Clinic, Rochester, Minnesota

ARJUN KHOSLA, MD
Division of Urology, Department of Surgery, Beth Israel Deaconess Medical Center, Instructor In Surgery, Harvard Medical School, Boston, Massachusetts

URSZULA KOWALIK, MD
Urology Resident, University of Vermont Medical Center, Burlington, Vermont

AMY E. KRAMBECK, MD
Professor, Department of Urology, Mayo Clinic, Rochester, Minnesota

GARJAE LAVIEN, MD
Fellow, Genitourinary Cancer Survivorship, Genitourinary Survivorship Program, Division of Urology, Duke University Medical Center, Durham, North Carolina

ADAM E. LUDVIGSON, MD
Resident, Division of Urology, Maine Medical Center, Portland, Maine

JESSICA MANDEVILLE, MD
Department of Urology, Lahey Hospital and Medical Center, Burlington, Massachusetts

ROBERT C. McDONOUGH III, MD
Division of Urology, Maine Medical Center, Assistant Clinical Professor, Tufts University School of Medicine, Portland, Maine

ARTHUR MOURTZINOS, MD, MBA
Department of Urology, Lahey Hospital and Medical Center, Burlington, Massachusetts

PATRICK MURRAY, MD
Division of Urology, Maine Medical Center, Resident, Tufts University School of Medicine, Portland, Maine

VERNON M. PAIS Jr, MD
Associate Professor, Section of Urology, Department of Surgery, Geisel School of Medicine at Dartmouth, Hanover, New Hampshire; Section of Urology, Dartmouth Hitchcock Medical Center, Lebanon, New Hampshire

ANDREW C. PETERSON, MD
Associate Professor of Surgery, Genitourinary Survivorship Program, Division of Urology, Duke University Medical Center, Durham, North Carolina

MARK K. PLANTE, MD, FRCS(C), FACS
Chief, Division of Urology, Department of Surgery, University of Vermont Medical Center, Urology Residency Program Director, Director of Urologic Research, Associate Professor of Surgery, University of Vermont College of Medicine, Burlington, Vermont

STEPHEN T. RYAN, MD
Resident, Division of Urology, Maine Medical Center, Portland, Maine

ALEX J. VANNI, MD, FACS
Department of Urology, Lahey Hospital and Medical Center, Assistant Professor, Tufts University School of Medicine, Burlington, Massachusetts

VIJAYA M. VEMULAKONDA, MD, JD
Department of Pediatric Urology, Children's Hospital Colorado, Aurora, Colorado

GRAHAM T. VERLEE, MD
Division of Urology, Maine Medical Center, Assistant Clinical Professor, Tufts University School of Medicine, Portland, Maine

ANDREW A. WAGNER, MD
Division of Urology, Department of Surgery, Beth Israel Deaconess Medical Center, Assistant Professor of Surgery, Harvard Medical School, Boston, Massachusetts

DAVID S. WANG, MD
Associate Professor, Department of Urology, Boston Medical Center, Boston University School of Medicine, Boston, Massachusetts

UWAIS ZAID, MD
Fellow, Genitourinary Reconstruction, Genitourinary Survivorship Program, Division of Urology, Duke University Medical Center, Durham, North Carolina

LEONARD N. ZINMAN, MD
Department of Urology, Lahey Hospital and Medical Center, Professor, Tufts University School of Medicine, Burlington, Massachusetts

Contents

expedient bladder decompression is important for long-term outcomes. Age, benign prostatic hyperplasia, and lower urinary tract symptoms are patient factors that predispose to retention. Surgery-related factors include operative time, intravenous fluid administration, type of anesthesia, and procedure type. The mainstay for treatment in the acute setting is Foley catheter placement. Starting alpha-blockers in men is also indicated as they increase voiding trial success. Long-term solutions for chronic retention include a variety of surgeries, with transurethral prostatectomy as the gold standard.

Surgical intervention for female voiding dysfunction is common, involving a single or multifaceted approach affecting multiple organ systems in the pelvis. Surgical success relies on knowledge of surgical history, anatomic approaches, and judicious use of supports or materials. Due to the varied repairs used over the last few decades, it is important for the general surgeon to understand both current and historic approaches. This understanding will help in planning future pelvic surgery as well as in evaluating current ramifications of prior surgery.

 Video content accompanies this article at http://www.surgical. theclinics.com

Benign prostatic hypertrophy (BPH) is a common cause of voiding dysfunction. BPH may lead to bladder outlet obstruction and resultant troublesome lower urinary tract symptoms. Initial management of BPH and bladder outlet obstruction is typically conservative. However, when symptoms are severe or refractory to medical therapy or when urinary retention, bladder stone formation, recurrent urinary tract infections, or upper urinary tract deterioration occur, surgical intervention is often necessary. Numerous options are available for surgical management of BPH ranging from simple office-based procedures to transurethral operative procedures and even open and robotic surgeries. This article reviews the current, most commonly used techniques available for surgical management of BPH.

Microscopic and gross hematuria present unique and difficult diagnostic and management challenges in the already complex general surgery patient. This article provides the general surgeon with relevant knowledge in the pathophysiology, anatomy, etiologies, workup, and treatments of hematuria. In addition common causes of hematuria that may be encountered by the general surgeon (including trauma, urinary tract infection, urolithiasis, and malignancy) are reviewed. Additionally, the difficult to manage clinical situation of clot urinary retention is presented. This article provides a urologic framework of thinking for the clinician to best manage a general surgery patient who has hematuria.

Nephrolithiasis is a common affliction, affecting approximately 10% of adults. Potentially presenting with acute abdominal or flank pain, nausea, or emesis, it may pose as a general surgical condition. Therefore, recognition, diagnosis, and management concerns are pertinent to the general surgeon. Furthermore, the risk of nephrolithiasis is increased in common general surgical conditions, including inflammatory bowel disease, hyperparathyroidism, and short gut. Nephrolithiasis may be induced as a result of general surgical interventions, including gastric bypass and bowel resection with ileostomy. An understanding of this common disease will improve coordination of patient care between urologists and general surgeons.

Genitourinary prosthetics are used for correction of functional deficits and to improve the quality of lives of affected patients. General surgeons must evaluate patients scheduled for nonurologic surgery with urologic devices that can impact their perioperative management. Lack of recognition of these prosthetics preoperatively can lead to unnecessary morbidity for the patient and have legal implications for the surgeon. Close consultation with a urologist may avoid common complications associated with these devices and allows for surgical assistance when operative misadventures do occur. This article reviews 3 common urologic prosthetics: testicular prosthesis, artificial urinary sphincter, and penile prosthesis.

Pediatric urology spans the neonatal period through the transition into early adulthood. There are a variety of common pediatric urologic conditions that overlap significantly with pediatric surgery. This article reviews the pertinent pathophysiology of a few key disease processes, including the pediatric inguinal hernia and/or hydrocele, cryptorchidism, and circumcision. General surgeons may find themselves in the position of managing these problems primarily, particularly in rural areas that may lack pediatric subspecialization. An understanding of the fundamentals can guide appropriate initial management. Additional focus is devoted to the management of genitourinary trauma to guide the general surgeon in more acute, emergent settings.

Intestinal surgery involves an operative space shared by both general surgeons and urologists and is a border region where these 2 surgical disciplines often intersect. Urologists routinely use both small and large bowel for reconstructive procedures and surgeons often encounter such reconstructions of the urinary tract. It is essential for surgeons to understand the

urologic indications for using intestinal segments for reconstructive procedures, the variety of such reconstructions, the anatomic landmarks and
potential pitfalls that should be considered when intraoperatively encountering such reconstructions, and the potential metabolic consequences of
the incorporation of bowel segments into the urinary collecting system.

Uroenteric fistulae can occur between any part of the urinary tract and the
small and large bowel. Classification is generally based on the organ of
origin in the urinary tract and the termination of the fistula in the segment
of the gastrointestinal tract. Surgery is often necessary. Congenital fistulae
are rare, with most being acquired. Uroenteric fistulae most frequently
occur in a setting of inflammatory bowel disease. Imaging often helps in
the diagnosis. Management of urinary fistulae includes adequate nutrition,
diversion of the urinary tract, diversion of the gastrointestinal tract, treatment of underling inflammatory process or malignancy, and surgery.

Pain occurs in the male genitourinary organs as for any organ system in
response to traumatic, infectious, or irritative stimuli. A knowledge and
understanding of chronic genitourinary pain can be of great utility to practicing nonurologists. This article provides insight into the medical and surgical management of subacute and chronic male pelvic, inguinal, and
scrotal pain. The pathophysiology, diagnosis, and medical and surgical
treatment options of each are discussed.

Robot-assisted surgery offers the advantages of a minimally invasive
approach with greater technical ease and a shorter learning curve than
pure laparoscopy. Fueled by the success of the robot-assisted laparoscopic prostatectomy, urologists are increasingly using the robotic platform for other advanced operations involving the kidney, ureters,
bladder, and prostate. Robotic surgery has been shown to be safe and
effective, with good perioperative, functional, and oncologic outcomes.
Although cost continues to be a major concern regarding the use of robotic
technology, improved efficiency and reduced hospital stays associated
with the minimally invasive approach are allowing for better cost-
effectiveness.

SURGICAL CLINICS
OF NORTH AMERICA

THE CLINICS ARE AVAILABLE ONLINE!
Access your subscription at:
www.theclinics.com

Foreword

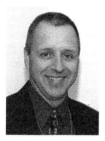

Ronald F. Martin, MD, FACS
Consulting Editor

During my residency, we all spent time on urology rotations during our first and second postgraduate years. I, for one, thought it was a great part of the training program for lots of reasons. Among them were that the urologists used different tools than we did at that time. They had cystoscopes, catheters, wire baskets, and shock-wave machines when all we had were knives, scissors, strings, and clamps. Of course, that was in the very last days of the pre-laparoscopic era for us general surgeons. The urologists under whom I trained practiced something that looked like surgery a little bit, looked like endoscopy a little bit, and looked like office medicine and minor procedures a little bit. It was very different from general surgery, as I knew it. And the urologists were very different in personality from the general surgeons I knew.

If one spends enough time listening to doctors, one hears a lot of bold statements. One also hears a lot of bold predictions; some of which come true. One of the urologists I worked with as a resident and became good friends with over the years was, to me, a larger-than-life demonstration of just how different urologists and general surgeons were—certainly not better or worse, just different. One day we were waiting to get some case started and he for no apparent reason that I could discern told me that he was only three drugs away from being out of a job. Other than my surprise at what sparked that particular declaration, I was even more surprised to think it could be true. I had not really considered that any of our "kind" of work or the need for it to exist could be eliminated by a drug. Parenthetically, I have thought about it every day since. When I asked him to further explain himself, he said that medical cures for renal carcinoma, benign prostatic hypertrophy, and renal lithiasis would or could basically put him out of a job. I remained astounded.

One can easily analyze my mentor's prediction and conclude that there would still be a need for urologists if all those conditions were to become manageable by nonoperative means. Even so, his assertion that he would be out of a job was probably accurate. It was the first time I had to consider us surgeons as a commodity product as well as a profession. It was also the first time I probably wrestled with the concept of how many people have to get sick and require certain kinds of care to keep a surgeon employed. It made me think about what makes "bread and butter" what it is.

Surg Clin N Am 96 (2016) xiii–xiv
http://dx.doi.org/10.1016/j.suc.2016.04.001
0039-6109/16/$ – see front matter © 2016 Published by Elsevier Inc.

surgical.theclinics.com

A casual perusal of this issue of the *Surgical Clinics of North America* by Drs Beaule and Hansen should be enough to allay anyone's fears that urologists are about to go out of business. Since the time of my conversation with my old boss and friend, the discipline of urology has markedly expanded their capabilities to help the suffering, and medicines to replace operative management have not completely appeared yet. No doubt, the medial management of many of the above problems has become much more sophisticated, especially as regards renal cell carcinoma, but not to the point of eliminating urologic surgery.

General surgeons have many good reasons to want to be well-versed in matters that are usually dealt with by our urology brethren. Some of the more trying aspects of complex abdominal operations relate to trying to protect the kidneys and ureters, just for openers. Having to deal with genitourinary injuries and concerns when no urology support is immediately available, as was common when operating in Iraq and Afghanistan, and may be common in austere environments right here in the United States is also a good reason. Last, if one lives long enough, there is a significant likelihood that one will become a patient in need of urologic services for one reason or another. Though the list above is not exhaustive, they are all good reasons to wish to be informed.

We at the *Surgical Clinics of North America* continue to value a comprehensive approach to the topics that address the knowledge-based needs of general surgeons of all kinds. We are deeply indebted to Drs Beaule and Hansen and their colleagues for generating this collective series of reviews with an aim to giving the general surgeon the information she or he needs to best care for the surgical patient.

My friend and mentor may not have predicted the end to a need for his services in a timely manner, but his assessment that we all serve a role in the grand scheme was spot on. Also, his awareness that all such roles are potentially transient was spot on. We should all challenge ourselves to view what we do through the prism of whether or not what we offer is the best solution for the patient. It remains more important to do things for people as opposed to do things to people. Also, we shouldn't fear that we might give something up; we usually wind up generating far more to do by other means anyway.

Ronald F. Martin, MD, FACS
York Hospital System
16 Hospital Drive, Suite A
York, ME 03909, USA

E-mail address:
rmartin@yorkhospital.com

Preface

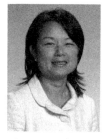
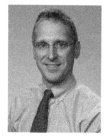

Lisa T. Beaule, MD   Moritz H. Hansen, MD
Editors

With the foundation of the American Urologic Association in 1902, urology emerged as a specialty distinct from general surgery. However, these two specialties remain closely associated, and, of all of the surgical subspecialties, urology has perhaps the closest kinship to general surgery. Despite the remarkable technical advances over the past century, the abdominal, inguinal, perineal, and scrotal regions remain the operative spaces shared by both urologists and general surgeons. And it is in these shared border regions where these two surgical disciplines often intersect.

The practice of modern urology has evolved to include a variety of surgical approaches to include endoscopy, laparoscopy, robotics, and laser surgery for nephrolithiasis, in addition to open surgery for a broad range of extirpative as well as reconstructive procedures. Urology encompasses oncologic procedures, pediatric urology, stone surgery, female pelvic floor reconstruction, male prosthetic surgery, inguinal and pelvic pain, urologic emergencies, and trauma. Because of our shared operative spaces, it is important for the general surgeon to recognize and understand common urologic procedures that may impact surgical planning, and to understand surgical anatomy following urologic reconstructive procedures.

In this issue of the *Surgical Clinics of North America*, we review common urologic conditions (urinary retention, voiding dysfunction), complex reconstructions involving bowel and prosthetics, as well as urgent urologic conditions (Fournier gangrene, testicular torsion, genitourinary trauma) that may be encountered by the general surgeon. Tips and tricks for diagnosis and treatment are included throughout.

We are indebted to the contributing authors and grateful for their experience, expertise, and wisdom. We hope that this issue will be of help to the general surgeon who is planning surgery on a patient who has had a previous urologic procedure, or who may not have ready access to a urologist when encountering a patient with prior urologic surgery, or when managing an acute urologic emergency.

Surg Clin N Am 96 (2016) xv–xvi
http://dx.doi.org/10.1016/j.suc.2016.03.016
0039-6109/16/$ – see front matter © 2016 Published by Elsevier Inc.

surgical.theclinics.com

It has truly been a privilege to serve as guest editors of this issue and to have participated in this endeavor.

Lisa T. Beaule, MD
Tufts University School of Medicine
Maine Medical Center
22 Bramhall Street
Portland, ME 04015, USA

Moritz H. Hansen, MD
Tufts University School of Medicine
Maine Medical Center
22 Bramhall Street
Portland, ME 04015, USA

E-mail addresses:
beaull@mmc.org (L.T. Beaule)
hansemo@mmc.org (M.H. Hansen)

Urologic Emergencies

Adam E. Ludvigson, MD[a], Lisa T. Beaule, MD[b],*

KEYWORDS

- Urologic emergencies • Testicular torsion • Acute urinary retention • Paraphimosis
- Obstructed pyonephrosis • Fournier gangrene • Ischemic priapism

KEY POINTS

- Urologic emergencies must be identified in a timely fashion.
- Optimal management strategy should be determined when urologic services are not available.
- An understanding of the pathophysiology of acute urologic emergencies is crucial.

ACUTE URINARY RETENTION

Overview

Urinary retention is one of the most common medical problems encountered in clinical practice, and most health care professionals will be involved in its treatment at one time or another. Acute and chronic urinary retention, however, are different clinical entities that demand differing courses of treatment. Acute urinary retention (AUR) requires prompt recognition and reversal by medical staff of all levels, whereas chronic urinary retention is by definition a less immediately severe condition.

Causes/Pathophysiology

Stated broadly, AUR is the sudden inability of the bladder to empty itself of urine, whether due to a blocked outflow tract or intrinsic abnormality of the bladder (or both). Using this definition, AUR can be divided into obstructive and dysfunctional categories.

In all obstructive causes of AUR, the underlying cause of retention is the physical obstruction of the outflow tract, that is, the bladder neck or urethra. This obstruction is most commonly due to benign prostatic hyperplasia (BPH), a common condition among older men. As men age, the central zone of the prostate (the area lining the urethra) undergoes a slow but steady enlargement, causing progressive narrowing of the urethra. Because the onset is insidious, a patient may chronically retain increasing

There are no disclosures to report.
[a] Division of Urology, Maine Medical Center, 100 Brickhill Ave., South Portland, Maine 04106, USA; [b] Division of Urology, Maine Medical Center, Tufts University School of Medicine, 100 Brickhill Ave., South Portland, Maine 04106, USA
* Corresponding author.
E-mail address: beaull@mmc.org

Surg Clin N Am 96 (2016) 407–424
http://dx.doi.org/10.1016/j.suc.2016.02.001 surgical.theclinics.com
0039-6109/16/$ – see front matter © 2016 Elsevier Inc. All rights reserved.

amounts of urine for many years before a precipitating event suddenly leads to the complete inability to urinate. The inciting event can be infection, medications, recent trauma (such as urethral catheter insertion), locoregional anesthesia, or idiopathic. Once in retention, the bladder becomes over-distended such that the sarcomeres of the smooth muscle cells in the bladder wall cannot properly engage one another, and the contractile force of the bladder is diminished, worsening the problem.

Any other process that causes urethral narrowing can produce difficulty emptying the bladder, such as urethral stricture or bladder neck contracture. Urethral strictures and bladder neck contractures are typically sequelae of urologic procedures, such as traumatic urethral instrumentation or previous prostate surgery, straddle injuries, or sexually transmitted infection. However, they may be congenital, and patients may not be aware of them at the time of presentation.

Urine outflow can also be blocked by a foreign object. The most common cause is a blood clot formed within the bladder of a patient with significant gross hematuria, whether from bladder cancer, traumatic urethral catheter insertion, or recent surgery. Any recent urologic surgery or procedure is a risk factor for hematuria. Other foreign objects can block urine outflow as well, such as bladder or kidney stones, or material left over from urologic procedures that involve resection of tissue.

In addition, intrinsic bladder dysfunction can produce urinary retention every bit as acutely as a physical blockage and can worsen any underlying low-level physical blockage as well. Common causes for bladder dysfunction include medications (anticholinergics in particular), nerve damage due to diabetes or congenital defect, and, as previously discussed, simple over-distention due to other causes[1] (**Box 1**).

Diagnosis

The diagnosis of AUR is straightforward in theory, but occasionally challenging in practice. Patients with AUR will usually complain of suprapubic pain/pressure, urinary frequency, urgency, voiding in small amounts, bladder spasms, penile pain, and inability to urinate, but some patients may be unable to relate their symptoms, or may actually be asymptomatic. If patients have diminished bladder sensation, their symptoms can be nonspecific: these patients often present with only shortness of breath and diaphoresis.

A bladder scanner may be used to quantify the amount of urine present in the bladder to aid diagnosis, but the results should be interpreted carefully. The bladder scanner is frequently fooled by the presence of intra-abdominal fluid, oddly shaped

---

Box 1
Common drugs leading to bladder dysfunction

Benadryl (diphenhydramine)

General/locoregional anesthetics

Opioids

Alcohol intoxication

Antidepressants (tricyclics especially)

Decongestants

Muscle relaxants

Adapted from Vilke GM, Ufberg JW, Harrigan RA, et al. Evaluation and treatment of acute urinary retention. J Emerg Med 2008;35(2):194.

bladders, and recent surgeries causing inflammation in the area, which leads to estimates of urine that are too high or too low. The bladder scanner should never be used to follow urine output if the patient's fluid status is in doubt. Absent any indications that the number may be inaccurate, and assuming the patient is not chronically retentive of large volumes of urine, a bladder scanner reading of 400 mL or higher should prompt catheterization.

If a dedicated bladder scanner is not available, simple ultrasonography can be used to directly visualize the bladder. Physical examination will frequently reveal a palpable bladder above the pubic bone as well as suprapubic tenderness. A digital rectal examination can identify prostatic enlargement or tenderness. A basic metabolic panel (BMP) should be obtained to rule out electrolyte disturbances, and a complete blood count (CBC) should be obtained if hematuria is the presenting complaint, because patients can lose a surprising amount of blood via this mechanism.

Patient history should focus on the length of time since the last void, the color and consistency of the urine, and baseline voiding characteristics. The clinician should ascertain whether the patient has trouble emptying their bladder normally and inquire specifically as to any recent or past urologic interventions. A suprapubic or midline abdominal incision or radiation tattoos may be associated with prior prostate or bladder surgery or radiation therapy; in this instance, a smaller catheter should be considered, as the cause is less likely to be BPH and more likely to be urethral stricture of bladder neck contracture. Special attention should be paid to any scrotal prosthesis that may represent a pump for an artificial urinary sphincter (AUS). In this case, urologic consultation should always be obtained before placement of a urethral catheter to deactivate the AUS in order to avoid erosion and damage to the device (**Box 2**; **Fig. 1**).

Treatment

The initial management of urinary retention is always drainage of the bladder. In the vast majority of cases, this is accomplished by the insertion of a urethral catheter. Any clinician who is treating a patient with AUR should first attempt placement of a urethral catheter, unless there is some obvious anatomic complication that necessitates the involvement of Urology. In general, if the urethral meatus is visible, urethral placement should be attempted through it at least once.[2]

Urethral catheter placement technique

The first consideration is the size of the catheter, measured in the French catheter scale. A catheter's size in French is exactly 3 times its outer diameter in millimeters (therefore, its circumference is slightly larger, because the circumference is the diameter times pi). For example, an 18-French catheter has an outer diameter of 6 mm. Outer diameter is stressed here to emphasize that a regular and 3-way 20-French

---

Box 2
Workup of acute urinary retention

Review of surgical history (especially urologic)

Assess baseline voiding function

Bladder scan

Basic metabolic panel (BMP)

Complete blood count (CBC) if hematuria

Digital rectal examination (DRE)

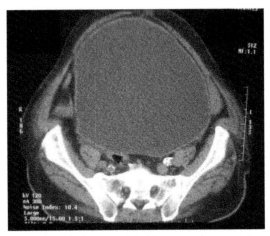

Fig. 1. CT scan: severely distended urinary bladder secondary to urinary retention. (*From* Sharma A, Naraynsingh V. Distended bladder presenting with constipation and venous obstruction: a case report. J Med Case Rep 2012;6:34.)

catheter will have different internal diameters, because a 3-way catheter must incorporate 3 internal channels into the same outer tube.

When trying to pass a urethral catheter through a large prostate, a larger catheter should be used, rather than a smaller one. Many insertion attempts fail because a small catheter was used, which lacks the stiffness necessary to push past the lobes of an enlarged prostate. A reasonable starting point is 18 French. If resistance is consistently encountered, further attempts should be abandoned to avoid the possibility of creating a false passage that will hinder further attempts. A Coudé (French for "elbow") catheter, a catheter with an upwards bend at the tip, can and should be used if BPH is suspected. The catheter is inserted perpendicular to the patient as with a normal catheter placement and then lowered toward the bed when resistance is encountered at the prostate, allowing the bent tip to negotiate the enlarged prostate (**Box 3**; **Fig. 2**).

If urethral catheter placement is not possible, a flexible cystoscope can be used to gain access to the bladder under direct visualization in order to place a wire for guidance. In some cases, the wire can be placed blindly, although this should be done with extreme caution. The urethral stricture can then be serially dilated with sounds as needed to facilitate urethral catheter placement. If all else fails, the bladder can be drained directly via suprapubic decompression or formal suprapubic tube placement. Ultrasound guidance, which is available in most emergency departments, can be helpful and safer than blind placement.

If the patient is in clot retention (that is, blood clots are blocking urine flow), the best catheter to place is a large-bore single-channel catheter, such as a silastic or 6-eye

---

Box 3
Common catheter choices

BPH: 18-French Coudé catheter

Clot retention: 22- to 24-French silastic catheter, 22-French 6-eye if unavailable

Continuous bladder irrigation: 20- to 24-French 3-way catheter

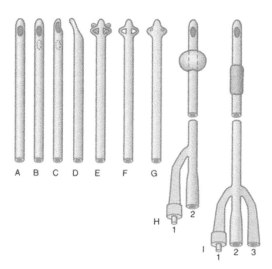

Fig. 2. Large-diameter catheters. *A*, Conical-tip urethral catheter. *B*, Robinson urethral catheter. *C*, Whistle-tip urethral catheter. *D*, Coudé hollow olive-tip catheter. *E*, Malecot self-retaining, four-wing urethral catheter. *F*, Malecot self-retaining, two-wing urethral catheter. *G*, Pezzer self-retaining drain, open-end head, used for cystostomy drainage. *H*, Foley-type balloon catheter. *I*, Foley-type, three-way balloon catheter, one limb of distal end for balloon inflation (*1*), one for drainage (*2*), and one to infuse irrigating solution to prevent clot formation within the bladder (*3*). (*From* Thompson JR. Bladder catheterization. In: Stehr W, editor. The Mont Reid surgical handbook. 6th edition. Philadelphia: Saunders; 2008. p. 839–48; with permission.)

catheter, because the patient will need his or her bladder irrigated thoroughly to remove the clots. Although a 3-way catheter will eventually need to be placed to allow continuous bladder irrigation to stop more clots from forming, this catheter cannot be hand-irrigated well and should only be placed once clots have been evacuated from the bladder, not before.

FOURNIER GANGRENE
Overview

Fournier gangrene is a term given to a severe and rapidly progressive necrotizing infection of the skin and soft tissue of the perineal region, including the genitalia. It is one of the few true urologic emergencies and prompt recognition is critical in order to save as much tissue as possible (as well as the patient's life). Morbidity is significant; however, in the modern era with rapid surgical intervention and broad-spectrum antibiotics, the mortality has decreased somewhat. Treatment remains invariably morbid, and a multidisciplinary approach is required to manage the myriad clinical challenges that arise both during and after the acute treatment period.

Causes/Pathophysiology

The exact cause of Fournier gangrene is not known presently, although most patients have comorbid factors that predispose them to infection and skin breakdown (eg, obesity, diabetes, immune compromise, or perirectal abscess). Bacterial isolates from patients frequently reveal a polymicrobial milieu involving both anaerobic and aerobic bacteria. A common event to all cases appears to be bacterial access to the deep fascial planes, whereby rapid necrosis of tissue causes an ideal anaerobic environment for proliferation of still more bacteria. Once established, the infection spreads very rapidly, due to the causative organisms' secretion of various tissue toxins and virulence factors. Mortality varies according to numerous factors and has been associated most closely with hypertension, congestive heart failure, renal failure, and coagulopathy.[3] The same study reported an overall mortality of 7.5%, and centers with experience in treating this condition have been shown to have significantly improved outcomes (**Box 4**).

Diagnosis

Patients will usually present with complaints of severe perineal pain. As with necrotizing fasciitis, this pain is out of proportion to any external signs. Erythema is often present, progressing rapidly to dark or black necrosis and sloughing of tissue. Patients may report tightness and discomfort in the perineal/genital region before the onset of pain. Clinical suspicion should remain high for patients with the appropriate risk factors who exhibit these symptoms, especially given the dramatically high rate of progression once an infection begins. Crepitus, or a computed tomographic (CT) scan finding of subcutaneous air, is pathognomonic, although operative management should under no circumstances be delayed for definitive imaging. Patients may become hemodynamically unstable very quickly as tissue death accelerates (**Figs. 3–5**).

The use of serum markers of infection is usually low-yield, because the disease invariably declares itself very rapidly. Electrolytes should by all means be monitored closely, but these tend to serve as a guide for the management of severe sepsis as one would for any patient and do not exhibit derangements specific to Fournier.

Treatment

The first step of treatment is initiation of broad-spectrum antibiotics, chosen according to the hospital's antibiogram. However, antibiotics only serve to halt the spread of systemic illness. The only definitive treatment option for Fournier gangrene is swift and aggressive debridement of all affected tissue. Tissue is excised sharply until bleeding is encountered; this is usually the indication that healthy, viable tissue has been reached. Tissue Gram stain and culture can be helpful in directing ongoing antimicrobial treatment. Hemostasis can be achieved via liberal use of cautery, tying off larger vessels as necessary. In men, the scrotal skin is frequently involved, and at times almost none of it can be saved—however, the testicles are rarely involved and are often left exposed at the conclusion of debridement. Testicular thigh pouches can be created in subsequent procedures to maintain the testicles and to facilitate dressing changes, but wet-to-dry packing is all that is required to protect them in the short term.

Box 4
Risk factors for Fournier gangrene

Diabetes

Immunosuppression

Obesity

Pre-existing perineal soft tissue infection

Liver disease

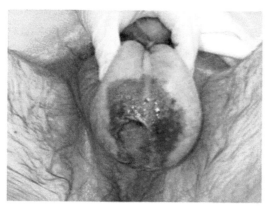

Fig. 3. Fournier gangrene demonstrating dark, necrotic skin and soft tissue involving the right hemiscrotum and extending into the left hemiscrotum and perineum. (*From* Kessler CS, Bauml J. Non-traumatic urologic emergencies in men: a clinical review. West J Emerg Med 2009;10(4):286.)

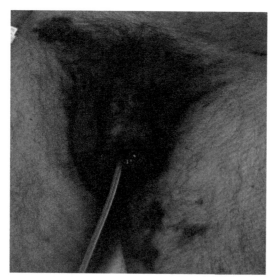

Fig. 4. Fournier gangrene demonstrating expanding necrotic tissue involving the genitalia, right inguinal region, and left inner thigh. (*From* Kim DJ, Kendall JL. Fournier's gangrene and its characteristic ultrasound findings. J Emerg Med 2013;44(1):e100; with permission.)

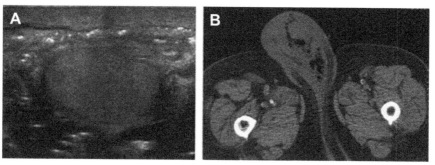

Fig. 5. Subcutaneous gas in Fournier gangrene on scrotal ultrasound (*A*) and CT scan of scrotum (*B*). (*From* Mirochnik B, Bhargava P, Dighe MK, et al. Ultrasound evaluation of scrotal pathology. Radiol Clin North Am 2012;50(2):319, vi; with permission.)

If enough penile tissue remains, a urethral catheter is left in place to prevent urine drainage onto open wounds. In some cases, it may be necessary to place a suprapubic tube to allow perineal and penile tissues to heal appropriately.

Under no circumstances should attempts be made to reconstruct a scrotum at the time of initial debridement, because the wound is still actively infected, and the patient is unlikely to tolerate lengthy surgery. Once the infection has been adequately treated and all necrotic tissue has been debrided, attention can be turned to reconstruction. Plastic surgery consultation is often useful, because muscle flap rotations are sometimes needed to fill in the large defects left after aggressive debridement.

Patients will almost invariably require treatment in an intensive care unit following surgery, because they are very often systemically ill—most deaths occur late in this postoperative period, not during the initial acute surgically managed phase.[3]

ISCHEMIC PRIAPISM
Overview

Priapism is an uncommon urologic emergency that presents as an unwanted erection that persists longer than 4 hours. This condition is subdivided into ischemic, or low-flow, priapism; and non-ischemic, or high-flow, priapism. Ischemic priapism is the focus of this section, because its treatment should be as urgent as possible to prevent possible long-term sequelae, whereas nonischemic priapism can be treated far less urgently and portends no loss of tissue or function. Although only male priapism will be discussed here, it is important to note that clitoral priapism can occur in very rare cases as well, due to the presence of erectile tissue.[4]

Causes/pathophysiology

An erection is produced by the corpora cavernosa, two tubelike structures that run the length of the shaft of the penis and project into the pelvis for anchoring purposes. Each corporal body consists of a spongy mass of highly vascularized tissue surrounded by a tough fibrous coating. During sexual arousal, the vessels feeding the corpora dilate under autonomic control, allowing more blood into the corpora; this in turn tamponades the outflow vessels. The result is that the spongy tissue within each corporal body expands against the inflexible fibrous sheath, producing rigidity. During detumescence, the inflow vessels constrict again, allowing a net amount of blood to leave the corpora, which reduces the tamponade of the outflow vessels, which allows more blood to leave, and so on.

However, if this process is interrupted, the corpora can enter a state of sustained engorgement that quickly becomes painful and begins to threaten tissue—it is essentially a compartment syndrome of the penis.[5] The physiologic internal pressure of the corpora, in addition to preventing venous outflow, begins to impede inflow as well, leading to tissue ischemia and eventually necrosis. For this reason, any erection that has persisted longer than 4 hours should be dealt with promptly to prevent serious immediate or future complications.

This disruption is often related to medications, especially those with α-adrenergic effects. Oral erectile dysfunction agents are rarely implicated, and in fact, extremely high doses of these medications can be ingested without producing priapism.[6] Blood disorders such as sickle cell anemia, which causes clogging of the outflow vessels and persistence of the erection, is a significant risk factor; this is in contrast to high-flow or nonischemic priapism, in which fistulization between arterial and venous systems within the penis produces erection through too-rapid inflow of arterial blood into the corpora. Although the erection is persistent, it is the result of an overabundance of well-oxygenated blood, and therefore, is neither painful nor an emergency (**Box 5**).

> **Box 5**
> **Pharmacologic agents leading to ischemic priapism**
>
> Vasoactive agents used for erectile dysfunction (eg, phentolamine, prostaglandin E1)
>
> α-Blocking agents (eg, prazosin, terazosin, tamsulosin)
>
> Hydroxyzine
>
> Antidepressants and antipsychotics
>
> Certain antihypertensives (eg, hydralazine, propranolol, labetolol)
>
> Cocaine
>
> Ethanol
>
> *Adapted from* Anele UA, Le BV, Resar LM, et al. How I treat priapism. Blood 2015;125(23):3553.

The incidence of priapism has been shown to be bimodal, with most patients presenting between 5 to 10 and 20 to 50 years of age. The incidence is much higher in those affected by sickle cell anemia, for previously discussed reasons. For this patient population, lifetime incidence can reach as high as 42%, with significant clinical sequelae.[7]

Diagnosis

The patient should be asked if he has a history of priapism, sickle cell disease, or trauma to the penis. An adequate history of present illness (HPI) is important as the length of time the erection has persisted is a critical piece of information. High-flow priapism will present as a persistent erection that is not rigid and is not painful. Patients will frequently present very late in the time course of this process because of this characteristic lack of pain.

The diagnosis of ischemic priapism can usually be made clinically. Patients almost always present with a very rigid, painful erection that has persisted much longer than 4 hours (acute embarrassment often prevents a more timely visit to the hospital). The glans penis is usually not engorged. Skin changes, if present, are an ominous sign.

Even if clinical suspicion is high, a penile blood gas should be drawn to ensure accurate diagnosis, because performing a procedure to reverse ischemic priapism carries certain risks and should never be undertaken for high-flow priapism. This procedure is performed by using a large-bore intravenous needle with an angiocatheter to access the corporal body (after the injection of local anesthesia) and gently draw off 5 to 10 mL of blood for analysis. Withdrawing too hard will collapse the surrounding veins and prevent aspiration. The angiocatheter should be left in place to assist with future irrigation. Blood gas analysis in ischemic priapism usually reveals acidosis, hypoxia, and hypercapnia; values consistent with arterial blood indicate high-flow priapism instead. Color Doppler ultrasonography can be used as well, although penile blood gas analysis is more common and is generally sufficient to make the diagnosis (**Fig. 6**).

Treatment

Treatment of ischemic priapism hinges on the removal of accumulated blood and clot from within the corpora, and reversal of the underlying cause. The mainstay of treatment in the emergency room is injection of an α-agonist agent, usually phenylephrine, to produce vasoconstriction of the inflow channels and allow blood to drain passively from the corpora. Sometimes, a single injection is sufficient to achieve detumescence; however, penile irrigation is often required in conjunction. This is accomplished by the

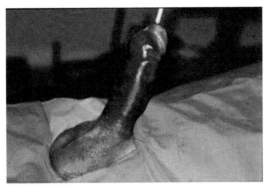

Fig. 6. Ischemic priapism. Ecchymosis (from attempted corporal injection of α-adrenergic agonist and aspiration) spares the glans penis. (*From* Ralph DJ, Garaffa G, Muneer A, et al. The immediate insertion of a penile prosthesis for acute ischaemic priapism. Eur Urol 2009;56(6):1035; with permission.)

placement of a single large-bore angiocatheter into the corpora to allow instillation and aspiration of saline solution. Placement of the angiocatheter is sufficient to correct the problem in most cases and rarely results in significant complications (aside from the complications inherent to the condition itself).

If priapistic episodes recur, the surgeon may elect to perform a shunting procedure to reduce the likelihood of future events. Shunt placement consists simply of creating a defect in the corpora, to improve the ability of blood to drain out. Shunts can be created between the corpora and either the glans, corpus spongiosum, or dorsal vein of the penis; they are preferably created as distally as possible to minimize the chances of erectile dysfunction. The preferred approach (for which multiple technical methods exist) is to insert a large-bore needle or scalpel through the glans into the tip of each of the corpora, creating a passage for blood into the tissue of the glans. Proximal shunts, if necessary, can be a morbid procedure[8] (**Fig. 7**).

Long-term sequelae of recurrent or long-lasting priapistic episodes can include erectile dysfunction and scarring of the corpora, leading to penile curvature and

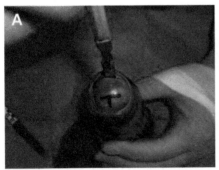
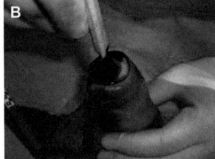

Fig. 7. T-shunt technique, a type of distal glandulocavernosal shunt, used to treat ischemic priapism that is unresponsive to corporal irrigation and injection. (*A*) Initial incision and markings, (*B*) completed procedure with brisk outflow of blood. (*From* Zacharakis E, Raheem AA, Freeman A, et al. The efficacy of the T-shunt procedure and intracavernous tunneling (snake maneuver) for refractory ischemic priapism. J Urol 2014;191(1):165; with permission.)

painful erections. These conditions can sometimes be corrected with future proce-dures, but return to normal function is far from assured.

OBSTRUCTIVE PYONEPHROSIS
Introduction

Although nephrolithiasis may be a painful condition, it rarely has the potential to cause serious medical harm. An obstructing, infected stone is another matter entirely, how-ever. When infection develops behind an obstructing ureteral stone, the resulting illness can progress very rapidly, and for this reason, any patient with findings indica-tive of infection along with a kidney stone is treated promptly. The term obstructive pyonephrosis refers to a severe infection in a hydronephrotic or obstructed kidney that can lead to parenchymal destruction and loss of function; it is a more severe form of urosepsis and can be clinically indistinguishable.

Causes/Pathophysiology

Renal stones are present in many asymptomatic individuals, who may go their entire lives without having an attack of renal colic. Men tend to be affected more than women, and Caucasians more often than Hispanics, Asians, and African Americans, in descending order.[9] Stone disease before age 20 is rare, with rates increasing until about the fourth to sixth decade of life.[10]

When a renal stone migrates into the ureter and causes obstruction, distention of the urothelial tract produces intense pain. Imaging will usually demonstrate hydronephrosis (dilation of the renal pelvis) in this case. If symptoms of flank pain are well-controlled on oral pain medications, and there is no associated infection, intractable emesis, or acute renal injury, then a trial of medical expulsive therapy is reasonable. This usually consists of hydration, an α-adrenergic blocker such as tamsulosin (Flomax), and narcotic pain control. Notably, there is increasing evidence that tamsulosin does not affect the suc-cess rate; however, it can improve ureteral pain.[11] If hydronephrosis is prolonged or se-vere, forniceal rupture can occur, which refers to extravasation of urine through the junction of the distal convoluted tubule and collecting duct of the kidney. This rupture is a normal physiologic pressure-release mechanism of the kidney. CT and ultrasound will show a perinephric fluid collection in this case, but no specific surgical intervention or antibiotics are required—treatment of the obstruction is sufficient, as discussed later[12] (**Fig. 8**).

When a stone obstructs the ureter, the buildup of urine behind it is susceptible to infection. If this occurs, the condition is known as obstructive pyonephrosis. Because infected urine can reflux directly into the bloodstream, patients can become septic very rapidly and require aggressive medical treatment. Drainage of the infected urine is imperative and is the mainstay of therapy, aside from appropriate antibiotic treatment.

Obstructive pyonephrosis can develop immediately in response to a stone, or it can develop as a chronic stone progresses to complete obstruction. The stone itself can serve as a nidus of infection. Infection with certain types of bacteria, particularly the Proteus genus, can lead to large and rapid accumulations of struvite stone, which can fill the entire collecting system and result in a "staghorn calculus."

Diagnosis

A high degree of clinical suspicion is necessary to successfully treat this condition, because the patient's condition can worsen rapidly. Urinalysis (UA) should be ob-tained, and urine sent empirically for culture. The clinician should keep in mind that if the stone is completely obstructing, infected urine may not reach the bladder, and

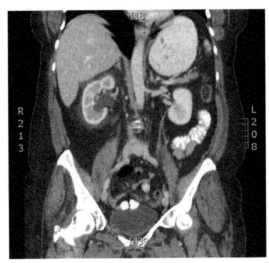

Fig. 8. Forniceal rupture with resulting fluid around right kidney associated with moderate hydronephrosis (personal patient).

a UA may therefore be normal. Negative test results should not delay treatment if the overall clinical picture suggests infection.

Imaging, whether CT or ultrasound, can help confirm the presence and severity of obstruction. Findings of hydronephrosis along with any findings suggestive of infection indicate urgent treatment. If obstruction due to kidney stone is suspected, no contrast is necessary for CT imaging; in fact, the lack of contrast enhances the ability to locate small stones.

Urinalysis interpretation

Interpreting UA results can be difficult at times. The most important test results when assessing a patient for infection in the setting of ureteral obstruction are leukocyte esterase, leukocytes, erythrocytes, nitrites, and bacteria. The presence of an indwelling ureteral stent can cloud the picture, because the stent itself will lead to hematuria and leukocytes in the urine. However, very high leukocyte esterase values (greater than 400), or the presence of nitrites, are rarely due to ureteral stents and should be treated as infection. As previously discussed, a negative UA should not delay treatment if infection is suspected on a clinical basis, because infected urine cannot drain to the bladder in the setting of complete obstruction.

Treatment

Prompt drainage is the only treatment option for obstructive pyonephrosis. Ideally, this can be accomplished by placing a ureteral stent, allowing infected urine to bypass the obstruction and temporizing the patient so that definitive treatment can be performed when infection has cleared. Kidney stones themselves are never treated or removed in the setting of infection, because the trauma to the urothelium can introduce bacteria into the bloodstream and worsen the patient's illness. During placement of the stent, urine can be obtained directly from the renal pelvis using a ureteral catheter, allowing an accurate urine culture to be sent. This ureteral catheter is especially helpful if the blockage is complete enough to prevent any infected urine from draining into the bladder.

If ureteral stenting is not possible or if the patient is showing signs of hemodynamic instability, a percutaneous nephrostomy tube should be placed by an Interventional

Radiologist or qualified Urologist without delay. Definitive treatment of the stone or other obstruction is then scheduled once the patient has recovered sufficiently.

PARAPHIMOSIS
Introduction

Paraphimosis is a painful and potentially serious condition characterized by the inability to return the foreskin to its normal position after it is retracted. It is usually seen in the hospital or chronic care setting following insertion of a urethral catheter into an uncircumcised male patient, during which the foreskin is retracted, allowing it to become entrapped in that position. If left untreated, paraphimosis has the potential to lead to tissue ischemia and necrosis—it should therefore be reduced as soon as possible.

Pathophysiology

A normal foreskin can be easily retracted back over the glans and returns to its normal position without difficulty. However, men may have a narrow band of tissue in the foreskin, called a phimotic ring, that can make retraction of the foreskin difficult. Men may not be aware of this condition, because they may seldom or never retract their foreskin completely, or it may not interfere sufficiently with their normal life to warrant correction. When the foreskin and its phimotic ring are retracted, a biological tourniquet is applied to the penis, causing edema to develop distally and making reduction of the foreskin increasingly difficult.[13]

Even an otherwise normal penis can develop enough edema in this state to cause paraphimosis. If a urinary catheter is in place providing an additional source of tension, or if injury, illness, fluid overload, or other medical conditions contribute to tissue edema, the problem is compounded.

Diagnosis

The diagnosis is usually made clinically, by physical examination, and by patient interview. Patients experience increasing pain as the tissue edema progresses and will be unable to reduce their foreskin. Patients with dementia may exhibit increasing agitation, prompting a physical examination and discovery of the problem. Sedated or noncommunicative patients, and those with neurologic conditions affecting their penile sensation, are particularly dangerous, because their condition may not be noted for some time. Over a period of hours, the affected tissue may become so edematous as to impede blood flow, leading to tissue loss and necrosis. If a urinary catheter is not present, patients may develop urinary retention as well (see **Fig. 8**).

Treatment

Several techniques exist for reducing paraphimosis; treatment is largely dictated by provider preference.[5,14] The singular goal is to return the foreskin to its normal position and allow the patient's edema to recede, but frequently the anatomy is so distorted that even identification of foreskin, penis, and glans may be very difficult.

The authors' preferred method is to use gentle, constantly increasing pressure to gradually reduce edema enough to allow reduction of the foreskin. This method can be accomplished by simply squeezing the penis firmly until the foreskin can be retracted; alternatively, a simple compressive dressing can be applied for 10 to 15 minutes before reduction is attempted.[15] Although one hand is applying steady pressure, the other should be used to gently squeeze and push the glans until it can be slid through the phimotic ring. In some cases, it may be easier to grasp the foreskin with both hands and use the thumbs to gently push the glans back through the phimotic ring. If using a compressive dressing, the dressing can be removed and reapplied/tightened as necessary (**Figs. 9–11**).

The amount of pressure that can be brought to bear is often limited by the patient's discomfort, which can obviously be significant. Liberal use of narcotic pain medication and/or sedation may be necessary in severe cases. Topical anesthetics are often not effective, especially in adult patients, but ice can both provide analgesia and reduce edema. Patience is essential; an extended period of firm pressure is frequently required to reverse enough of the tissue edema to allow a successful reduction.

If all attempts to reduce the foreskin at the bedside fail, surgical intervention is indicated to prevent tissue loss. Circumcision is usually required in this instance, because the phimotic ring must be incised sharply to relieve the pressure.

TESTICULAR TORSION
Introduction

Testicular torsion is another of the true urologic emergencies, and prognosis is strongly determined by time to surgical intervention. The signs and symptoms of torsion are often unambiguous enough to establish the diagnosis without imaging or further tests, although these are certainly useful. However, no test should ever delay progression to the operating room if torsion is suspected. If recognized and treated in a prompt manner, torsion has a good prognosis, but the risk of sequelae is present regardless.

Pathophysiology

Testicular torsion cases peak between 12 and 16 years of age and are usually not associated with any significant past medical history; however, the presence of mass or malignancy on the cord, such as lymphoma, can predispose to torsion and compromise of vascular supply. Cold weather has been shown to increase incidence

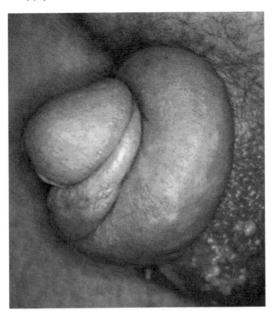

Fig. 9. Paraphimosis with severe edema of distal penile shaft and proximal tight phimotic ring (not seen in photo). (*From* Kessler CS, Bauml J. Non-traumatic urologic emergencies in men: a clinical review. West J Emerg Med 2009;10(4):283.)

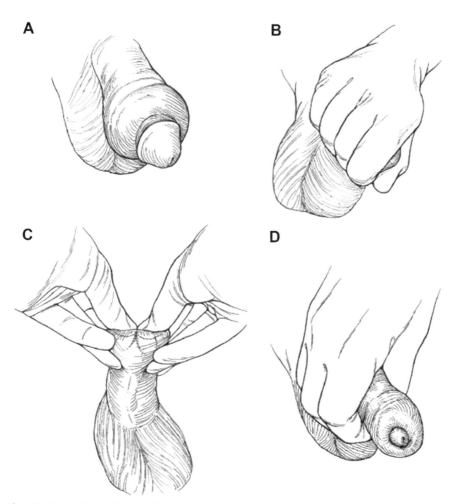

Fig. 10. Reduction of paraphimosis. Reduce edema of distal penile skin with manual compression to allow for replacement of distal penile preputial tissue over the glans penis. (*A*) Typical appearance of edematous penis with paraphimosis, (*B*) Firm manual pressure is applied to reduce edema, (*C*) Gentle counter-traction is applied to reduce foreskin, (*D*) Fully reduced paraphimosis with normal appearance of the penis. (*From* Vilke GM, Ufberg JW, Harrigan RA, et al. Evaluation and treatment of acute urinary retention. J Emerg Med 2008;35(2):196; with permission.)

somewhat, possibly due to the increased tone of dartos and cremasteric fibers, but this hypothesis is controversial.[16]

The most common type of testicular torsion encountered by surgeons is intravaginal torsion, wherein the testicle rotates within the tunica vaginalis. Intravaginal torsion is usually due to a congenital deformity known as bell clapper deformity.[17] A normal testicle is prevented from rotating within the tunica vaginalis by a broad fusion of the parietal and visceral layers along the epididymis; however, in a significant portion of men, the area of fusion is smaller than usual, predisposing the testicle to rotation around this narrowed axis. The compression of arterial inflow to the testicle produces ischemia and intense pain.

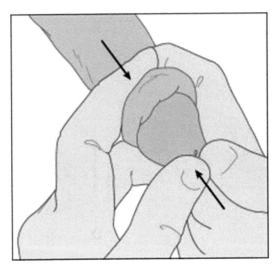

Fig. 11. Reduction of paraphimosis. (*From* Buttaravoli P. Chapter 81: Phimosis and paraphimosis. In: Buttaravoli P, editor. Minor emergencies. 2nd edition. Philadelphia: Mosby; 2007. p. 330; with permission.)

In comparison, extravaginal torsion, the twisting of the entire tunica vaginalis and spermatic cord, is primarily a perinatal event that presents as a painless, "vanishing" testicle in a newborn baby, or as a painless swollen and discolored hemiscrotum at birth. It is not a surgical emergency, because the window for salvage has almost always already passed by the time torsion is recognized.[18]

Diagnosis

The primary symptom of torsion is intense, sudden pain in the affected testicle. The severity of the pain means patients rarely delay seeking treatment, and therefore, often present well within the window of treatment. On physical examination, edema may be present, and the testicle may be observed or palpated (if allowed by the patient) higher than usual in the scrotum. The cremasteric reflex, upward movement of the affected testis elicited by lightly stroking the ipsilateral medial thigh, can be a helpful diagnostic test, because the presence of a functioning reflex is strongly correlated with intact blood flow. A UA may be obtained if the clinical picture is not completely indicative of torsion and there is suspicion for an infectious process —for example, if pain is relatively mild and urinary frequency, urinary urgency, or dysuria is present.

The mainstay of diagnostic tests for testicular torsion in recent years is the scrotal Doppler ultrasound, which can unequivocally demonstrate lack of blood flow to the testicle and confirm the diagnosis.[19] The presence of blood flow should be compared with the contralateral testicle, because blood flow can be reduced rather than completely eliminated in some cases (**Fig. 12**).

It must be stressed: no diagnostic test should delay surgical exploration of the scrotum if torsion is strongly suspected. Urologic consultation should be obtained immediately at the same time confirmatory tests are being ordered. In an adolescent patient with severe, sudden-onset testicular pain, very little clinical information would be sufficient to warrant delaying surgery. If testicular torsion is recognized less than 6 hours after the onset of pain, the rate of testicular salvage is 95%. This rate drops to 80% after 7 hours, and 60% after 12 hours. After 12 hours, loss of the testicle is more likely than not.[20]

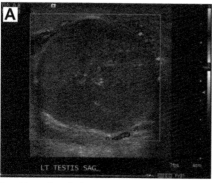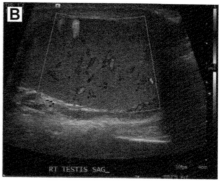

Fig. 12. Left-sided testicular torsion as demonstrated by absence of intratesticular Doppler flow on scrotal ultrasound. The right testis demonstrates normal blood flow. (*A*) Left testicle, which demonstrates no flow on Doppler ultrasound, (*B*) The normal contralateral testicle with intact bloodflow. (*From* Wang J-H. Testicular torsion. Urological Science (Urol Sci) 2012;23(3):85; with permission.)

Treatment

Manual detorsion can sometimes be accomplished, which may improve salvage rates until surgical exploration is available; again, this should never delay the operating room, as even a successfully detorsed testicle must be surgically explored.[20] The affected testicle should be rotated "away" from midline, as if one is opening a book, because approximately two-thirds of torsion cases prove to be rotated in a medial direction.[19,20] Patients who are premedicated with narcotics will better tolerate bedside detorsion.

Surgical detorsion and orchiopexy are accomplished through a midline incision at the median raphe. After delivering the testicle, it is untwisted and observed closely to determine its viability. It is common to find an inflammatory hydrocele. If the testicle shows signs of adequate reperfusion (tissue viability, robust Doppler flow within the spermatic cord), it is sutured in a 3-point fixation to the scrotum with nonabsorbable suture to prevent future torsion events. If it appears necrotic or does not reperfuse after detorsion, orchiectomy is indicated. A concomitant contralateral orchiopexy should be performed to ensure no future events, especially if an orchiectomy was necessary.

Assuming all goes well in surgery, the long-term sequelae of testicular torsion is somewhat unclear. Oxidative stress has been shown to impair testicular functioning in animal models,[21] but it is difficult to generalize these results to humans, and no study has conclusively linked fertility problems to past episodes of torsion (assuming both testicles remain intact).

REFERENCES

1. Fitzpatrick JM, Desgrandchamps F, Adjali K, et al, Reten-World Study Group. Management of acute urinary retention: a worldwide survey of 6074 men with benign prostatic hyperplasia. BJU Int 2012;109(1):88–95.
2. Bacsu C, Van Zyl S, Rourke KF. A prospective analysis of consultation for difficult urinary catheter insertion at tertiary care centres in Northern Alberta. Can Urol Assoc J 2013;7(9–10):343–7.
3. Sorensen MD, Krieger JN, Rivara FP, et al. Fournier's gangrene: management and mortality predictors in a population based study. J Urol 2009;182(6):2742–7.

4. Goldstein I. Medical and surgical management of clitoral priapism. J Sex Med 2014;11(12):2838–41.
5. Dubin J, Davis JE. Penile emergencies. Emerg Med Clin North Am 2011;29(3): 485–99.
6. Matheeussen V, Maudens KE, Anseeuw K, et al. A non-fatal self-poisoning attempt with sildenafil. J Anal Toxicol 2015;39(7):572–6.
7. Levey HR, Segal RL, Bivalacqua TJ. Management of priapism: an update for clinicians. Ther Adv Urol 2014;6(6):230–44.
8. Chen W, Sun SB, Sun LA, et al. Modified technique in treating recurrent priapism: a technique report. Asian J Androl 2015;17(2):329–31.
9. Soucie JM, Thun MJ, Coates RJ, et al. Demographic and geographic variability of kidney stones in the United States. Kidney Int 1994;46(3):893–9.
10. Hiatt RA, Friedman GD. The frequency of kidney and urinary tract diseases in a defined population. Kidney Int 1982;22(1):63–8.
11. Pickard R, Starr K, MacLennan G, et al. Use of drug therapy in the management of symptomatic ureteric stones in hospitalised adults: a multicentre, placebo-controlled, randomised controlled trial and cost-effectiveness analysis of a calcium channel blocker (nifedipine) and an alpha-blocker (tamsulosin) (the SUSPEND trial). Health Technol Assess 2015;19(63):1–172.
12. Gulati A, Prakash M, Bhatia A, et al. Spontaneous rupture of renal pelvis. Am J Emerg Med 2013;31(4):762.e1–3.
13. Barkin J, Rosenberg MT, Miner M. A guide to the management of urologic dilemmas for the primary care physician (PCP). Can J Urol 2014;21(Suppl 2): 55–63.
14. Hayashi Y, Kojima Y, Mizuno K, et al. Prepuce: phimosis, paraphimosis, and circumcision. Sci World J 2011;11:289–301.
15. Pohlman GD, Phillips JM, Wilcox DT. Simple method of paraphimosis reduction revisited: point of technique and review of the literature. J Pediatr Urol 2013; 9(1):104–7.
16. Korkes F, Cabral PR, Alves CD, et al. Testicular torsion and weather conditions: analysis of 21,289 cases in Brazil. Int Braz J Urol 2012;38(2):222–8 [discussion: 228–9].
17. Sharp VJ, Kieran K, Arlen AM. Testicular torsion: diagnosis, evaluation, and management. Am Fam Physician 2013;88(12):835–40.
18. Callewaert PR, Van Kerrebroeck P. New insights into perinatal testicular torsion. Eur J Pediatr 2010;169(6):705–12.
19. Avery LL, Scheinfeld MH. Imaging of penile and scrotal emergencies. Radiographics 2013;33(3):721–40.
20. Sessions AE, Rabinowitz R, Hulbert WC, et al. Testicular torsion: direction, degree, duration and disinformation. J Urol 2003;169(2):663–5.
21. Turner TT, Bang HJ, Lysiak JL. The molecular pathology of experimental testicular torsion suggests adjunct therapy to surgical repair. J Urol 2004;172(6 Pt 2): 2574–8.

Surgical Management of Urologic Trauma and Iatrogenic Injuries

Leonard N. Zinman, MD*, Alex J. Vanni, MD*

KEYWORDS

- Trauma • Kidney • Bladder • Urethra • Ureter • Genitalia

KEY POINTS

- Trauma patients requiring urologic-specific evaluation must be identified.
- The most efficient means of diagnosing urologic trauma should be determined based on the mechanism of injury.
- The optimal management strategy is based on the location and degree of urologic injury and patient stability.

INTRODUCTION

Genitourinary injuries may be seen as a sequel to both blunt and penetrating trauma occurring in approximately 10% of all patients admitted to an emergency department. Trauma is the number one cause of death in patients aged 1 to 44 and accounts for more than 120,000 deaths per year in the United States, 10% of which have a concomitant component of genitourinary origin with the kidney as the most frequently involved organ.[1,2] These injuries may be quite elusive, concealed anatomically in the relatively nonresponsive retroperitoneal and pelvic locations where even intravenous (IV) contrast computed tomography (CT) might not identify them clearly. Urogenital trauma is rarely fatal, but may ultimately become the basis for significant short- and long-term morbidity, if not recognized early during its course. The major causes of genitourinary trauma are motor vehicles accidents, deceleration injuries, and penetrating firearm assault violence, all of which are on the increase.[3]

Blood in the urine signifies a urogenital injury. However, this is neither specific for location of injury nor a prognosticator for the severity of injury.[4,5] Blunt trauma with associated hematuria requires evaluation of both the upper and the lower genitourinary system, as forces associated with high-speed motor vehicle collisions can

Disclosures: The authors have nothing to disclose.
Department of Urology, Lahey Hospital and Medical Center, Tufts University School of Medicine, 41 Mall Road, Burlington, MA 01805, USA
* Corresponding authors.
E-mail addresses: Leonard.N.Zinman@Lahey.org; Alex.J.Vanni@Lahey.org

Surg Clin N Am 96 (2016) 425–439
http://dx.doi.org/10.1016/j.suc.2016.02.002
0039-6109/16/$ – see front matter © 2016 Elsevier Inc. All rights reserved.

surgical.theclinics.com

produce significant injury to the entire genitourinary system. Hematuria in patients suffering penetrating abdominal trauma indicates possible urologic injury to the kidneys, ureters, or bladder.

Genitourinary trauma usually occurs in the setting of multisystem trauma. Timely evaluation and management of the trauma patient have the potential to minimize urologic morbidity and mortality. In what follows, each of the major urogenital organs is treated separately. New imaging modalities and a growing emphasis on nonoperative expectant management of both upper and lower urinary tract injuries have changed the field of urologic trauma. Concomitant injury to both the upper and the lower urinary tract is rare, but careful evaluation is critical to identify these devastating injuries.

RENAL INJURY
Initial Evaluation

Blunt renal trauma constitutes the most common genitourinary organ injury and is the result of motor vehicle collision, falls from heights, a sustained direct blow to the flank, lower rib fractures, or a complication of elective renal surgery from percutaneous stone surgery or partial nephrectomy. In a large population study, the incidence of trauma patients in the United States who had renal injuries was 1.2% with 14,000 patients hospitalized in the United States with renal trauma alone.[2] In addition, 24% of all solid abdominal organ injuries involve the kidneys.[6]

The presenting signs and symptoms of blunt trauma may include flank or abdominal pain and bruising, hematuria, hemodynamic instability, flank hematoma (expanding and pulsatile), and sepsis or ileus from urinary extravasation, which may not be recognized initially and may require delayed recognition and intervention.

Penetrating abdominal injuries as a result of gunshot or stab wounds should always alert the physician to possible renal injury. A thorough physical examination of the abdomen, chest, and back must be performed because gunshot wounds may be misleading because of the small entrance defects and may not initially reveal the extent of tissue damage. To identify the location and extent of the penetration with imaging, a paper-clip marker may be placed at the entrance and exit sites to help define the damage during all imaging techniques, because most penetrating injuries will require surgical exploration.[7]

Contrast CT with delayed imaging of the ureters is the gold-standard imaging modality to evaluate the entire urinary tract as well as the anatomy and function of the kidney. The American Association for the Surgery of Trauma (AAST) Organ Injury Scale is used to classify blunt and penetrating renal injuries and corresponds closely to the appearance of the kidney on CT (**Table 1**).[8] Renal injuries may be classified as renal contusions, renal lacerations with or without collecting system injury, renal pedicle avulsion, and vascular disruption, renal artery thrombosis, injury to the renal pelvis or ureteropelvic junction disruption.

CT should be performed in all cases of suspected renal trauma in hemodynamically stable patients. The standard protocol includes helical (spiral) CT with a portal venous phase (from the diaphragm to the ischial tuberosities) to survey lower genitourinary structures or the presence of active arterial bleeding, followed after 10 minutes by delayed images to identify the presence of urinary contrast extravasation. CT should not be used as the primary evaluation tool in hemodynamically unstable patients, because these patients should be managed operatively, and other diagnostic tests, such as diagnostic peritoneal lavage or ultrasound, should initiate the evaluation because the critical need of immediate surgical control of bleeding is crucial.

Most blunt renal injuries are minor with contusions that account for 64% to 81% of cases. Wessels[9] in a multicenter study of 6892 patients with renal trauma found

Table 1
American Association for the Surgery of Trauma organ injury scales for renal injury

AAST Grade	Characteristics of Injury	AIS-90 Score
I	Contusion with microscopic or gross hematuria, urologic studies, normal, nonexpanding subcapsular hematoma without parenchymal laceration	2;2
II	Nonexpanding perirenal hematoma confined to renal retroperitoneum; laceration <1 cm parenchymal depth of renal cortex without urinary extravasation	2;2
III	Laceration >1 cm parenchymal depth of renal cortex without collecting system rupture or urinary extravasation	3
IV	Parenchymal laceration extending through renal cortex, medulla, and collecting system; injury to main renal artery or vein with contained hemorrhage	4;4
V	Completely shattered kidney; avulsion of renal hilum that devascularizes kidney	5;5

Abbreviation: AIS, abbreviated injury scale.

contusion or hematomas in 64.2%, grade II or III lacerations in 24.8%, grade IV injury in 7.7%, and grade V injury in 3.3% of cases.[10]

Contemporary CT imaging with support of the grading system has provided a platform for the management of renal trauma and helps dictate the options of nonoperative and angiographic approaches and has been pivotal in decreasing surgical intervention and nephrectomy.[11]

Angiography is rarely performed, but can be a valuable tool to both diagnose and treat renal injury via transcatheter embolization for active arterial bleeding, a pseudoaneurysm, or an arteriovenous fistula. Because the most common form of surgical management of renal injury is nephrectomy, angioembolization, when feasible, has been shown to decrease the rate of nephrectomy and increase renal salvage.[9,12–14]

A rare but serious complication of renal arterial thrombosis and embolization with ischemic parenchyma is the development of renovascular hypertension. Development of renovascular hypertension has been documented in 0.2% of cases and is mediated by the renin-angiotensin system and can be managed by a delayed laparoscopic nephrectomy. Long-term follow-up is critical to identify this systemic event, which may develop in a delayed fashion.

Management

The goal of renal trauma management is to preserve the maximal number of renal units in as safe a manner as feasible. Thus, the management of blunt and penetrating renal injury varies greatly.

Nonoperative

There is an established and sustained shift in the renal injury therapeutic paradigm with an increasing nonoperative approach that involves close monitoring, bed rest, serial hemoglobin/hematocrit measurement with transfusions if necessary, and selective repeat CT imaging. Virtually all grade I–IV renal injuries and a select group of grade V injuries are now initially managed conservatively.[13,15] The accuracy and rapidity of helical CT, combined with improvement in renal reconstruction, have decreased the number of renal explorations and nephrectomies performed over past 2 decades.[12] Fewer than 5% of blunt injuries and 36% of all penetrating renal injuries are undergoing operative management.[9] Ongoing arterial bleeding in hemodynamically stable patients may be treated with angiography and selective embolization.[16,17] Thrombosis of the renal artery or its branches is managed expectantly.

Bed rest is maintained until the urine becomes grossly clear. The urethral catheter can be removed when the patient is stable and can spontaneously void.

All grade IV–V renal injuries that involve urinary extravasation managed nonoperatively should initially have a repeat CT scan at 48 to 72 hours to re-evaluate the degree of urine extravasation. If the degree of extravasation has not diminished, ureteral stenting is indicated, and the bladder should be decompressed with a urethral catheter.[17–19] Patients with increasing white blood cell count, fevers, increasing flank pain, or ongoing blood loss should have a repeat CT scan. Percutaneous drainage is performed if an infected hematoma or urinoma is detected.

Operative

The only absolute indication for surgical exploration in renal trauma is persistent life-threatening hemorrhage from a severe parenchymal disruption or "shattered kidney," renal pedicle transection, or an uncontained expanding hematoma in a patient clinically in shock and in need of a lifesaving nephrectomy.[14] Relative indications for renal explorations include patients who have failed conservative management with persistent bleeding, ongoing urinary extravasation, the critically ill patient with multiple associated intraperitoneal injuries, or penetrating trauma. Although most kidney explorations result in nephrectomy, early renal hilum vascular control has been advocated to reduce the need for nephrectomy. Voelzke and McAninch[20] reported a series of penetrating injuries to 206 renal units that were successfully managed expectantly with a salvage rate of 80%.

The strongest predictor for nephrectomy is the grade of renal injury. A significant number of patients with penetrating injury and a minority of those with blunt injury require immediate laparotomy before radiographic evaluation.[9,21] The use of IV urography is currently used as an intraoperative one-shot study with contrast when emergency exploration is needed to assess the presence of a contralateral kidney before possible nephrectomy. A plain abdominal film is obtained 10 minutes after injection of a 150-mL bolus of iodinated contrast material.[22,23] In critically ill patients with multiple injuries, renal exploration should only be undertaken if a pulsatile or expanding retroperitoneal hematoma is identified. If exploration is not performed, CT staging of the renal injury is performed once the patient is stabilized.[16,24,25]

Operative Technique

A midline transabdominal incision extending from the xiphoid process to the pubic symphysis allows exploration of the kidneys with optimal access to the renal hilum. Preliminary isolation of the renal artery and vein may be achieved before Gerota fascia is opened to minimize blood loss. Early vascular control with isolation of the vessels has demonstrated potential renal salvage with expected functional restoration of 85%.[14,20,26] Proximal vascular control is achieved by placing the transverse colon on the chest and the small intestine in a Lahey bag (BectonDickson, Franklin Lakes, NJ) and to the right. This placement will expose the root of the mesentery, the ligament of Treitz, and the underlying great vessels. The retroperitoneal incision is made over the aorta superior to the inferior mesenteric artery, extending up to the ligament of Treitz. If a large retroperitoneal hematoma prevents easy feel of the aorta at the level of the ligament, then the incision should be made medial to the inferior mesenteric vein. This vein runs a few centimeters to the left of the aorta, where you can dissect superiorly along the anterior aortic wall until you see the renal vein crossing over the aorta. Place a vessel loop around the renal vein, which then permits you a guide to the remaining renal vessels, which are then also encircled, but not occluded, unless heavy bleeding is relentless, and then clamping with mannitol should be limited to 30 minutes of warm ischemic time. Most bleeding at this point is managed manually. The kidney is then exposed laterally by mobilizing the colon along the white line of Toldt to shift the colon medially. Open Gerota fascia along the lateral aspect and expose the kidney without incising the capsule. Once hemostasis is achieved, sharp debridement of nonviable parenchyma is performed, and the collecting system is scrutinized for leakage sites. Injection of 2 or 3 mL of diluted methylene blue into the renal pelvis with a 30-gauge needle may help identify openings that are not covered by parenchyma, which will usually seal the tear, if present. The open pelvis defect and open calyces can be closed with 4-0 absorbable sutures. Kidney lacerations are closed by renorrhaphy after suturing identified vessels with 4-0 absorbable suture on the parenchymal surface. FloSeal or Gelfom bolsters can be placed between the lacerated renal surfaces and the renal parenchymal edge followed by closure of the capsule if viable, using 3-0 monofilament absorbable mattress sutures.[27–29] An omental flap can be sutured to a kidney defect or to wrap the kidney and is guided through a paracolic gutter to reach the reconstructed kidney. In the case of a shattered kidney or multiple lacerations, an envelope of Vicryl mesh may also be placed around the kidney to help maintain the repair. A Jackson-Pratt closed suction drain is placed away from suture lines, and the kidney is placed in a loosely closed Gerota capsule. In the presence of a concurrent injury to the pancreas and left kidney, multiple drains and an interposition of omentum should be placed between the 2 structures.

An injury to the main renal vein will require a repair. Segmental veins can safely be ligated, but the main vein may need repair with a 5-0 Prolene closure of the vein wall laceration. The patient will require bed rest and catheter drainage until gross hematuria clears and is mobile enough to void. Imaging with CT scan and a nuclear functional scan is required at 3 months to evaluate renal function of the injured kidney. Postoperative hemorrhage is rare if the injured parenchyma has been adequately debrided and repaired. If recurrent bleeding occurs, it is best evaluated and managed by angiography.

Complications

The reported complication rate following renal injury ranges between 3% and 20%. Patients with fever, increasing flank pain, and elevated white blood cell count should have a CT scan to evaluate for an infected retroperitoneal hematoma or urinoma.[17,18] These fluid collections are usually managed by percutaneous drainage ± endoscopic stenting as previously described. Delayed bleeding is a rare and life-threatening complication that is more commonly associated with penetrating injury. Angiography will diagnose and treat possible arteriovenous fistulas or pseudoaneurysm formation.

INJURY TO THE URETER
Initial Evaluation

Ureteral trauma occurs in less than 1% of genitourinary injuries, and thus, the trauma surgeon must maintain a high degree of suspicion when evaluating the trauma patient. Injury to the ureter should be suspected with multisystem trauma involving the bowel, bladder, or vascular injury, deceleration injury, and any penetrating injury near the ureter.[30] Hematuria is present in 25% to 83% of patients. Most injuries result from penetrating trauma, with only 4% to 20% of injuries occurring due to blunt trauma.[31,32] Children are at an increased risk of ureteropelvic junction disruption, which typically occurs with severe deceleration injury.[33] In stable patients, a CT scan with delayed images should be performed to evaluate the ureter. Unrecognized injury can result in urinoma, sepsis, and nephrectomy.[30,31]

Management

Ureteral injuries should be repaired surgically unless the diagnosis is made in a delayed fashion. If an abscess or urinoma is present, a percutaneous nephrostomy is placed and periureteral drainage is performed.[34,35] If an incomplete ureteral injury is identified, retrograde ureteral stenting may be attempted. If unsuccessful, a nephrostomy tube is placed.

Surgical Exploration

In stable patients, ureteral injuries should be surgically reconstructed according to the location of the injury. Injuries above the pelvic brim, including ureteropelvic junction disruption, should be debrided, spatulated, and repaired with a primary anastomosis. The ureter must be mobilized sufficiently, but with care to avoid injuring the blood supply. Interrupted absorbable sutures (4-0 or 5-0) are used, and a double-J ureteral stent is placed. If there is a bowel injury adjacent to the repair, omentum can be used to cover the repair. Injuries of the distal ureter (distal to the iliac vessels) can be managed by reimplantation into the bladder. Reimplantation can be performed either in an extravesical approach or by opening the bladder in the midline and bringing the ureter through the bladder wall in a new hiatus on the posterior aspect of the wall. The ureter should be spatulated and anchored to the bladder with 3-0 or 4-0 absorbable sutures. A double-J ureteral stent should be placed. The bladder is then closed in 2 layers with absorbable sutures. A closed suction drain and urethral catheter are placed.

In situations whereby the ureteral defect is too large for primary anastomosis, a psoas hitch or Boari flap may be performed. A psoas hitch involves mobilizing the bladder (dividing the contralateral superior vesical artery may be required) and anchoring it to the psoas tendon. In addition, a Boari flap may be required if the defect is too long for a psoas hitch. Defects in which either a Boari flap or bowel interposition is required should be performed in a delayed fashion.

If the patient is unstable, if the surgeon is unfamiliar with ureteral reconstruction techniques, or if the defect is too long for acute reconstruction, the ureter should be ligated proximal to the injury, a nephrostomy tube place, and delayed reconstruction performed.

Retroperitoneal drains are removed after 2 to 3 days unless the output is consistent with urine. The urethral catheter can be removed after 7 days. The double-J ureteral stent is removed cystoscopically 4 to 6 weeks after repair, preferably with a retrograde pyelogram to ensure proper healing. A nuclear medicine renal scan, IV pyelogram, or CT scan with delayed images is performed 3 months after stent removal to evaluate for asymptomatic obstruction.

BLADDER INJURY
Initial Evaluation

Blunt trauma is responsible for most bladder injuries, with penetrating events accounting for 14% to 33% of all injuries.[36,37] Twenty-nine percent of patients with a pelvic fracture in combination with gross hematuria have a bladder injury, and thus, any type of pelvic fracture and hematuria warrants investigation for a potential bladder injury.[38] A high index of suspicion needs to be present with intoxicated individuals who have a full bladder and sustain even mild trauma and complain of abdominal pain because they may have ruptured their bladder. Bladder perforations may also be due to iatrogenic instrumentation–related trauma. Approximately two-thirds of patients with a bladder injury are extraperitoneal, and one-third are intraperitoneal, a distinction that typically determines whether the injury is surgically repaired.

The signs and symptoms of bladder injury are generally nonspecific, although 95% of patients present with gross hematuria. The patients may complain of suprapubic pain, dysuria, or inability to void, and on physical examination, may reveal tenderness in the suprapubic region, ileus, or an acute abdomen.[38–40]

Because of its established accuracy, CT cystography is the test of choice to investigate bladder wall integrity.[41,42] Indications for cystography include pelvic fracture with gross hematuria, blunt trauma with gross hematuria, and low-density free abdominal fluid on CT (<25 HU), blunt trauma with a pelvic ring fracture and greater than 30 red blood cells per high power field, penetrating trauma with any degree of hematuria, and an injury to the pelvis. Once patent urethral continuity is determined to be intact, bladder catheterization is performed and the bladder is filled with 300 mL of iodinated contrast. The sensitivity and specificity of CT cystography for bladder rupture are 95% and 100%, respectively.[43] Because of the high incidence of concomitant urethral injury seen in bladder rupture (5%–29%), confirmation of urethral integrity is important before catheterization.[36,43,44] Confirmation will provide efficient and timely evaluation in the multitrauma patient in whom CT cystography adds to the standard abdominal and pelvic trauma CT imaging. This type of combined imaging has the advantage of rapidly acquired information without transferring the patient while offering the potential to diagnose additional injuries.

Extraperitoneal bladder rupture is nearly always associated with pelvic fractures caused by a burst or shearing mechanism with a subsequent anterolateral wall laceration during traumatic deformation of the bony pelvis. The classic CT finding of extraperitoneal bladder rupture is contrast extravasation around the base of the bladder confined to perivesicular and space of Retzius with fluid seen anterior and lateral to the bladder. A CT cystogram may also be able to image and identify bladder neck injury, which needs immediate reconstruction to preserve continence.[45]

Management

Nonoperative
Accurate classification of bladder injury is vital to enable optimal management. Extraperitoneal ruptures are managed conservatively with placement of a urethral catheter or suprapubic cystotomy if there is a coexisting urethral injury.[44,46,47] Contraindications to nonoperative management include urinary infection, pelvic fractures requiring internal fixation, the presence of bony fragments in the bladder, bladder neck injury (that may compromise continence), rectal injuries, and female urethral or vaginal lacerations associated with pelvic fractures. CT or conventional cystography is performed in 10 to 14 days to document healing. Once the extravasation has resolved, catheter removal can be based on the patient's overall status and mobility. Open repair may be required if ongoing extravasation persists more than 4 weeks.[45]

Operative
All penetrating and intraperitoneal ruptures of the bladder are managed by means of exploration and repair. If the patient requires laparotomy for associated injuries and can tolerate the extra operating time, surgical repair of extraperitoneal bladder injuries is also prudent. Conversely, in severely unstable patients, catheter drainage can be used as a temporizing measure until the patient is able to undergo exploration.

Bladder exploration can be performed via an intraperitoneal approach or by entering the extraperitoneal space of Retzius in the anterior pelvis. Intraperitoneal injuries present as a stellate rupture of the dome of the bladder, and by enlarging this opening, one can inspect the interior of the bladder to exclude extraperitoneal injuries and evaluate the bladder neck.[48] In cases involving orthopedic reconstruction of the pelvis, the bladder may be approached extraperitoneally through the incision used to expose the pubic symphysis. Although extensive hemorrhage has been described in this scenario, it is a rare event. Most extraperitoneal bladder injuries associated with pelvic fractures are anteriorly located, small in size, and easily closed without a more extensive bladder exploration.

Penetrating injuries and unrecognized blunt bladder injuries discovered at laparotomy without prior CT cystography call for a careful evaluation. By opening the bladder vertically at the dome or along the anterior surface, one can identify sites of injury intravesically and inspect the ureteral orifices and the bladder neck.[48] Lacerations are closed with 3-0 absorbable sutures, which approximate detrusor muscle and mucosa in one layer and provide hemostasis. In patients with penetrating injuries, entrance and exit sites must be identified. The cystotomy is then closed with 2 layers of continuous 3-0 slowly absorbable sutures.

Postoperatively, adequate urinary drainage is essential to successful healing of the repaired bladder, and there is no evidence that suprapubic catheters are superior to urethral catheters in this context.[47,49] The catheter placed during trauma resuscitation is often not of sufficient caliber to allow easy bladder decompression; therefore, a 20-French urethral catheter should be substituted at the end of the operation. A closed suction drain near the bladder closure, but not on the suture line, is a necessity. A suprapubic cystotomy is rarely necessary, but may be an important adjunct if bleeding with clot formation needs irrigation for proper bladder decompression. CT or conventional cystography is performed in 10 to 14 days to document healing. Once the extravasation has resolved, catheter removal can be based on the patient's overall status and mobility.

URETHRAL INJURIES
Initial Evaluation

Urethral injuries are very uncommon in the genitourinary trauma population, and most are due to blunt trauma. Pelvic fracture urethral injuries (PFUI) occur with an approximate 1.5% to 5% incidence in patients with pelvic fractures.[36,50] Although these injuries are rare, they have the potential of incurring substantial long-term morbidity of recurrent stricture disease, incontinence, and erectile dysfunction. For every 1-mm increase of pubic symphysis diastasis, the risk of urethral injury increases 10%.[51] Anterior (penile and bulbar) urethral injuries are most commonly the result of fall-astride, or straddle injuries, but can also occur infrequently as a result of penile fracture or penetrating injury to the genitalia.

Blood at the meatus (37%–93% of patients) is the classic sign of injury to the male urethra and always warrants retrograde urethrography (RUG).[52] Patients may also present with inability to void, or a "high-riding" prostate gland on digital rectal examination, which should immediately warrant the need for urethrography before any attempt to insert a catheter, which can convert an incomplete injury to a complete transection. Contrast extravasation on RUG demonstrates injury. If a catheter has been placed, cystography can confirm placement. If a PFUI has occurred, a suprapubic tube should be placed and the bladder evaluated with cystography to exclude a concomitant bladder injury.

Management

Pelvic fracture urethral injury

The recommended treatment of traumatic urethral injuries is based on the location and mechanism of injury. They have been traditionally managed by means of suprapubic cystotomy with delayed reconstruction in 3 to 6 months. Partial disruption is typically cared for nonoperatively with a suprapubic or urethral catheter and is associated with a low risk of stricture formation. In contrast, complete disruption of the prostatomembranous urethra by pelvic fracture is managed surgically with either endoscopic realignment or suprapubic cystostomy placement and delayed urethroplasty. Controversy remains regarding the best initial management strategy of traumatic urethral distraction injuries.[53,54] A recent study reported 27 patients undergoing primary alignment with 14 patients managed by suprapubic cystotomy and delayed urethral reconstruction at a mean follow-up of 40 months.[55] Realignment was successful in 37% of patients, whereas 11 patients with suprapubic tube went on to urethroplasty in a shorter time with 100% success of functional outcome, concluding that endoscopic realignment offers definitive therapy in approximately one-third of treated patients. Primary realignment is performed through the previously placed suprapubic tube site, which allows antegrade passage of instruments through the bladder at the same time as retrograde instrumentation per urethral meatus. Flexible cystoscopes or magnetic-tipped catheters advanced under fluoroscopy guidance can help place a wire into the bladder beyond the injury, and a Council-tip urethral catheter is then advanced over the wire without any attempt to create a direct anastomosis.

Suprapubic cystotomy still remains the simplest approach, placed percutaneously or at laparotomy with an inevitable urethral obliteration outcome. This procedure allows the patient time to recover and to undergo urethral reconstruction in a specialist center by an experienced reconstructive surgeon. All patients who suffer a PFUI should be followed for at least 1 year for development of a urethral stricture, erectile dysfunction, or urinary incontinence.[45]

Anterior urethra injury

Straddle injury to the bulbar urethra is usually managed with a suprapubic cystostomy and delayed repair unless the injury permits passage of a urethral catheter. Surgical repair of the anterior urethra is preferred in cases of penetrating trauma or those associated with penile fracture. Gunshot wounds that result in large defects greater than 2 cm or associated with other major injuries should be treated with a suprapubic cystostomy tube with subsequent reconstruction at a tertiary center.

PENILE INJURY
Initial Evaluation

Penile trauma is unusual with variable cause, but still comprises 10%–16% of genitourinary injuries reported by several single-institution series.[56] Injury to the flaccid penis is rare, occurring mainly as a result of penetrating or self-mutilation cause. Penetrating and gunshot injuries are uncommon outside of a battlefield setting.

Penile fracture is an uncommon injury that results from disruption of the tunica albuginea. It is probably an underreported injury, accounting for 1 in every 175,000 emergency room visits.[57] A large number of the cases reported in the literature are from the Mediterranean region, where there is an increased incidence of "Tagaandan." Tagaandan is a sexual practice where the erect penis is forcibly pushed down to achieve detumescence.[58] In the United States and Europe, most fractures occur after the penis slips out of the vagina during intercourse and thrusts against the perineum or pubic symphysis.[59,60] A retrospective report of 16 patients with penile fracture found that intercourse in stressful situations, such as out of the ordinary locations (6.8%) and extramarital affair (43.8%), appears to have a relationship to the injury.[61]

The clinical picture of a penile fracture includes a missed intromission, acute bending of the penis, and a snapping sound followed by acute pain and immediate detumescence. There is often a delay in presentation attributable to the embarrassment of the social implications.

Penetrating injuries to the penis may result from deliberate attempts at mutilation as well as from accidental firearm injury. Penile swelling is limited to the penis by Buck fascia, but scrotal and perineal ecchymosis will develop, if the deep investing fascia of the penis is disrupted. The inability to void, gross hematuria, and blood at the meatus will strongly point to a urethral injury that warrants further investigation.

Urethral injury is seen in 10% to 22% of penile fracture cases and in 11% to 29% of penetrating penile injuries.[62,63] RUG and cystoscopy before surgical exploration are means of identifying concomitant urethral injuries sustained during a penile fracture or penetrating penile injury.[45]

Management

A circumferential, preputial, subcoronal incision with degloving blunt dissection of the skin and dartos fascia to the base of the penis will provide good exposure for penile fracture and most penetrating injuries. Tunica albuginea fractures are usually transversely oriented and may extend ventrally behind the corpus spongiosum, which presents a deeper injury that will require mobilization and retraction of the urethra to visualize the defect. The tunica albuginea rupture should be closed with interrupted 3-0 polydioxanone absorbable sutures. Even in cases of penetrating injury, most defects can be closed. In circumstances of large tissue loss, the wound may need to be managed in a staged fashion. Once the tunica albuginea has been closed, the dartos and skin are closed with fine suture. A lightly compressive circumferential dressing is placed.

PENILE AMPUTATION

Penile amputation is a true emergent catastrophe that is burdened by time-dependent reconstruction by a surgical team with a microvascular and urologic surgeon. Successful restoration of erectile, neurosensory, vascular, and urethral function is dependent on proper preservation of the amputated organ. The amputated part should be placed in saline-soaked gauze and a plastic bag. This bag should then be placed in a second bag containing slushed ice. Cold ischemia times longer than 24 hours are acceptable to allow transport to tertiary centers for replantation. Replantation after 16 hours of warm ischemia has been described.[64]

The creation of an intact microvascular circulation will improve the potential for a viable shaft skin, a sensate glans, and normal orgasmic function and should be performed if possible. Once the urethra is mobilized sufficiently, it is reanastomosed in 2 layers and a catheter placed. The septum of the corpora cavernosa is then connected and the tunica albuginea reanastomosed. The restored cavernosa blood flow preserves the distal corpora, the glans, and the urethra. Ischemic skin loss is expected without reanastomosis of the dorsal artery and vein. When the dorsal arteries, dorsal nerves, and deep dorsal vein are each reanastomosed by an experienced microvascular surgeon and the dartos and skin are closed, preservation of anatomy and function is remarkably high. Postoperative management includes catheter diversion, bed rest, anticoagulation, hydration, and monitoring distal penile arterial flow.

SCROTAL AND TESTICULAR INJURY
Initial Evaluation

Traumatic injuries to the scrotum and testes commonly occur in young men between the ages of 15 and 40 years old, resulting from either blunt or penetrating insults, degloving injuries, and electric burns. Penetrating scrotal injuries commonly involve not only the testes but also the corpora cavernosa, the urethra, and the spermatic cord.[65]

Clinical presentation of a ruptured testicle can be elusive, but is usually immediately painful, with rapid onset of swelling, tenderness, and ecchymosis. Injury to the scrotal wall or tunica vaginalis may cause significant swelling without rupture of the tunica albuginea of the testis. Testicular torsion should be included in the differential in cases of testicular trauma. A pelvic hematoma caused by pelvic fracture can also result in massive scrotal swelling, so that blunt scrotal injuries need careful scrutiny by ultrasound.

High-frequency ultrasonography with high-resolution images using a 7- to 14-MHz linear array transducer is the optimal imaging technique and a key to accurate evaluation of scrotal trauma, because evaluating the testicles on physical examination after trauma is difficult. As a result, all cases of scrotal blunt trauma should be evaluated with an ultrasound unless the clinical examintaion is completely normal. It is ideal for noninvasive evaluation of the scrotal contents, including testicular integrity, blood flow, hematoma, fluid collections, and foreign bodies.[65]

Blunt trauma is the most commonly seen form of trauma and is usually the result of an athletic injury (50%), a motor vehicle collision (9%–17%), or a violent assault.[66] Penetrating trauma is usually due to gunshot wounds and stab wounds, animal attacks, and self-mutilation. In a machine injury, degloving or avulsion injury may occur, which may result in the need of a split skin graft replacement.

Management

Scrotal exploration should be performed by making a midline vertical incision along the median raphe. This incision allows for access to both testicles through the same incision. If injury to the spermatic cord is suspected, the incision can be carried toward the groin for better exposure. The objective of exploration is to preserve testicle parenchyma (for endocrine and cosmetic purposes). In addition, large hematomas can be evacuated, thereby shortening the patient's recovery time.

The tunica vaginalis is opened to allow complete inspection of the tunica albuginea. If a tunica albuginea rupture is present, sharp debridement of any necrotic, nonviable tissue and extruded seminiferous tubules is performed, and the easily identified tunica rents are closed with running 4-0 monocryl sutures. The testis is placed into the scrotum with fixation sutures to the dartos, and a 2-layer closure of the scrotum is carried out with 4-0 absorbable suture. A Penrose drain is placed through a separate incision and removed when drainage stops. Ice, elevation, and anti-inflammatory medication should be started promptly.

Most testicular ruptures can be reconstructed by primary closure of the tunica envelope. Although most testicular ruptures can be closed primarily, a tunica vaginalis graft of the exposed testicular parenchyma may be used if the defect is too large for primary closure.[45]

Scrotal skin lacerations can usually be closed primarily unless there is prolonged delay before surgical care or there is a grossly contaminated wound associated with a rectal injury. Hemostasis in the scrotum needs much more intense meticulous attention because there is a higher incidence of delayed bleeding in such hypervascular mobile tissue. The skin and tunica dartos require separate 2-layer closure with a Penrose drain, placed through a dependent stab wound. The scrotum should be elevated and dressed with a firm compression dressing.

In the event of a scrotal avulsion injury from motor vehicle or a high-speed, rotating, machinery mechanism, an extensive debridement, followed by delay with wet to dry dressings, should be applied while awaiting healthy granulation tissue if there is concern about immediate wound management. The defect size and location will dictate the specific tissue transfer mode used, which may include primary closure, meshed split thickness skin grafts, placement of testes in subcutaneous pouches in thigh or abdomen, or the use of Singapore, anteromedial thigh flaps, or an inferior gluteal posterior thigh fasciocutaneous flap.[67]

REFERENCES

1. Centers for Disease Control and Prevention: Injury prevention & control: data & statistics. 2013. Available at: http://www.cdc.gov/injury/lc-charts/leading_causes_of_death_by_age_group_2013. Accessed August 8, 2015.
2. Wessells H, Suh D, Porter JR, et al. Renal injury and operative management in the United States: results of a population-based study. J Trauma 2003;54:423–30.
3. World Health Organization: Global burden of disease. 2015. Available at: http://www.who.int/healthinfo/global_burden_disease/en. Accessed August 8, 2015.
4. Bright TC, White K, Peters PC. Significance of hematuria after trauma. J Urol 1978;120:455–6.
5. Miller KS, McAninch JW. Radiographic assessment of renal trauma: our 15-year experience. J Urol 1995;154:352–5.
6. Smith J, Caldwell E, D'Amours S, et al. Abdominal trauma: a disease in evolution. ANZ J Surg 2005;75:790–4.
7. Meng MV, Brandes SB, McAninch JW. Renal trauma: indications and techniques for surgical exploration. World J Urol 1999;17:71–7.
8. Moore EE, Shackford SR, Pachter HL, et al. Organ injury scaling: spleen, liver, and kidney. J Trauma 1989;29:1664–6.
9. Wright JL, Nathens AB, Rivara FP, et al. Renal and extrarenal predictors of nephrectomy from the national trauma data bank. J Urol 2006;175:970–5 [discussion: 975].
10. Shewakramani S, Reed KC. Genitourinary trauma. Emerg Med Clin North Am 2011;29:501–18.
11. Buckley JC, McAninch JW. Revision of current American Association for the Surgery of Trauma renal injury grading system. J Trauma 2011;70:35–7.
12. Hammer CC, Santucci RA. Effect of an institutional policy of nonoperative treatment of grades I to IV renal injuries. J Urol 2003;169:1751–3.
13. Dugi DD 3rd, Morey AF, Gupta A, et al. American Association for the Surgery of Trauma grade 4 renal injury substratification into grades 4a (low risk) and 4b (high risk). J Urol 2010;183:592–7.
14. Santucci RA, Wessells H, Bartsch G, et al. Evaluation and management of renal injuries: consensus statement of the renal trauma subcommittee. BJU Int 2004; 93:937–54.
15. Simmons JD, Haraway AN, Schmieg RE Jr, et al. Blunt renal trauma and the predictors of failure of non-operative management. J Miss State Med Assoc 2010;51: 131–3.

16. Breyer BN, McAninch JW, Elliott SP, et al. Minimally invasive endovascular techniques to treat acute renal hemorrhage. J Urol 2008;179:2248–52 [discussion: 2253].

17. Buckley JC, McAninch JW. Selective management of isolated and nonisolated grade IV renal injuries. J Urol 2006;176:2498–502 [discussion: 2502].

18. Alsikafi NF, McAninch JW, Elliott SP, et al. Nonoperative management outcomes of isolated urinary extravasation following renal lacerations due to external trauma. J Urol 2006;176:2494–7.

19. Fiard G, Rambeaud JJ, Descotes JL, et al. Long-term renal function assessment with dimercapto-succinic acid scintigraphy after conservative treatment of major renal trauma. J Urol 2012;187:1306–9.

20. Voelzke BB, McAninch JW. Renal gunshot wounds: clinical management and outcome. J Trauma 2009;66:593–600 [discussion: 600–1].

21. Davis KA, Reed RL 2nd, Santaniello J, et al. Predictors of the need for nephrectomy after renal trauma. J Trauma 2006;60:164–9 [discussion: 169–70].

22. Morey AF, McAninch JW, Tiller BK, et al. Single shot intraoperative excretory urography for the immediate evaluation of renal trauma. J Urol 1999;161:1088–92.

23. Patel VG, Walker ML. The role of "one-shot" intravenous pyelogram in evaluation of penetrating abdominal trauma. Am Surg 1997;63:350–3.

24. Miller DC, Forauer A, Faerber GJ. Successful angioembolization of renal artery pseudoaneurysms after blunt abdominal trauma. Urology 2002;59:444.

25. Umbreit EC, Routh JC, Husmann DA. Nonoperative management of nonvascular grade IV blunt renal trauma in children: meta-analysis and systematic review. Urology 2009;74:579–82.

26. McAninch JW, Carroll PR. Renal trauma: kidney preservation through improved vascular control—a refined approach. J Trauma 1982;22:285–90.

27. Ramakumar S, Roberts WW, Fugita OE, et al. Local hemostasis during laparoscopic partial nephrectomy using biodegradable hydrogels: initial porcine results. J Endourol 2002;16:489–94.

28. Richter F, Tullmann ME, Turk I, et al. Improvement of hemostasis in laparoscopic and open partial nephrectomy with gelatin thrombin matrix (FloSeal). Urologe A 2003;42:338–46 [in German].

29. User HM, Nadler RB. Applications of FloSeal in nephron-sparing surgery. Urology 2003;62:342–3.

30. Siram SM, Gerald SZ, Greene WR, et al. Ureteral trauma: patterns and mechanisms of injury of an uncommon condition. Am J Surg 2010;199:566–70.

31. Elliott SP, McAninch JW. Ureteral injuries from external violence: the 25-year experience at San Francisco General Hospital. J Urol 2003;170:1213–6.

32. Best CD, Petrone P, Buscarini M, et al. Traumatic ureteral injuries: a single institution experience validating the American Association for the Surgery of Trauma-Organ Injury Scale grading scale. J Urol 2005;173:1202–5.

33. Sonmez K, Karabulut R, Turkyilmaz Z, et al. Bilateral ureteropelvic junction disruption in a 5-year-old boy. J Pediatr Surg 2008;43:e35–7.

34. Koukouras D, Petsas T, Liatsikos E, et al. Percutaneous minimally invasive management of iatrogenic ureteral injuries. J Endourol 2010;24:1921–7.

35. Liatsikos EN, Karnabatidis D, Katsanos K, et al. Ureteral injuries during gynecologic surgery: treatment with a minimally invasive approach. J Endourol 2006;20:1062–7.

36. Bjurlin MA, Fantus RJ, Mellett MM, et al. Genitourinary injuries in pelvic fracture morbidity and mortality using the National Trauma Data Bank. J Trauma 2009;67:1033–9.

37. Aihara R, Blansfield JS, Millham FH, et al. Fracture locations influence the likelihood of rectal and lower urinary tract injuries in patients sustaining pelvic fractures. J Trauma 2002;52:205–8 [discussion: 208–9].

38. Morey AF, Iverson AJ, Swan A, et al. Bladder rupture after blunt trauma: guidelines for diagnostic imaging. J Trauma 2001;51:683–6.

39. Hsieh CH, Chen RJ, Fang JF, et al. Diagnosis and management of bladder injury by trauma surgeons. Am J Surg 2002;184:143–7.

40. Avey G, Blackmore CC, Wessells H, et al. Radiographic and clinical predictors of bladder rupture in blunt trauma patients with pelvic fracture. Acad Radiol 2006; 13:573–9.

41. Wirth GJ, Peter R, Poletti PA, et al. Advances in the management of blunt traumatic bladder rupture: experience with 36 cases. BJU Int 2010;106:1344–9.

42. Quagliano PV, Delair SM, Malhotra AK. Diagnosis of blunt bladder injury: a prospective comparative study of computed tomography cystography and conventional retrograde cystography. J Trauma 2006;61:410–21 [discussion: 421–2].

43. Deck AJ, Shaves S, Talner L, et al. Computerized tomography cystography for the diagnosis of traumatic bladder rupture. J Urol 2000;164:43–6.

44. Cass AS. Diagnostic studies in bladder rupture. Indications and techniques. Urol Clin North Am 1989;16:267–73.

45. Morey AF, Brandes S, Dugi DD 3rd, et al. Urotrauma: AUA guideline. J Urol 2014; 192:327–35.

46. Kotkin L, Koch MO. Morbidity associated with nonoperative management of extraperitoneal bladder injuries. J Trauma 1995;38:895–8.

47. Parry NG, Rozycki GS, Feliciano DV, et al. Traumatic rupture of the urinary bladder: is the suprapubic tube necessary? J Trauma 2003;54:431–6.

48. Corriere JN Jr, Sandler CM. Bladder rupture from external trauma: diagnosis and management. World J Urol 1999;17:84–9.

49. Alli MO, Singh B, Moodley J, et al. Prospective evaluation of combined suprapubic and urethral catheterization to urethral drainage alone for intraperitoneal bladder injuries. J Trauma 2003;55:1152–4.

50. Brandes S, Borrelli J Jr. Pelvic fracture and associated urologic injuries. World J Surg 2001;25:1578–87.

51. Basta AM, Blackmore CC, Wessells H. Predicting urethral injury from pelvic fracture patterns in male patients with blunt trauma. J Urol 2007;177:571–5.

52. Martinez-Pineiro L, Djakovic N, Plas E, et al. EAU guidelines on urethral trauma. Eur Urol 2010;57:791–803.

53. Hadjizacharia P, Inaba K, Teixeira PG, et al. Evaluation of immediate endoscopic realignment as a treatment modality for traumatic urethral injuries. J Trauma 2008; 64:1443–9 [discussion: 1449–50].

54. Leddy LS, Vanni AJ, Wessells H, et al. Outcomes of endoscopic realignment of pelvic fracture associated urethral injuries at a level 1 trauma center. J Urol 2012;188:174–8.

55. Johnsen NV, Dmochowski RR, Mock S, et al. Primary endoscopic realignment of urethral disruption injuries—a double-edged sword? J Urol 2015;194:1022–6.

56. Cerwinka WH, Block NL. Civilian gunshot injuries of the penis: the Miami experience. Urology 2009;73:877–80.

57. Aaronson DS, Shindel AW. U.S. national statistics on penile fracture. J Sex Med 2010;7:3226.

58. el-Sherif AE, Dauleh M, Allowneh N, et al. Management of fracture of the penis in Qatar. Br J Urol 1991;68:622–5.

59. Mydlo JH. Surgeon experience with penile fracture. J Urol 2001;166:526–8 [discussion: 528–9].
60. Koifman L, Barros R, Junior RA, et al. Penile fracture: diagnosis, treatment and outcomes of 150 patients. Urology 2010;76:1488–92.
61. Kramer AC. Penile fracture seems more likely during sex under stressful situations. J Sex Med 2011;8:3414–7.
62. Phonsombat S, Master VA, McAninch JW. Penetrating external genital trauma: a 30-year single institution experience. J Urol 2008;180:192–5 [discussion: 195–6].
63. Tsang T, Demby AM. Penile fracture with urethral injury. J Urol 1992;147:466–8.
64. Jezior JR, Brady JD, Schlossberg SM. Management of penile amputation injuries. World J Surg 2001;25:1602–9.
65. Buckley JC, McAninch JW. Diagnosis and management of testicular ruptures. Urol Clin North Am 2006;33:111–6, vii.
66. Dogra VS, Gottlieb RH, Oka M, et al. Sonography of the scrotum. Radiology 2003; 227:18–36.
67. Wessells H. Genital skin loss: unified reconstructive approach to a heterogeneous entity. World J Urol 1999;17:107–14.

Diagnosis and Management of Lower Urinary Tract Dysfunction

Robert C. McDonough III, MD[a],*, Stephen T. Ryan, MD[b]

KEYWORDS

- Urodynamics • Lower urinary tract dysfunction • Neurogenic bladder

KEY POINTS

- The function of the lower urinary tract is a complex system involving both the end organs of the bladder and the urinary sphincter as well as multiple areas of the nervous system.
- Urodynamics is a broad term that describes multiple studies that can assist the urologist in the classification and treatment of various lower urinary tract disorders.
- Many lower urinary tract disorders do not require surgery for treatment, but are amenable to treatment through medical and behavioral means.

INTRODUCTION

Lower urinary tract dysfunction involves a broad spectrum of disease, ranging from the bladder that is unable to empty to one that is unable to store urine appropriately. Effective treatment of these symptoms may lead to surgery; however, the clinician can often manage the patient with medical or behavioral intervention alone. In some cases the cause of the dysfunction may be quite complex and necessitates diagnostic testing to ensure proper therapy. Urologists will often use a set of tests known as urodynamics to further characterize the patient's urinary function. This article reviews function of both the normal and the abnormal bladder, the role of urodynamics in evaluation of lower urinary tract dysfunction, and the medical and behavioral management of some of these disorders.

NORMAL BLADDER PHYSIOLOGY

The normal bladder cycles through 2 phases: filling and emptying. The filling (or storage) phase allows for the bladder to passively fill with urine. The viscoelastic properties of the bladder should allow for large urinary volumes to be stored at low bladder

[a] Division of Urology, Maine Medical Center, Tufts University School of Medicine, Portland, ME 04105, USA; [b] Division of Urology, Maine Medical Center, Portland, ME 04105, USA
* Corresponding author.
E-mail address: mcdonr@mmc.org

Surg Clin N Am 96 (2016) 441–452
http://dx.doi.org/10.1016/j.suc.2016.02.003
0039-6109/16/$ – see front matter © 2016 Elsevier Inc. All rights reserved.

surgical.theclinics.com

pressures. This process is mediated by sympathetic neural input to the bladder via β3 receptors that allow for relaxation of the detrusor muscle.[1] During bladder filling, there should be no involuntary bladder contractions. The bladder outlet should also remain closed at rest.

Emptying of the bladder is accomplished by contraction of the bladder detrusor muscle. The bladder outlet should relax in a coordinated fashion before bladder contraction to ensure no obstruction to urinary flow. The outlet consists of both an external sphincter (under somatic control via the pudendal nerve) and an internal sphincter at the bladder neck. Relaxation of the internal sphincter and contraction of the bladder are both mediated by parasympathetic cholinergic stimulation. In normal voiding, there should also be no physical obstruction to urinary flow along the length of the urethra.

The neural control of this process is presented in **Fig. 1**.[2] Afferent and efferent nerves arising from the S2-4 nerve roots serve as a closed reflex loop: when the bladder meets a certain volume threshold, a reflex contraction is initiated. This contraction is poorly coordinated, however. To compensate, afferent input is transmitted through the spinal cord to the pontine micturition center (PMC) located in the brainstem. Efferent signals from the PMC are then relayed down the spinal cord to allow for coordinated contraction and appropriate relaxation of the sphincteric complex. Finally, the cortex of the brain provides social control over the entire reflex mechanism through input to the PMC. If a reflex contraction is signaled at a socially

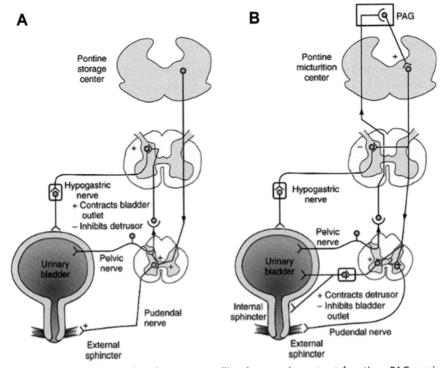

Fig. 1. Schematic of neural pathways controlling lower urinary tract function. PAG, periaqueductal gray. (*From* Yoshimura N, Chancellor MB. Physiology and pharmacology of the bladder and urethra. In: Wein AJ, Kavoussi LE, Campbell MF, editors. Campbell-Walsh Urology. 10th edition. Philadelphia: Elsevier; 2012; with permission.)

inappropriate time, the cortex can suppress the reflex to allow for voiding later. This reflex suppression is often mediated by what is known as the guarding reflex: an increase in activity of the external urinary sphincter, accompanied by a brief increase in intravesical pressure followed by an abrupt cessation of detrusor activity.[3]

LOWER URINARY TRACT PATHOPHYSIOLOGY

Lower urinary tract disorders can easily be categorized by dysfunction of either of the main functions of the bladder, either storage or emptying. Furthermore, each of these categories can be further divided depending on the anatomic source of the problem in the lower urinary tract—the bladder itself or the bladder outlet.[4] Examples of these are listed in **Table 1**.

By thinking of these problems in these broad terms, the clinician is able to focus on the underlying problem in addition to the cause. Some causes of lower urinary tract dysfunction are not necessarily treatable in and of themselves, but the sequelae can be addressed directly.

LOWER URINARY TRACT DYSFUNCTION: PATIENT EVALUATION

As with any patient, the workup begins with a complete and thorough history to best understand the nature of the patient's complaints. The clinician should enquire about the specific symptoms: frequency, urgency, urge or stress incontinence, bladder pain, hematuria, dysuria, or retention. The duration of symptoms, severity, and degree of bother should also be determined. Review of surgical and medical history may reveal disease processes that are directly related to the patient complaints. Accurate determination of the patient's medications is also crucial, because many medications can have a direct impact on the function of the lower urinary tract. In female patients, a complete obstetric and menstrual history should also be obtained. Standardized validated questionnaires are available as excellent tools to help in determining symptoms, degree of bother, and impact on quality of life.[5]

Relevant physical examination includes assessment of the abdomen, genitalia, perineum, rectum, and back. One should also perform a limited neurologic examination consisting of evaluation of mental status, gait, physical dexterity and mobility, and extremity weakness. Key points of the physical examination for both sexes are listed in **Box 1**.

Laboratory examination for most patients with lower urinary tract dysfunction is primarily limited to urinalysis. Possible findings of infection, glucosuria, pyuria,

Table 1
Common lower urinary tract disorders characterized by type of dysfunction and location of disorder

	Failure to Store	Failure to Empty
Because of bladder	Overactivity • Neurologic injury • Hypertrophy Hypersensitivity • Inflammation/infection • Psychological	Neurologic • Neurologic injury • Pharmacologic Myogenic • Acontractile bladder
Because of outlet	SUI • Pelvic floor laxity • Lack of urethral support Intrinsic sphincter deficiency	Prostatic obstruction Bladder neck contracture Urethral stricture Striated sphincter dyssynergia

> **Box 1**
> **Important points of physical examination for patients with lower urinary tract dysfunction**
>
> *Male*
> - Abdomen: Suprapubic fullness, or pain with pressure to suggest a full bladder
> - Genitalia: Appearance, lesions, hair distribution
> - Urethral meatus: Caliber and location
> - Urethra: Masses, tenderness, scarring
> - Digital rectal examination: Sphincter tone, masses, and prostatic size, prostatic tenderness
>
> *Female*
> - Abdomen: Suprapubic fullness, or pain with pressure to suggest a full bladder
> - Genitalia: Appearance, assess for atrophy/hair distribution
> - Urethra: Location, caliber, prolapse
> - Vaginal introitus: Discharge, lesions, atrophy, prolapse with strain (consider split speculum)
> - Speculum examination: Cervix appearance/discharge or lesions.
> - Bimanual examination to assess uterus (size, mobility), adenexa (masses, tenderness)
> - Digital rectal examination to assess for sphincteric tone

proteinuria, or hematuria all have relevance to the patient with bladder issues. Urine culture is warranted in any patient with concern for infection. Microscopic hematuria should not be ignored and may warrant a full urologic workup. The basic metabolic profile is also important in a select group of patients, as some severe bladder dysfunction can result in renal impairment.

A voiding diary is also highly recommended (**Fig. 2**). With this tool, the clinician can better understand how the patient functions outside of the doctor's office. Urinary frequency, urgency, incontinence, intake, and possible polyuria can all be examined. The voiding diary has also been demonstrated to be useful as a tool to assess treatment efficacy.[6] Last, the highest voided volume on the patient's diary has been shown to correlate well with the patient's cystometric capacity on urodynamics.[7]

Imaging has little role in the vast majority of patients with lower urinary tract dysfunction. The upper tracts should be evaluated in patients wherein the bladder puts them at risk as well as in patients with hematuria. Specific imaging may also be indicated by associated comorbidities.

URODYNAMICS

Urodynamics is a collective term that describes several studies that are used to assess the function of the lower urinary tract. Urodynamic studies attempt to mimic normal bladder filling and emptying while monitoring various parameters that can characterize how the lower urinary tract works in real time. Descriptions of the various urodynamic studies follow.

Noninvasive Uroflowmetry

The patient presents with a full bladder and then voids into a measuring device that is able to quantify flow rate. Maximum and average flow rates can be determined, along with voided volume, length of time to void, and the shape of the voiding curve. A few examples are provided in **Fig. 3**. Noninvasive uroflowmetry is often accompanied by

INTAKE & VOIDING DIARY

This is a chart to record your fluid intake, voiding (urination) and urine leakage. Choose two days (entire 24 hour days) to complete this record. The two days do not need to be in a row. Pick days in which it will be convenient for you to measure EVERY void. Bring completed diary to your next visit.

Instuctions:

1. Begin recording upon rising in the morning, and continue for a full 24 hours.

2. Record separate lines for voids, leaks and fluid intake.

3. Measure voids in "cc's" or in ounces.

4. Measure fluid intake in ounces.

5. When recording a leak, please indicate the volume (on a 1, 2 or 3 scale), your activity during the leak, and if you had an urge ("yes" or "no") at the time of leakage.

DATE #1 _____

Time	Amount Voided (in cc's or ounces)	Leak volume 1 = drops/damp 2 = wet 3 = bladder emptied	Activity during leak	Urge? Yes/No	Fluid Intake (amount in ounces/type)

Fig. 2. Sample intake/voiding diary. (*Courtesy of* Robert C. McDonough III, MD, Portland, ME.)

an after-void residual assessment, which can be accomplished in a noninvasive fashion with ultrasound. Although easy for the patient to perform, this study is limited by lack of data on bladder pressure. Low flow rates can be a result of either detrusor failure or obstruction to urinary flow.

The upper image indicates a normal tracing, whereas the lower image shows decreased flow rates and a prolonged voiding time possibly consistent with bladder outlet obstruction.

Multichannel Urodynamics

By using a pressure transducer to measure bladder pressure, more information can be obtained. A specialized catheter can be placed in the bladder lumen, which allows the bladder to be filled with fluid at a controlled rate while simultaneously measuring

A

B

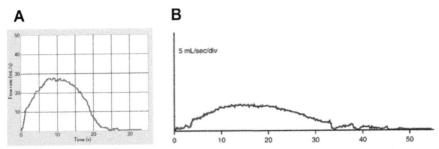

Fig. 3. (A and B) Sample uroflow tracings. (From Herschorn S. Urodynamic evaluation of the patient with prolapse. Female urology. 3rd edition. Philadelphia: Elsevier; 2008; and Boone TB, Kim YH. Uroflowmetry. In: Nitti VW, editor. Practical urodynamics. Philadelphia: WB Saunders; 1998. p. 28–51; with permission.)

pressure. However, the pressure measured in the bladder is a combined result of true detrusor contraction as well as any intra-abdominal pressure external to the bladder. To compensate for this, a secondary pressure transducer is placed in the abdominal cavity; this can be accomplished through placing the secondary catheter in the rectum in all patients or the vagina in women. In patients with bowel diversions, the ostomy can also be used. Detrusor pressure is calculated by subtracting the measured abdominal pressure from the measured vesicular pressure. A sample urodynamic tracing is provided in **Fig. 4.**

Multichannel urodynamics is typically broken up into 2 major components—the cystometrogram (CMG) and the pressure flow study (PFS). These multichannel urody-namics assess the filling and emptying functions of the bladder, respectively. For the CMG, the bladder is filled at a controlled rate while the patient reports any sensation of fullness or need to void. Bladder sensation, capacity, compliance, and stability can all be measured in this fashion. In addition, the patient can be asked to cough or perform Valsalva to look for leakage pressures. For the PFS, true detrusor pressure is measured while the patient voids into a flowmeter (as with noninvasive uroflow). High pressures with low flow are typically associated with obstruction, whereas low pressures with low flow would indicate detrusor failure. A calculated residual volume can be obtained by comparing the measured amount voided to the amount instilled in the bladder.

Electromyogram

Electromyogram (EMG) is used to evaluate function of the external urinary sphincter, a striated muscle under voluntary control. EMG may be done with either needle or pad electrodes and is also measured simultaneously with filling and emptying. EMG is somewhat limited by a high amount of artifact, generally associated with patient movement.

Video Urodynamics

If the urodynamics suite is capable of fluoroscopy, then this can also be done selec-tively during the procedure if contrast is used as the instillation fluid. Real-time imaging can help better define sphincteric function and also can help define other anomalies such as vesicoureteral reflux, cystocele, or ureteroceles.

Recommendations on Use

Urodynamics can be extremely helpful in the diagnosis of multiple conditions related to dysfunction of the lower urinary tract. However, the study is somewhat invasive and

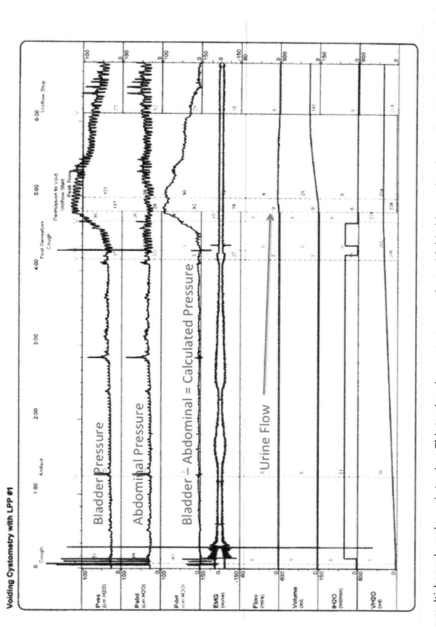

Fig. 4. Sample multichannel urodynamic tracing. This tracing demonstrates a patient with bladder outlet obstruction. Note the high calculated detrusor pressure seen on the upper right, which corresponds with a low flow rate further below on the image. LPP, leak point pressure.

involves the risk of radiation exposure to the patient and clinician if fluoroscopy is used. Several societies have published guidelines on the proper use of urodynamics. The following is a summary of those recommendations.[8–13]

Urodynamics required

Urodynamics are essential in the patient population with neurologic bladder dysfunction or "neurogenic bladder." These studies allow the clinician to develop a baseline of bladder function in patients who will likely need long-term urologic care. Findings that may put the kidneys at risk in the long term can be identified and corrected. In addition, bladder symptoms in these often complex patients can be better analyzed to help guide therapy. Urodynamic studies should also be strongly considered in any patient who is to undergo an invasive procedure for the treatment of incontinence, pelvic floor prolapse, or lower urinary tract symptoms. Finally, pressure flow studies should be obtained in any patient undergoing surgery to relieve bladder outlet obstruction in whom the clinician is unsure of the quality of the patient's underlying bladder function.

Urodynamics helpful

In patients with uncertain diagnoses after initial clinical workup, urodynamics may be of assistance in better characterizing the patient's problem. In addition, these studies can be of great assistance when the patient's complaints are not in accordance with the objective clinical findings. Urodynamics may assist the clinician in patient counseling regarding expectations from a planned procedure or treatment. Last, postoperative urodynamic studies can provide a helpful point of comparison to preoperative data in the case of unexpected or failed treatment outcome for lower urinary tract disorders.

Urodynamics unnecessary

Urodynamic studies are not required in female patients with uncomplicated stress incontinence demonstrable in the office setting. Also, if the clinician is sure in a particular diagnosis and is considering a noninvasive conservative treatment option, then invasive urodynamics are also not needed. Some patients with neurogenic bladder (such as stroke patients) have predictable lower urinary tract function and are low risk for damage to the upper urinary tract. Urodynamics can safely be avoided in these patients as well.

MEDICAL AND BEHAVIORAL MANAGEMENT OF LOWER URINARY TRACT DYSFUNCTION

Regardless of the myriad of causes that can lead to lower urinary tract dysfunction, nonoperative management is often guided by the end result—either failure to store or empty urine. Although the urologic surgeon cannot correct the underlying problem of spinal cord injury or diabetic neuropathy for example, he can often manage the bladder without the need for surgical intervention.

Failure to Empty Due to Bladder

Currently, there are limited options for pharmaceutical treatment of detrusor failure. Bethanechol (Urecholine), a muscarinic cholinergic agonist, is the only medication available. Unfortunately, the results of this medication are often disappointing. A recent review showed no consistent evidence to support the use of parasympathomimetic agents for the treatment of detrusor failure.[14]

Mechanical drainage via catheter is generally the treatment of choice for this patient population. Mechanical drainage via catheter can be accomplished with an indwelling urethral or suprapubic catheter, or through clean intermittent catheterization (CIC). All these choices carry a risk of urinary tract infection, and most patients using these methods will develop asymptomatic bacteriuria from colonization. One fundamental difference between indwelling catheters and CIC is that chronic indwelling catheters carry an estimated lifetime risk of bladder carcinoma of 8% to 10%.[15] Intermittent catheterization does not have this risk, but does require a motivated patient (or supportive care) with the ability to do the procedure.

Failure to Empty Due to Outlet

Outlet obstruction from mechanical sources such as urethral strictures generally will require operative intervention. However, if the source of obstruction is from poor relaxation of the sphincteric complex, medical therapy can be of some utility.

Contraction of the internal smooth muscle sphincter is mediated primarily by α-A1 adrenergic receptors. Several α-adrenergic antagonists are commercially available. Newer agents such as alfuzosin (Uroxatral) and tamsulosin (Flomax) are highly α-a1 selective and are less likely to cause orthostatic hypotension from less influence on vascular smooth muscle tone.[16] Unfortunately, there are no selective medicines for the treatment of spasticity of the striated external sphincter, although benzodiazepines, dantrolene, and baclofen have all been used with varying degrees of success.[17] Of course, mechanical drainage can also be used in those who fail medical therapy.

Failure to Store Due to Bladder

Detrusor overactivity is the end result of not just disease processes but also several additional factors. Environmental influences, diet, and abnormal learned behavior all contribute to the severity of the patient's condition. With that in mind, treatment of detrusor overactivity necessitates a multimodal approach. The vast majority of patients will experience symptomatic relief through behavioral and dietary modification along with the potential addition of pharmaceutical intervention.

Dietary modification for the overactive bladder involves the elimination or reduction of substances that are known bladder irritants. High acid loads, caffeine, and theophylline are all examples of such irritants. The authors currently recommend limiting intake of vitamin C and protein, reducing intake of citrus fruits, and eliminating caffeinated coffee/tea as well as chocolate.[18] Patients should also carefully examine their overall fluid intake: if input is excessive, more urine typically would be excreted and would exacerbate the overactivity through sheer overproduction of volume.[19] Smoking cessation also reduces the bladder irritant load.

Pelvic floor physical therapy can play a major role in helping this patient population. Setting a timed voiding schedule can help the patient regulate their voiding patterns. Regular Kegel exercises can help reinforce the natural guarding reflex, which will help to abate urinary urgency. Finally, distraction exercises can help the patient suppress the need to void until a more appropriate time.[20–22]

Medical management of the overactive bladder has traditionally been treated by anticholinergic medications. Of the 5 muscarinic receptor subtypes, 2 are predominantly present and functional in the bladder: M2 and M3. Numerous drugs are available with varying degrees of selectivity for either the M2 or the M3 receptors, but all generally are relatively clinically equivalent in patient efficacy.[23] Many of the side effects of these drugs are directly related to the cross-reactivity with muscarinic receptors on nontarget organs such as the salivary glands or the bowels. In fact, the primary side effects of these medications are dry mouth and constipation from blocking cholinergic muscarinic input to these organs. Despite this, they do remarkably well at treating symptoms, and the American Urological Association Best Practice Guidelines for Overactive Bladder recommend attempting to manage the side effects separately instead of abandoning the medication if the side effects are problematic.[24]

Anticholinergic effects can cause cognitive impairment in some elderly patients, so one should be cautious in that patient population. Patients with already decreased gut motility or concurrent detrusor weakness should be carefully followed. Last, this drug class should be avoided in patients with acute narrow angle glaucoma.

Recently, a new drug option has become available. Rather than anticholinergic blockade of bladder contraction, β-3 agonists cause direct relaxation of the bladder and have been shown to improve bladder overactivity symptoms.[25,26] Currently, myrabegron (Myrbetriq) is the only available β-3 agonist in the United States. Because of cross-reactivity with vascular β-receptors, this drug can increase vascular tone leading to an increase in baseline blood pressure. Patients with hypertension should be monitored to ensure the impact of this is not significant. As with anticholinergics, the clinician should also exercise caution in using this medication in patients who also have poor detrusor function.

Failure to Store Due to Bladder Outlet

Failure to store due to the outlet is generally a failure of the sphincteric complex that leads to stress urinary incontinence (SUI). Kegel exercises are of great help to the patient here by strengthening those muscles. If the patient is able to anticipate an action that will lead to stress incontinence, conscious activation of the sphincteric complex may prevent leakage. Physical therapy here can also be of great assistance in reinforcing this.[27]

Beyond behavioral therapy, there are no effective medical options available for treatment; this is primarily a surgical disorder. α-Agonists and estrogens (in women) have been tried with disappointing results. Duloxetine (Cymbalta) showed some promise at one point, but this medication was not approved for SUI due to its adverse effects.[28]

SUMMARY

Lower urinary tract dysfunction can be the result of many causes: anatomic, neurologic, pharmaceutical, and myogenic failure to name a few broad categories. The simplest way to approach lower urinary tract dysfunction is either failure to store urine or failure to empty the bladder appropriately. Every patient should receive the same evaluation that they would receive for any complaint, a history of present illness, and a focused physical examination. Urologists sometimes use urodynamics to help guide management of complex patients.

Keeping a focus as to the main precipitating cause, either failure to store or failure to empty urine can help guide management without necessarily needing urodynamics. Taking that one step further, the surgeon should then consider if the problem is due to the bladder or the bladder outlet. Combining these 2 crucial factors can guide a physician into understanding the root of patients' problems and focus on effective behavioral and medical solutions.

REFERENCES

1. Andersson KE, Martin N, Nitti V. Selective β_3-adrenoceptor agonists for the treatment of overactive bladder [Review]. J Urol 2013;190(4):1173–80.

2. Yoshimura N, Chancellor MB. "Chp 60 physiology and pharmacology of the bladder and urethra." Campbell-Walsh Urology. 10th edition. Philadelphia: Elsevier; 2012.

3. Park JM, Bloom DA, McGuire EJ. The guarding reflex revisited. Br J Urol 1997;80: 940–5.

4. Wein A. "Pathophysiology and classification of lower urinary tract dysfunction." Campbell-Walsh Urology. 10th edition. Philadelphia: Elsevier; 2012.
5. van de Vaart H, Falconer C, Quail D, et al. Patient reported outcomes tools in an observational study of female stress urinary incontinence. Neurourol Urodyn 2010;29(3):348–53.
6. Hseih CH, Chang ST, Hsieh CJ, et al. Treatment of interstitial cystitis with hydro-distention and bladder training. Int Urogynecol J Pelvic Floor Dysfunct 2008; 81(2):153–9.
7. Diokno AC, Wells TJ, Brink CA. Comparison of self-reported volume with cysto-metric bladder capacity. J Urol 1987;137(4):698–700.
8. Collins CW, Winters JC. AUA/SUFU adult urodynamics guideline: a clinical review. Urol Clin North Am 2014;41(3):353–62.
9. Smith A, Bevan D, Douglas HR, et al. Management of urinary incontinence in women: summary of updated NICE guidance. BMJ 2013;347:f5170.
10. Swain S, Hughes R, Perry M, et al. Management of lower urinary tract dysfunction in neurological disease: summary of NICE guidance. BMJ 2012;345:e5074.
11. Gammie A, Clarkson B, Constantinou C, et al. International Continence Society guidelines on urodynamic equipment performance. Neurourol Urodyn 2014; 33(4):370–9.
12. Winters JC, Dmochowski RR, Goldman HB, et al. Urodynamic studies in adults: AUA/SUFU guideline. J Urol 2012;188(6 Suppl):2464–72.
13. Nager CW, Brubaker L, Litman HJ, et al. A randomized trial of urodynamic testing before stress-incontinence surgery. N Engl J Med 2012;366(21):1987–97.
14. Barendrecht MM, Oelke M, Laguna MP, et al. Is the use of parasympathomimetics for treating an underactive urinary bladder evidence-based? BJU Int 2007;99: 749–52.
15. Delnay K, Stonehill W, Goldman H, et al. Bladder histological changes associated with chronic indwelling urinary catheter. J Urol 1999;161:1106–9.
16. Djavan B, Chapple C, Milani S, et al. State of the art on the efficacy and tolerability of alpha1-adrenoceptor antagonists in patients with lower urinary tract symptoms suggestive of benign prostatic hyperplasia. Urology 2004;64(6):1081–8.
17. Andersson K, Wein A. "Pharmacologic management of lower urinary tract storage and emptying failure." Campbell-Walsh Urology. 10th edition. Philadelphia: Elsevier; 2012.
18. Bryant CM, Dowell CJ, Fairbrother G. Caffeine reduction education to improve urinary symptoms. Br J Nurs 2002;11:560.
19. Hashim H, Abrams P. How should patients with an overactive bladder manipulate their fluid intake? BJU Int 2008;102:62.
20. Burgio KL, Goode PS, Johnson TM 2nd, et al. Behavioral versus drug treatment for overactive bladder in men: the Male Overactive bladder treatment in veterans (MOTIVE) trial. J Am Geriatr Soc 2011;59:2209.
21. Wyman JF, Fantl JA, McClish DK, et al. Comparative efficacy of behavioral interventions in the management of female urinary incontinence. Continence Program for Women Research Group. Am J Obstet Gynecol 1998;179:999.
22. Burgio KL, Goode PS, Locher JL, et al. Behavioral training with and without biofeedback in the treatment of urge incontinence in older women: a randomized controlled trial. JAMA 2002;288:2293.
23. Abrams P, Andersson KE, Buccafusco JJ, et al. Muscarinic receptors: their distribution and function in body systems, and the implications for treating overactive bladder. Br J Pharmacol 2006;148:565.

24. Gormley E, Lightner D, Burgio K, et al. Diagnosis and treatment of overactive bladder (non-neurogenic) in adults: AUA/SUFU guideline. J Urol 2015;193(5): 1572–80.

25. Khullar V, Amarenco G, Angulo JC, et al. Efficacy and tolerability of mirabegron, a beta(3)-adrenoceptor agonist, in patients with overactive bladder: results from a randomised European-Australian phase 3 trial. Eur Urol 2013;63:2.

26. Nitti VW, Auerbach S, Martin N, et al. Results of a randomized phase III trial of mirabegron in patients with overactive bladder. J Urol 2013;189:4.

27. Fantyl JA, Wyman JF, McLish DK, et al. Efficacy of bladder training in older women with urinary incontinence. JAMA 1991;265:609–13.

28. Dmochowski RR, Miklos JR, Norton PA, et al. Duloxetine versus placebo for the treatment of North American women with stress urinary incontinence. J Urol 2003;170(4 Pt 1):1259–63.

Urinary Retention in Surgical Patients

Urszula Kowalik, MD[a], Mark K. Plante, MD, FRCS(C)[b],*

KEYWORDS

- Urinary retention • Postoperative • Surgery • Bladder function

KEY POINTS

- Urinary retention, in some cases, is a preventable complication in general surgical patients in the postoperative setting.
- Urinary retention can be secondary to outlet obstruction, disruption of innervation to the bladder, or bladder overdistention.
- The goals for prevention should include identification of patients at risk. Risk factors known to be associated with increased risk of acute retention are age, medications, anesthetics, benign prostatic hyperplasia/lower urinary tract symptoms, and surgery-related factors, including operating room time, intravenous fluids, and procedure type.
- Diagnosis of urinary retention is best confirmed by bladder scan, as symptoms, such as pain and urge to void, are unreliable.
- The mainstay of initial management of urinary retention is placement of a Foley catheter. Alpha-blockers should be started, as they increase the likelihood of a successful voiding trial.

URINARY RETENTION

Urinary retention in surgical patients is a common source of morbidity and can result in added costs that can potentially be avoided. Over the years, the urologic, general surgical, orthopedic, and anesthesia literature have addressed the problem; however, the definitions remain unclear with few if any guidelines for prevention and management. Recommendations for patients with increased baseline risk, that is, patients with known benign prostatic hyperplasia (BPH), are scarce as well. Studies on the topic are generally very heterogeneous with varying populations, operative conditions, and notably what constitutes retention. This article mainly focuses on the risk factors

Disclosure Statement: The authors have nothing to disclose.
[a] University of Vermont Medical Center, 111 Colchester Avenue, Mailstop 222WP2, Burlington, VT 05401, USA; [b] Division of Urology, Department of Surgery, University of Vermont Medical Center, University of Vermont College of Medicine, 111 Colchester Avenue, Mailstop 320FL4, Burlington, VT 05401, USA
* Corresponding author.
E-mail address: mark.plante@med.uvm.edu

Surg Clin N Am 96 (2016) 453–467
http://dx.doi.org/10.1016/j.suc.2016.02.004
0039-6109/16/$ – see front matter © 2016 Elsevier Inc. All rights reserved.

surgical.theclinics.com

for and subsequent management of postoperative urinary retention (POUR) as it is commonly encountered by the general surgeon and has been shown to be responsible for up to 20% to 25% of unplanned admissions after ambulatory surgery.[1,2]

Definitions

Urinary retention has taken on many definitions in the literature but can be best described as the inability to spontaneously and adequately empty the bladder. This definition is broad as it encompasses what has been described as acute versus chronic as well as complete versus incomplete retention. The categories are not mutually exclusive as both acute and chronic retention can be complete or incomplete and the literature has used a combination of other varying definitions making it very difficult to compare studies.

Acute urinary retention (AUR) is one of the few true urologic emergencies. The International Continence Society (ICS) defines AUR as a "painful, palpable or percussible bladder, when the patient is unable to pass any urine."[3] It can be spontaneous or secondary to surgery, medications, BPH, cerebrovascular accident, immobility, or anesthesia. In the case of BPH-related AUR, McNeil[4] found that differentiating between spontaneous and precipitated AUR was not important as the management did not change, whereas precipitated AUR unrelated to BPH may require altered management.

Chronic urinary retention is described by the ICS as "a non-painful bladder, which remains palpable or percussible after the patient has passed urine."[3] This definition includes patients with high postvoid residuals (PVRs) as well as those who fail a trial of voiding without a catheter placed for AUR. These patients often times require surgical intervention; however, given that long-term complication rates related to the retention are low,[5] conservative management may be considered based on unique patient factors.

At present, no precise definition of POUR exists, even among urologists. It is also very important to note that most cases of urinary retention are not associated with either a palpable or percussible bladder.

Epidemiology

AUR is reported to occur in 0.2% to 0.6% of the general population.[6,7] This number increases to 2.0% to 3.8% in the general surgical population.[8,9] Several recent studies have reported POUR rates of up 14% to 16% in surgical patients overall. These differences may best be explained by the heterogeneity of surgical patient populations and the overall operative conditions as some types of procedures have drastically increased rates of POUR as compared with those evidenced in the general population. Two examples of these much higher rates of POUR are anorectal surgeries and total joint arthroplasties with reported rates of retention ranging from 20% to 48%[10–12] and 0% to 75%,[13] respectively.

Pathophysiology

Normal bladder function

Normal bladder function involves both the storage and emptying of urine. It is controlled by supraspinal and medullary centers via autonomic and somatic pathways (**Fig. 1**).

In order for micturition to occur, the external sphincter must relax via quiescence of the somatic innervation (pudendal nerve S2–S4) and the detrusor must then contract which requires activation of the parasympathetics (pelvic nerve S2–S4) and inhibition of sympathetics (hypogastric nerve T10–L2). During micturition, parasympathetic innervation also allows for urethral smooth muscle to relax.[14]

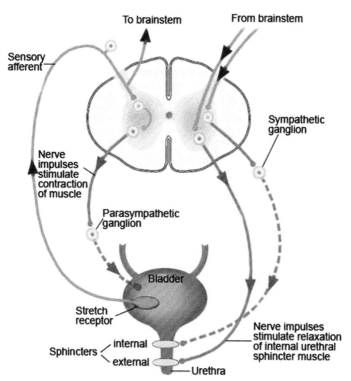

Fig. 1. Micturition reflex pathway. (*Courtesy of* the McGill Molson Medical Informatics Project, Montreal, Quebec, Canada, with permission.)

Normal bladder capacity of an adult is 400 to 600 mL. The first need to void is usually experienced at 150 mL, and the urge to void is experienced by 300 mL. In general, PVRs should be less than 10% of bladder capacity. Studies evaluating voiding trials have used a variety of definitions; however, no consensus exists as to what maximum PVR is acceptable in order to still have a trial void without catheter to be deemed successful.

Cause of retention

The exact mechanisms that contribute to urinary retention have yet to be established, although 3 causes have been suggested as likely candidates.

Obstruction: either mechanical or dynamic Mechanical obstruction may be either due to urethral strictures or possibly a change in bladder position and/or edema in the pelvis after surgery. It has long been thought that BPH with a large, ball-valving median lobe and/or, more recently, intravesical prostatic protrusion can contribute; however, no studies have clearly established this relationship and further investigation is warranted.

Dynamic obstruction can be secondary to increased tone. For instance, anorectal stimulation during surgery can increase alpha-adrenergic activity, which causes bladder outlet obstruction.[15]

Disruption of the innervation: sensory and motor pathways Drugs inhibiting detrusor contraction, spinal anesthetics inhibiting the sacral reflex micturition loop, and injury to the nerves during pelvic surgery can all play a role. For instance, during rectal cancer surgery, autonomic nerve damage during total mesorectal excision or lymph node dissection can cause urinary dysfunction.[15]

Overdistention: myogenic failure Overfilling of the bladder during surgery can lead to overstretching of the smooth muscle detrusor fibers in addition to possible muscle fatigue, ischemia, and even axonal degeneration. Myogenic failure is directly influenced by both intravenous (IV) fluid administration and the total anesthesia/surgery time.

Risk Factors

Because of the enormous variability of the patient populations studied, mixed results exist on which risk factors are most relevant to predisposing to urinary retention. Furthermore, some risk factors may be more important in certain types of procedures while seemingly having little to no impact on others.

Age

Degeneration of neural pathways involved with bladder function is thought to be responsible for the increased risk of POUR in older patients. A recent meta-analysis of 21 studies, involving 7802 patients, found that increased age significantly increased the risk of POUR with an odds ratio (OR) of 2.11 for those patients older than 60 years.[16,17] Other studies have suggested that as early older than 50 years is a significant risk factor.[18,19]

Sex

Sex has been clearly shown to be a risk factor for urinary retention not related to surgery given many men have BPH, which is clearly a risk factor for lower urinary tract dysfunction and retention. Importantly, however, this association has not been as strongly elucidated for POUR.[17,18,20] Mason and colleagues[16] found no association in a meta-analysis of 10 studies, including 5624 patients, between sex and POUR.

Medications

- Anticholinergics and medications with anticholinergic properties (antipsychotics, antihistamines, antiemetics, antidepressants, sedatives) can directly inhibit detrusor contractility as well as promote sedation, delirium, and constipation (**Table 1**).
- Alpha-adrenergic agonists can directly increase urinary sphincter tone.
- Opiates decrease both bladder contractility and the sensation for urge in a dose-dependent fashion with recovery of function varying on the specific opiate's properties.[21] The incidence of opioid precipitated retention in the postoperative setting has been found to be as high as 25%.[22]
- Nonsteroidal antiinflammatories (NSAIDs) are thought to reduce bladder contractility via cyclooxygenase-2 inhibition, which, in turn, inhibits prostaglandins that play an important role in detrusor contraction. A population-based case-control study found that patients taking NSAIDs had a 2-fold increased risk of developing AUR compared with controls postoperatively.[23]
- Calcium-channel blockers and beta-adrenergic agonists relax the detrusor muscle.

Anesthesia

- General anesthetics cause bladder atony by acting as smooth muscle relaxants and by directly interfering with autonomic regulation of detrusor tone, thereby predisposing patients to bladder overdistention and subsequent retention.

Table 1
Medications associated with retention

Medication	Examples	Medication	Examples
Anticholinergics	Atropine Darifenacin Dicyclomine Disopyramide Fesoterodine Glycopyrrolate Oxybutynin Propantheline Solifenacin Tolterodine Trospium	Antidepressants (TCAs/SSRIs)	Amitriptyline Imipramine Citalopram Escitalopram Fluoxetine paroxetine Sertraline
Calcium channel blockers	Amlodipine Diltiazem Nifedipine Verapamil	Alpha-adrenergic agonists	Ephedrine Pseudoephedrine Phenylpropamine Midrinone
Antihistamines	Diphenhydramine	Beta-adrenergic agonists	Isoproterenol Terbutaline
Antipsychotics	Haloperidol	NSAIDs	Ibuprofen Naproxen
Sedatives	Benzodiazepines	Narcotics	Morphine Hydromorphone Oxycodone

Abbreviations: NSAIDs, nonsteroidal antiinflammatory drugs; SSRIs, selective serotonin reuptake inhibitors; TCAs, tricyclic antidepressants.

- Spinal anesthesia results in a blockade of the micturition reflex. Using urodynamic monitoring during surgery, Kamphuis and colleagues[24] showed that the urge to void disappeared immediately after injection of spinal anesthetic. Detrusor blockade lasted longer than motor blockade. Furthermore, the detrusor blockade lasted until spinal anesthetic regressed to S3, which translated into higher accumulated bladder volumes with longer-acting anesthetics like bupivacaine as compared with lidocaine.
- Multiple studies have looked at rates of retention following spinal versus general anesthesia with a consensus that spinal anesthesia has a higher risk of POUR.[17,18]
- In contrast, a meta-analysis of 70 inguinal hernia studies, only 2 of which were randomized, general anesthesia had the highest rate of retention at 3% as compared with regional and local anesthesia with retention rates of 2.42% versus 0.37%, respectively.[25]
- A prospective trial looking at patients undergoing thoracotomy using a bupivacaine/hydromorphone epidural postoperatively for pain control found that urinary retention rates were 26.0% as compared with 12.4% for those patients who did not receive an epidural.[26]

Benign prostatic hyperplasia

- Studies assessing the relationship between urinary retention and preoperative voiding symptoms have had mixed results, likely because some studies found that, for patients presenting with AUR, acute retention was the first symptoms of BPH in 49%.[27] It is generally accepted that men with BPH are at an increased risk of AUR, supported by a meta-analysis of 570 articles whereby it was found that lower urinary tract symptoms (LUTS) were significantly associated with an increased risk of urinary retention (OR 2.83).[16] Further, the Health Professionals Follow-up Study, including almost 6100 patients, found that two-thirds of patients that developed AUR had International Prostate Symptom Scores (IPSS) scores in the moderate to severe range.[28]

- In a 4-year longitudinal study, Jacobsen and colleagues[29] found that men with an IPSS greater than 7 had 4 times the risk of AUR compared with those with an IPSS score of 7 or less. Urinary symptoms in men have also been examined in the orthopedic literature with studies again showing that moderate to severe LUTS, established by IPSS score, increased the risk of retention in total joint replacements.[30] This association, however, has not been as clear for other surgeries, such as cataract replacement.[31]
- Studies using perioperative alpha-blockers to prevent POUR have shown mixed results, again with a difference seen with different surgeries. After herniorrhaphy, 2 placebo-controlled studies found that alpha-blocker use 24 hours preoperatively and continued postoperatively significantly reduced the rate of retention.[32,33] In contrast, however, 2 randomized controlled studies in anorectal surgery did not show any significant difference in postoperative retention rates.[34,35]

At this time, more studies are, therefore, required and alpha-blockers are not recommended for routine prophylaxis of POUR.

Surgery related

Operating room time
- Operative times longer than 120 minutes increased the risk of POUR 3-fold.[17] Another study of 352 patients undergoing rectal cancer surgery demonstrated an almost 3-fold increase risk of POUR for surgeries lasting greater than 240 minutes.[15]
- A single-institution review reported that for every 10-minute increase in operative time, an 11% increase in POUR is expected.[36]
- Given longer surgery times predispose patients to urinary retention, an accepted general rule suggests that for operative cases lasting longer than 3 hours, a Foley catheter should be inserted preoperatively.
- The association of total operating room time and POUR is compounded by the increased volumes of IV fluids administered as operating room time increases. No study, to date, has been able to clearly delineate which of the two has a stronger association.

Intravenous fluid
- The use of increased IV fluids intraoperatively has been shown to be an independent risk factor for POUR. Again, however, these studies have also noted that total operating room time consistently increases with the increased threshold volume. Bladder overdistention is likely responsible for this phenomenon.

Keita and colleagues[19] found that IV fluid infusion of greater than 750 mL more than doubled the risk of POUR. Similarly, in a retrospective review of 352 patients undergoing rectal cancer surgery, the administration of greater than 2000 mL of IV fluids intraoperatively was associated with a greater than 3-fold risk of POUR.[15] Furthermore, Kwaan and colleagues[11] showed that the risk of POUR increased by 20% for every liter of IV fluid given during rectal surgeries.

Procedure type

- Laparoscopic surgery was shown to be associated with more episodes of acute voiding difficulty in a prospectively randomized trial of 340 patients with T3 rectal cancer.[37] Voiding difficulty can be explained in part by possible neuropraxia caused by the need for increased retraction and instrument grasping, the effects of pneumoperitoneum on leading to lower urinary output intraoperatively secondary to decreased renal blood flow[38] which, in turn, may promote increased IV fluid administration with a and subsequent increase risk of bladder overdistention. Another study looked at 345 patients who underwent a hernia repair and found that laparoscopic repairs were associated with a 7.9% rate of POUR versus 1.1% for open procedures.[39] These findings were supported further by a prospective observational study of patients undergoing colorectal surgery whereby rates of retention using a laparoscopic approach were more than 3 times the rate seen in the open surgery group: 40% versus 12%.[40]
- Overall, it is also well established that anorectal surgeries are associated with high rates of POUR with the proposed mechanisms for this being alpha-adrenergic activation, a change in bladder position after surgery, and injury to autonomic nerves despite the surgical approach.
- Further, it has been noted that risk of POUR after lower limb arthroplasty is up to 20-fold higher than that in the general surgical population.[8] Sung and colleagues[41] examined 15,000 patients undergoing orthopedic surgery and found that total joint replacement had an increased risk of POUR compared with other orthopedic surgeries (OR 1.5). It is unclear why total joint surgery has higher rates of retention; however, it has been postulated that prolonged operative times, increased amounts of IV fluids, and higher doses of anesthetics and opiates likely play a role.
- In general, the placement of Foley catheters is recommended in these cases, although POUR remains a significant risk on their removal.

Women and children

- History and physical examination are usually not revealing for the risk of POUR cause in women and children with the cause unclear when it occurs. Urodynamic assessment (UDS), the objective studying bladder dynamics and function, may be indicated.
- Specific to children, dysfunctional voiding, occult spinal cord tethering, meatal stenosis, and urethral stricture are all possible causes of POUR in kids. After bladder decompression, pediatric urologic referral is encouraged.
- Outlet obstruction, also a cause of retention in women, may be secondary to pelvic organ and/or urethral prolapse or may be iatrogenic secondary to prior stress-incontinence procedures.
- Fowler syndrome, seen in women 15 to 30 years of age, is characterized by painless AUR with residual volumes of greater than 1 L. These patients typically have a history of voiding dysfunction, and UDS reveals impaired relaxation of the external sphincter.[42] Urologic referral is indicated for these patients.

Others

Perioperative voiding

- A series of 773 consecutive patients who were instructed to void both preoperatively and immediately postoperatively showed a significantly reduced risk of POUR.[18]

Elevated PVR in postanesthesia care unit

- A PVR of greater than 360 mL on arrival to the postanesthesia care unit has been found to be an independent risk factor for POUR with it occurring up to 9 times higher in these patients.[20] A second study found that the risk was almost 5 times higher for PVRs greater than 270 mL.[19]

Urinary tract infection, prior history of retention, diabetes mellitus

- Although mixed reports exist with respect to these factors, no clear association with POUR has been shown.[16]
- Even despite the well-recognized end-organ complication of uncontrolled diabetes mellitus of impairment of bladder sensation and contractility leading to increased risk of chronic retention, studies have failed to show increased rates of POUR.

Neurologic and neurosurgical causes

- Neurologic and neurosurgical pathologic conditions add a level of complexity for the cause of acute and chronic urinary retention. These conditions include but are not limited to stroke, multiple sclerosis, Parkinson disease, spinal cord injury, or spine surgery.
- Strokes can predispose patients to urinary retention in the acute setting. Depending on the level of insult, brainstem versus cortex, patients may experience either urinary retention or incontinence. Retention can also be seen after spine surgery, which has been found to be an independent risk factor of POUR in a prospective study of 137 neurosurgical patients.[43]
- Urinary dysfunction can take up to 1 year to stabilize or resolve. These patients should be referred to urology for urodynamic evaluation and long-term management.

Diagnosis

Associated signs and symptoms

- Associated acute autonomic dysfunction may be seen, including bradycardia, hypertension, cardiac arrhythmias, and less commonly tachycardia and asystole.
- Unfortunately pain and/or agitation are not very good predictors of POUR underlined by the fact that multiple studies have found that only about 40% of patients with POUR reported pain.
- Specifically, one study revealed that only 44% of patients with a PVR of greater than 500 mL felt the urge to void or that their bladder was full.[17]
- As already discussed, a palpable bladder is also an unreliable sign of retention given bladder volumes of 500 to 1000 mL are often times not palpable.
- Acute onset of frequency or continual, overflow incontinence can be a presenting symptom in patients with retention and provides further evidence that many patients do not experience pain or discomfort with acute retention.

Postvoid residual: how much is too much?

- Bladder scanning, using a self-contained ultrasonic device, has been found to be an accurate way to estimate bladder volume as compared with catheterization.[17,19,44]
- Very few studies have looked at a PVR cutoffs; currently no standard recommendations exist, with the more common cutoffs to diagnose retention being between 400 and 600 mL.[8,18,19] Notably, in a study of asymptomatic men, a PVR of greater than 180 mL, regardless of voided volume, had a positive predictive

value for associated urinary tract infection (UTI) of 87.0% and a negative predictive value of 94.7%.[45]

Complications of Retention

Although it is well known that long-term complications of urinary retention are generally rare, the acute complications contribute significantly to the psychological stress of patients, leading to increased morbidity and longer hospital stays. Avoiding these complications begins with identifying retention early and prompt decompression of the bladder.

- *Acute*: Gross hematuria, UTI, and urosepsis all increase morbidity.
- *Chronic*: decreased bladder sensation and contractility, incontinence, stones, hydronephrosis, and renal failure can occur in the long-term.
- In a large, worldwide study of greater than 6000 men assessing the conservative management of men with BPH and PVRs greater than 250 mL, the researchers found that complications, including renal failure, complete urinary retention, and UTIs, were uncommon.[46]
- *Postobstructive diuresis (POD)*[47]: This complication can occur in up to 50% of patients with significant and complete urinary tract obstruction. Characterized by urine outputs of greater than 200 mL/h over 2 hours or urine outputs greater than 3 L in 24 hours, POD occurs because of a combination of osmotic diuresis, physiologic diuresis in the setting of hypervolemia and, more rarely, nephrogenic diabetes insipidus. Management of established POD should include serum electrolytes monitoring twice daily with avoidance of IV fluid replacement as it will prolong and exacerbate the diuresis. Pathologic POD is continuous diuresis that lasts greater than 48 hours or that continues after patients are euvolemic and warrants nephrology consultation.

Treatment

Conservative

Hot pack/lukewarm-water-soaked gauze
- A randomized controlled trial of 126 patients with POUR revealed that, respectively, 59.5%, 71.4%, and 7.1% of patients using a hot pack, lukewarm-water-soaked gauze, or nothing had relief of urinary retention.[48] Unfortunately, the definition of retention in this study was subjective only, with no bladder scanning used to confirm high bladder volumes. Given the existence of some evidence supporting these noninvasive interventions, they may be considered in patients with moderate retention volumes of 200 to 400 mL and an inability to void. If unable to void with greater than 500 mL, intervention is indicated.
- Bladder decompression remains the mainstay for treatment of urinary retention in the acute setting. Historically, it was thought that gradual decompression of the bladder was preferable to rapid decompression to prevent circulatory collapse. This association has been disproven, and there are no significant differences in rapid versus gradual bladder decompression.[49] Regardless, vagal episodes can occur with catheter placement; patients exhibiting autonomic instability should be monitored closely after catheter placement.

Types of bladder drainage
- Urethral catheterization followed by a trial without catheter has become a standard worldwide.[46] It must, however, be noted that this is an invasive procedure with potential complications, including catheter-associated UTI (CAUTI), urethral trauma, and significant catheter-related pain; therefore, the decision to place a

Foley should not be taken lightly. The risk of CAUTI with short-term catheterization is reported to be 5% per day,[50] with bacterial colonization thought to be by way of retrograde ascent of perimeatal flora.

- Although Foley catheter placement should be the initial management option for patients with POUR, if persistent, clean intermittent catheterization and urologic evaluation should be considered.
- Large prospective studies looking to identify independent risk factors for CAUTI have shown that prolonged catheterization greater than 6 days is associated with a 5-fold increase in developing a UTI and that by 30 days CAUTI was nearly universal.[50]
- In the acute setting, suprapubic tube (SPT) placement should only be undertaken if urethral catheterization is not possible and urologic consultation for cystoscopic placement is unavailable. For patients with significant pelvic trauma, it may also be the preferred method of bladder drainage depending on the clinical situation. For SPT placement, ultrasound guidance of the initial needle placement is preferred if available but not absolutely necessary.
- Consideration needs to be given to avoid SPT placement in patients who are more likely to pull out the catheter themselves inadvertently either because of combative tendencies or dementia (**Fig. 2**).

Medications

- The advent and evolution of pharmacotherapy for BPH using alpha-blockers and 5-alpha-reductase inhibitors have largely replaced surgical therapy. In a prospective cross-sectional survey looking at men with acute retention and its

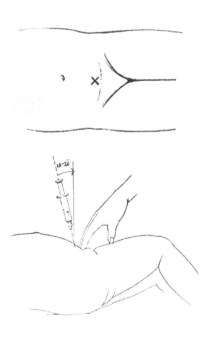

Percutaneous Suprapubic Tube Placement

1. Palpate the bladder
2. Prep and drape the infra-umbilical region
3. Inject local anesthetic into area 2 cm above pubic symphysis at midline.
4. Advance an 18-gauge hollow needle (spinal needle may be used) under continuous aspiration with a syringe until urine flashback appears at a 10–20 degree angle caudal.
5. Advance the needle 1 cm more, detach the syringe
6. Advance a floppy-tip guidewire (0.035 or 0.038 in Bentson) in Seldinger fashion until it coils in the bladder
7. Withdraw the needle and make a small incision on the anterior abdominal fascia
8. Dilate the tract with sequential graduated dilators to one size above desired catheter size
9. Advanced a Councill catheter over the guidewire and into the bladder.
10. Inflate balloon and/or suture tube to skin

Fig. 2. Percutaneous SPT placement.

management across 5 countries, Fitzpatrick and colleagues[46] found that starting alpha-blockers before a trial without catheter (TWOC) doubled the chances of success. These findings have been confirmed in several further studies; therefore, an alpha-blocker should be started in all patients who do not have a contraindication for several days before a TWOC.

- It has also been shown that the acute use of alpha-blockers in patients experiencing AUR may avoid the need for bladder catheterization. In a double-blinded randomized study of 360 men presenting to the emergency department with AUR, McNeill and colleagues[51] found that alfuzosin increased the likelihood of successful voiding in first-time AUR episodes, negating the need for acute catheterization, and that continuation of the medication decreased the need for surgical intervention at 6 months.
- A review of 42 studies found that alpha-blockers, alone or in combination with 5-alpha reductase inhibitors (5ARIs), generally reduce the incidence of AUR both short- and long-term. AUR rates with 5ARI monotherapy, in contrast, are higher in short-term studies (<12 months) but, similarly, lower in long-term studies (>12 months) compared with the untreated population.[52]

TWOC
- Delaying Foley removal has been associated with increased success rates for TWOC. This finding must be balanced, however, with the increasing risk of infection with every day that a catheter is left in place.
- Specifically relating to anorectal surgery, multiple studies have found that catheter removal less than 48 hours postoperatively was associated with an increased risk of retention.[11] One study in particular showed that patients who had their catheter removed on the first postoperative day had a 21.6% recurrent retention rate as compared with 7.8% if it was left until the second postoperative day.[15] For total joint arthroplasties populations, the reverse seems to be true whereby the risk of POUR was lowest when catheters were removed within 24 to 48 hours postoperatively.[53]
- Predictors of failure of TWOC include being older than 70 years, severe preexisting LUTS, and bladder volumes greater than 1000 mL at the time of catheter insertion.[46,54]
- No difference in outcomes have been shown for whether patients underwent a TWOC in the hospital as compared with being sent home with the Foley and following up as an outpatient for the TWOC.[55]

Women and children: special considerations
- For women with anatomic obstruction with associated prolapsed pelvic organs, their reduction and/or the use of a pessary use may be indicated in the acute setting. Conservative measures in both women and children include bowel medications for management of constipation and biofeedback with pelvic floor rehabilitation when necessary for the treatment and prevention of retention.

Urologic consultation
- Any patient thought to have a more complicated course, including those who fail TWOC, those with impaired renal function, and those having any prior history of urologic intervention, should be considered for referral for outpatient urologic follow-up.

Surgical intervention: overview
Surgery is mainly reserved to treat patients with chronic, recurrent urinary retention. Primarily, it is for those who have failed medical therapy and a, or several, TWOC.

Commonly, it is to provide outlet obstruction reduction, most commonly in male patients with BPH; but it can also be for the management of myogenic failure.

For obstruction from BPH, transurethral techniques are the current standard approach for most patients. Open simple prostatectomy remains an option reserved for patients with very large BPH glands.

Transurethral resection of the prostate
- Transurethral resection of the prostate (TURP) has for decades been considered to be and remains the gold standard for the treatment of lower urinary tract obstruction secondary to BPH.
- Other minimally invasive options, including transurethral needle ablation and transurethral microwave therapy, have been used, however, the symptom improvement and durability of relief from BPH-associated symptoms and have not been proven to be reliably commensurate with those seen with TURP.

Laser prostatectomy
- Numerous laser technologies have been developed in order to reduce outlet obstruction due to BPH in a more minimally invasive fashion. The techniques include coagulation, vaporization, resection, and enucleation of tissue using multiple different laser energy wavelengths. With the advances in laser technology, largely over the past decade, its use in BPH and growing clinical experience challenge TURP as the gold standard BPH treatment. To date, however, laser procedure outcomes and their ease of use has not been shown, again, to be as reliable as TURP.[56] The two most studied laser procedures, Greenlight and holmium enucleation of the prostate, have shown success in treating patients with retention with good short-term functional results and acceptable complication rates for patients in retention.[57–59]

Sacral neuromodulation
- Sacral neuromodulation, by way of an implantable pacemaker, has been shown to be an effective option for patients with nonobstructive urinary retention due to detrusor noncontractility, removing the need for chronic catheter use. Success rates have been reported ranging from 41% to 100%.[60]
- The principle behind sacral neuromodulation's success is thought to be due to the inhibition of somatic afferent sensory processing in the spinal cord. It is indicated in patients with nonobstructive urinary retention, including those with documented pelvic floor dysfunction.[14]

REFERENCES

1. Awan FN, Zulkifli MS, McCormack O, et al. Factors involved in unplanned admissions from general surgical day-care in a modern protected facility. Ir Med J 2013;106(5):153–4.
2. Lau H, Brooks DC. Predictive factors for unanticipated admissions after ambulatory laparoscopic cholecystectomy. Arch Surg 2001;136(10):1150–3.
3. Abrams P, Cardozo L, Fall M, et al. The standardisation of terminology in lower urinary tract function: report from the standardisation sub-committee of the International Continence Society. Urology 2003;61(1):37–49.
4. McNeil SA. Spontaneous versus precipitated AUR: the same? World J Urol 2006; 24(4):354–9.
5. Bates TS, Sugiono M, James ED, et al. Is the conservative management of chronic retention in men ever justified? BJU Int 2003;92(6):581–3.

6. Ugare UG, Bassey IA, Udosen EJ, et al. Management of lower urinary retention in a limited resource setting. Ethiop J Health Sci 2014;24(4):329–36.

7. Selius BA, Subedi R. Urinary retention in adults: diagnosis and initial management. Am Fam Physician 2008;77(5):643–50.

8. Baldini G, Bagry H, Aprikian A, et al. Postoperative urinary retention: anesthetic and perioperative considerations. Anesthesiology 2009;110(5):1139–57.

9. Wu AK, Auerbach AD, Aaronson DS. National incidence and outcomes of postoperative urinary retention in the Surgical Care Improvement Project. Am J Surg 2012;204(2):167–71.

10. Salvati EP, Kleckner MS. Urinary retention in anorectal and colonic surgery. Am J Surg 1957;94(1):114–7.

11. Kwaan MR, Lee JT, Rothenberger DA, et al. Early removal of urinary catheters after rectal surgery is associated with increased urinary retention. Dis Colon Rectum 2015;58(4):401–5.

12. Poylin V, Curran T, Cataldo T, et al. Perioperative use of tamsulosin significantly decreases rates of urinary retention in men undergoing pelvic surgery. Int J Colorectal Dis 2015;30(9):1223–8.

13. Balderi T, Carli F. Urinary retention after total hip and knee arthroplasty. Minerva Anestesiol 2010;76(2):120–30.

14. Yoshimura N, Chancellor MB. Physiology and pharmacology of the bladder and urethra. In: Wein AJ, Kavoussi LR, Campbell MF, editors. Campbell-Walsh urology. Philadelphia: Elsevier Saunders; 2012. p. 1755–85.

15. Lee SY, Kang SB, Kim DW, et al. Risk factors and preventive measures for acute urinary retention after rectal cancer surgery. World J Surg 2015;39(1):275–82.

16. Mason SE, Scott AJ, Mayer E, et al. Patient-related risk factors for urinary retention following ambulatory general surgery: a systematic review and meta-analysis. Am J Surg 2015. [Epub ahead of print].

17. Lamonerie L, Marret E, Deleuze A, et al. Prevalence of postoperative bladder distension and urinary retention detected by ultrasound measurement. Br J Anaesth 2004;92(4):544–6.

18. Hansen BS, Soreide E, Warland AM, et al. Risk factors of post-operative urinary retention in hospitalised patients. Acta Anaesthesiol Scand 2011;55(5):545–8.

19. Keita H, Diouf E, Tubach F, et al. Predictive factors of early postoperative urinary retention in the postanesthesia care unit. Anesth Analg 2005;101(2):592–6, table of contents.

20. Dal Mago AJ, Helayel PE, Bianchini E, et al. Prevalence and predictive factors of urinary retention assessed by ultrasound in the immediate post-anesthetic period. Rev Bras Anestesiol 2010;60(4):383–90.

21. Kuipers PW, Kamphuis ET, van Venrooij GE, et al. Intrathecal opioids and lower urinary tract function: a urodynamic evaluation. Anesthesiology 2004;100(6):1497–503.

22. Verhamme KM, Sturkenboom MC, Stricker BH, et al. Drug-induced urinary retention: incidence, management and prevention. Drug Saf 2008;31(5):373–88.

23. Verhamme KM, Dieleman JP, Van Wijk MA, et al. Nonsteroidal anti-inflammatory drugs and increased risk of acute urinary retention. Arch Intern Med 2005;165(13):1547–51.

24. Kamphuis ET, Ionescu TI, Kuipers PW, et al. Recovery of storage and emptying functions of the urinary bladder after spinal anesthesia with lidocaine and with bupivacaine in men. Anesthesiology 1998;88(2):310–6.

25. Jensen P, Mikkelsen T, Kehlet H. Postherniorrhaphy urinary retention–effect of local, regional, and general anesthesia: a review. Reg Anesth Pain Med 2002; 27(6):612–7.

26. Hu Y, Craig SJ, Rowlingson JC, et al. Early removal of urinary catheter after surgery requiring thoracic epidural: a prospective trial. J Cardiothorac Vasc Anesth 2014;28(5):1302–6.

27. Verhamme KM, Dieleman JP, van Wijk MA, et al. Low incidence of acute urinary retention in the general male population: the triumph project. Eur Urol 2005;47(4): 494–8.

28. Meigs JB, Barry MJ, Giovannucci E, et al. Incidence rates and risk factors for acute urinary retention: the health professionals follow-up study. J Urol 1999; 162(2):376–82.

29. Jacobsen SJ, Jacobson DJ, Girman CJ, et al. Natural history of prostatism: risk factors for acute urinary retention. J Urol 1997;158(2):481–7.

30. Elkhodair S, Parmar HV, Vanwaeyenbergh J. The role of the IPSS (international prostate symptoms score) in predicting acute retention of urine in patients undergoing major joint arthroplasty. Surgeon 2005;3(2):63–5.

31. Fazeli F, Gooran S, Taghvaei ME, et al. Evaluating international prostate symptom score (IPSS) in accuracy for predicting post-operative urinary retention after elective cataract surgery: a prospective study. Glob J Health Sci 2015;7(7):46885.

32. Mohammadi-Fallah M, Hamedanchi S, Tayyebi-Azar A. Preventive effect of tamsulosin on postoperative urinary retention. Korean J Urol 2012;53(6):419–23.

33. Gonullu NN, Dulger M, Utkan NZ, et al. Prevention of postherniorrhaphy urinary retention with prazosin. Am Surg 1999;65(1):55–8.

34. Cataldo PA, Senagore AJ. Does alpha sympathetic blockade prevent urinary retention following anorectal surgery? Dis Colon Rectum 1991;34(12):1113–6.

35. Jang JH, Kang SB, Lee SM, et al. Randomized controlled trial of tamsulosin for prevention of acute voiding difficulty after rectal cancer surgery. World J Surg 2012;36(11):2730–7.

36. Hudak KE, Frelich MJ, Rettenmaier CR, et al. Surgery duration predicts urinary retention after inguinal herniorrhaphy: a single institution review. Surg Endosc 2015;29(11):3246–50.

37. Kang SB, Park JW, Jeong SY, et al. Open versus laparoscopic surgery for mid or low rectal cancer after neoadjuvant chemoradiotherapy (COREAN trial): short-term outcomes of an open-label randomised controlled trial. Lancet Oncol 2010;11(7):637–45.

38. Demyttenaere S, Feldman LS, Fried GM. Effect of pneumoperitoneum on renal perfusion and function: a systematic review. Surg Endosc 2007;21(2):152–60.

39. Winslow ER, Quasebarth M, Brunt LM. Perioperative outcomes and complications of open vs. laparoscopic extraperitoneal inguinal hernia repair in a mature surgical practice. Surg Endosc 2004;18(2):221–7.

40. Kin C, Rhoads KF, Jalali M, et al. Predictors of postoperative urinary retention after colorectal surgery. Dis Colon Rectum 2013;56(6):738–46.

41. Sung KH, Lee KM, Chung CY, et al. What are the risk factors associated with urinary retention after orthopaedic surgery? Biomed Res Int 2015;2015:613216.

42. Fowler CJ, Christmas TJ, Chapple CR, et al. Abnormal electromyographic activity of the urethral sphincter, voiding dysfunction, and polycystic ovaries: a new syndrome? BMJ 1988;297(6661):1436–8.

43. Alsaidi M, Guanio J, Basheer A, et al. The incidence and risk factors for postoperative urinary retention in neurosurgical patients. Surg Neurol Int 2013;4:61.

44. Rosseland LA, Stubhaug A, Breivik H. Detecting postoperative urinary retention with an ultrasound scanner. Acta Anaesthesiol Scand 2002;46(3):279–82.

45. Truzzi JC, Almeida FM, Nunes EC, et al. Residual urinary volume and urinary tract infection–when are they linked? J Urol 2008;180(1):182–5.

46. Fitzpatrick JM, Desgrandchamps F, Adjali K, et al. Management of acute urinary retention: a worldwide survey of 6074 men with benign prostatic hyperplasia. BJU Int 2012;109(1):88–95.

47. Halbgewachs C, Domes T. Postobstructive diuresis: pay close attention to urinary retention. Can Fam Physician 2015;61(2):137–42.

48. Afazel MR, Jalali E, Sadat Z, et al. Comparing the effects of hot pack and lukewarm-water-soaked gauze on postoperative urinary retention; a randomized controlled clinical trial. Nurs Midwifery Stud 2014;3(4):e24606.

49. Boettcher S, Brandt AS, Roth S, et al. Urinary retention: benefit of gradual bladder decompression - myth or truth? A randomized controlled trial. Urol Int 2013;91(2): 140–4.

50. Maki DG, Tambyah PA. Engineering out the risk for infection with urinary catheters. Emerg Infect Dis 2001;7(2):342–7.

51. McNeill SA, Hargreave TB, Roehrborn CG, et al. Alfuzosin 10 mg once daily in the management of acute urinary retention: results of a double-blind placebo-controlled study. Urology 2005;65(1):83–9 [discussion: 89–90].

52. Oelke M, Speakman MJ, Desgrandchamps F, et al. Acute urinary retention rates in the general male population and in adult men with lower urinary tract symptoms participating in pharmacotherapy trials: a literature review. Urology 2015;86(4): 654–65.

53. Zhang W, Liu A, Hu D, et al. Indwelling versus intermittent urinary catheterization following total joint arthroplasty: a systematic review and meta-analysis. PLoS One 2015;10(7):e0130636.

54. Djavan B, Madersbacher S, Klingler C, et al. Urodynamic assessment of patients with acute urinary retention: is treatment failure after prostatectomy predictable? J Urol 1997;158(5):1829–33.

55. Pickard R, Emberton M, Neal DE. The management of men with acute urinary retention. National Prostatectomy Audit Steering Group. Br J Urol 1998;81(5): 712–20.

56. Gravas S, Bachmann A, Reich O, et al. Critical review of lasers in benign prostatic hyperplasia (BPH). BJU Int 2011;107(7):1030–43.

57. Ruszat R, Wyler S, Seifert HH, et al. Photoselective vaporization of the prostate: subgroup analysis of men with refractory urinary retention. Eur Urol 2006;50(5): 1040–9 [discussion: 9].

58. Elzayat EA, Habib EI, Elhilali MM. Holmium laser enucleation of prostate for patients in urinary retention. Urology 2005;66(4):789–93.

59. Peterson MD, Matlaga BR, Kim SC, et al. Holmium laser enucleation of the prostate for men with urinary retention. J Urol 2005;174(3):998–1001 [discussion: 1001].

60. Gaziev G, Topazio L, Iacovelli V, et al. Percutaneous tibial nerve stimulation (PTNS) efficacy in the treatment of lower urinary tract dysfunctions: a systematic review. BMC Urol 2013;13:61.

Surgical Management of Female Voiding Dysfunction

Ilija Aleksic, MD, Elise J.B. De, MD*

KEYWORDS

- Female incontinence • Pelvic organ prolapse surgery • Female voiding dysfunction
- Complications

KEY POINTS

- Correct preoperative diagnosis is key to the outcome of surgery for female voiding dysfunction. Patients should be evaluated for effective low-pressure storage, effective emptying, and lack of obstruction.
- Vaginal and abdominal approaches, or a combination, are used for incontinence and prolapse.
- Anatomic landmarks for repair of pelvic organ prolapse include the sacrum, sacrospinous ligament, uterosacral ligaments, iliococcygeus muscles, levator muscles, obturator fascia, and the arcus tendineus fascia pelvis.
- Common complications of vaginal repairs include ureter, nerve or vessel injury, urethral obstruction, mesh or graft erosion, and levator muscle spasm.
- A prior history of mesh should raise the index of suspicion for complications especially in the setting of pelvic pain, bleeding, or discharge.

INTRODUCTION

Voiding dysfunction, a multifactorial entity with a complex presentation, can be conceptualized more simply as a disorder of filling or emptying of the urinary bladder. The bladder functions to:

- Store volume at low pressures, a function dependent on compliance (the ability to stretch at low pressures), outlet resistance, and the absence of bladder contraction.
- Empty effectively, a function of adequate bladder contraction and absence of obstruction (such as bladder neck or external urethral sphincter obstruction, urethral stricture, obstructing cystocele, or sling).

Disclosure Statement: Dr I. Aleksic has nothing to disclose. Dr E.J.B. De: receives Bloomberg Foundation Grant for Fistula Work.
Division of Urology, Albany Medical College, 23 Hackett Boulevard MC 208, Albany, NY 12208, USA
* Corresponding author.
E-mail address: ede@communitycare.com

Compliance and contractility of the bladder change over time in response to:

- *Obstruction*: leading to hypertrophy with subsequent decompensation; examples include cystocele, detrusor sphincter dyssynergia, and prior antiincontinence surgery in the female.
- *Disinhibition*: upper motor neuron pathophysiology (eg, spinal cord injury or multiple sclerosis).
- *Denervation*: lower motor neuron pathophysiology (eg, abdominoperineal resection).

Successful surgical intervention for female voiding dysfunction depends on the proper preoperative diagnosis (See Robert C. McDonough III, Stephen T. Ryan: Diagnosis and Management of Voiding Dysfunction, in this issue). Due to the subjective and often confounding nature of urinary and pelvic symptoms, a considerable time investment in the clinic is required to diagnose and determine management. It is not uncommon for referral centers to evaluate patients considered refractory to surgical treatment who have simply been misdiagnosed. When conducted properly, surgery for female voiding dysfunction is directed toward restoring native anatomy (eg, reduction of cystocele) or circumventing impaired bladder function (eg, paralyzing a neurogenic overactive bladder with onabotulinumtoxin A and having the patient straight catheterize).

STRESS URINARY INCONTINENCE

Stress urinary incontinence (SUI) is defined as "the complaint of involuntary loss of urine on effort or physical exertion (eg, sporting activities), or on sneezing or coughing."[1] In patients with mixed-type incontinence, including urgency or unaware leakage, all types are addressed concurrently. Operative intervention for the stress component is still warranted if the stress component is predominant. Stress urinary incontinence occurs due to urethral hypermobility or intrinsic sphincter deficiency, and often both.

Urethral Hypermobility

Urethral hypermobility occurs as a continuum of anterior vaginal wall laxity.[2] Loss of the functional valve created by support at the level of the urethra results in leakage when there is an increase in intraabdominal pressure. Surgical intervention for urethral hypermobility aims to restore this natural hammocklike support.[3]

Intrinsic Sphincteric Deficiency

Intrinsic sphincteric deficiency refers to low pressure generation by the external urethral sphincter muscle itself.[4] Intervention involves increasing outlet resistance, accomplished by use of an injectable urethral bulking agent or a more obstructing surgical repair (eg, sling).[5]

STRESS URINARY INCONTINENCE PROCEDURES
Bulking Agents

A less invasive surgical therapy for stress urinary incontinence due to internal sphincter deficiency is the use of a urethral bulking agent. These are injected transurethrally or periurethrally. Injectable agents function mainly by increasing coaptation of the sphincter and providing a central volume that increases the functional length of the muscle.[6] This approach is best suited for:

- Stress urinary incontinence caused by intrinsic sphincter deficiency without hypermobility;
- Patients who are poor surgical candidates (because this procedure can be performed in the office under local anesthesia)[7]; and
- Residual incontinence after a sling or retropubic procedure.

Various agents have historically been used for their bulking effect. However, many are no longer available due to lack of efficacy or adverse effects such as particle migration and local inflammatory reactions. The materials of historical mention include Durasphere, Teflon, and Collagen. Current agents on the market are coaptite and Macroplastique.

Coaptite

Approved by the US Food and Drug Administration (FDA) in 2005, this bulking agent is composed of calcium hydroxylapatite, a principal constituent in bone, with a carrier made of carboxymethylcellulose.[8] Coaptite is considered nonantigenic and nonmigratory.

Macroplastique

Approved by the FDA in 2006, this bulking agent is composed of polydimethylsiloxane microparticles with a carrier made of polyvinylpyrrolidone gel.[9] Macroplastique is considered to be inert and nonmigratory, with no reports of urethral abscess or mass formation.

Technique

- Local anesthesia or monitored anesthesia care.
- Dorsal lithotomy position.
- A rigid 22-French cystoscope is inserted and the transurethral injection needle is angled toward the urethra at a 30° to 45° angle. The needle enters distal to the site of injection (either external sphincter or bladder neck).
  - Calcium hydroxylapatite: approximately 2 mL total of material is delivered underneath the urethral mucosa at 3 and 9 o'clock.
  - Polyvinylpyrrolidone gel: approximately 5 mL of material is delivered at 10, 2, and 6 o'clock.

Two major drawbacks to urethral injection therapy are a lower efficacy (19%–72%)[10] and the lack of long-term treatment effect, where patients have only temporary relief from symptoms. The majority of data is published on collagen and newer products show promise for better durability.

Considerations

- Injectable agents are appreciable on imaging and can be misinterpreted as a urethral stone or diverticulum.
- Complications include urinary tract infection, obstruction, vaginal mass, and (very rarely) abscess.

Open or Laparoscopic Surgical Intervention for Stress Urinary Incontinence

Open surgical intervention can be separated into historical and contemporary including mesh and native tissue. As described in the American Urological Association guidelines, in addition to injectables, there are 4 types of interventions available for stress incontinence: retropubic suspensions, laparoscopic suspensions, midurethral slings, and pubovaginal slings.[11]

Retropubic suspension

Marshall Marchetti Krantz procedure The *Marshall Marchetti Krantz* procedure was described in the 1940s as suspending the urethral wall and periurethral tissues (**Fig. 1**) to the pubic symphysis.[12] Long-term considerations include urethral devascularization, obstruction, secondary cystocele, and perioperative osteitis pubis.[13]

Burch colposuspension *Burch colposuspension* was introduced in the 1960s as anchoring the vaginal wall next to the bladder neck to Cooper's ligaments bilaterally to provide more reliable support and to avoid manipulation of the periurethral tissue (**Fig. 2**).[14] Long-term considerations include urethral obstruction and secondary cystocele. The procedure is still commonly performed either via retropubic or laparoscopic incisions.

Needle suspensions

These procedures involve a retropubic pass using a "needle" with varying risk of bladder injury and retropubic bleeding. Adopted from Takacs and Zimmern,[15] below is a brief list of suspensions.

Four-corner bladder neck (needle) suspension A 4-corner bladder neck (needle) suspension involves 2 sites of suspension on each side supporting both the bladder neck and the upper vagina with multiple suture passes (**Fig. 3**). Lateral support of the bladder base is restored and the vesicourethral junction into a high retropubic junction.[16] Suture pull-through led to lower success rates.

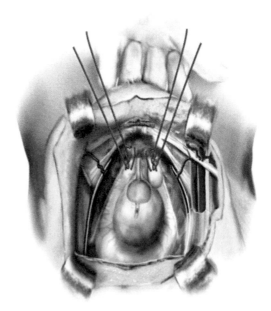

Fig. 1. Marshall–Marchetti–Krantz procedure. Suture placed bilaterally at the bladder neck, then through the pubic symphysis periosteum. (*From* Karram MM. Retropubic urethropexy for stress incontinence. In: Atlas of pelvic anatomy and gynecologic surgery. Philadelphia: Saunders; 2011. p. 423–6; with permission.)

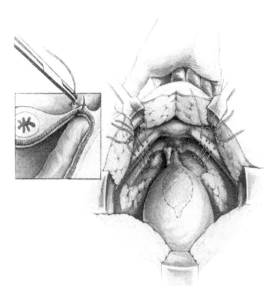

Fig. 2. Burch colposuspension technique. (*From* Walters MD. Retropubic operations for stress urinary incontinence, In: Walters MD, Karram MM, editors. Urogynecology and reconstructive pelvic surgery. 4th edition. Philadelphia: Elsevier Saunders; 2015; with permission.)

Anterior vaginal wall suspension Anterior vaginal wall suspension is a modification of the 4-corner bladder neck suspension. Helical sutures through the width of the anterior vaginal wall lead to lower potential for suture pull-through (**Fig. 4**). They are passed retropubic and tied off-tension overlying the rectus fascia.[17] This is a current procedure that allows for support of the anterior vaginal wall at the same time as correcting the hypermobility component of stress incontinence.

Pereyra Pereyra involves a small transverse suprapubic incision, stainless steel suture, 2 passes per side.[18] Suture pull-through impacted the success of this procedure.

Raz-modified Pereyra The Raz-modified Pereyra incorporated an inverted U incision, accessing the retropubic space for mobilization of the bladder neck and fingertip guidance during needle passage, and full-thickness vaginal wall helical anchoring sutures.[19]

Stamey The Stamey procedures includes the addition of a Dacron pledget to buttress the periurethral tissue, and performance of a concurrent cystoscopy during needle passage.[20]

Gittes The Gittes procedure is a no-incision, full-thickness "autologous pledget" tied suprapubically.[21]

Vaginal repair
Kelly-type plication The Kelly-type procedure includes plication of the pubocervical fascia (circular muscular layers of the vagina) overlying the bladder neck and urethra with imbricating sutures. No longer used as a primary procedure for stress incontinence due to low success rates. See Kelly Kennedy Plication.

Slings
According to the American Urogynecologic Society and the Society of Urodynamics, Female Pelvic Medicine and Urogenital Reconstruction, the polypropylene mesh

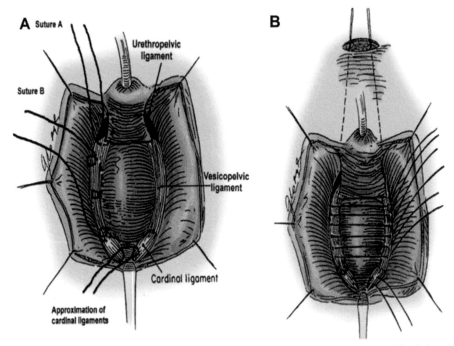

Fig. 3. (*A*) Four-corner suspension through goal-post incision. Suture A: periurethral tissue at mid urethra. Suture B: endopelvic fascia at bladder neck, perivesical fascia, and ipsilateral cardinal ligament. (*B*) Imbricating sutures to reduce the cystocele. Suspension sutures are transferred suprapubically. (*From* Karram M. Vaginal reconstructive surgery for sphincteric incontinence. In: Wein AJ, Kavoussi LR, Novick AC, et al, editors. Campbell-Walsh urology. Philadelphia: Saunders; 2007; with permission.)

midurethral (retropubic and transobturator) sling (**Fig. 5**) is now the recognized standard of care for the surgical treatment of stress urinary incontinence.[22] Because midurethral slings involve mesh, and due to anatomic concerns regarding long-term restoration of support, this recommendation is not universal.[5]

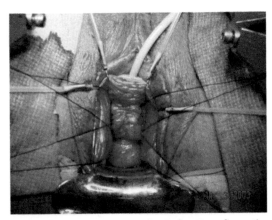

Fig. 4. Anterior vaginal wall suspension: "French window" configuration of helical sutures.

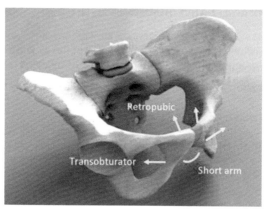

Fig. 5. Pelvic model. The *arrows* indicate the location of the retropubic sling, the transobturator sling and the short-arm sling. (*From* Riss P, Hinterholzer S. Maintaining standards for surgery for female urinary incontinence. Maturitas 2010;65(1):5–10; with permission.)

Retropubic midurethral mesh slings Trocars traverse the suprapubic area, the retropubic space, and the mid urethra. Severe vascular or nerve injury and bowel perforation as well as death have been reported due to injury along the trajectory of the trocars. Bladder perforation is a more common and less serious consequence.

Transobturator midurethral mesh sling Trocars traverse the obturator foramen at the junction of the inferior pubic ramus with the pubic symphysis via the notch posterior to the insertion of the adductor longus tendon and a vaginal incision along the mid urethra. The obturator nerve provides adduction (adductor muscles), lateral rotation of the hip (gracilis muscle), and sensory innervation of the inner side of the thigh and knee. Injury can impact adduction and leg crossing, leading to pain and parasthesias. There can also be anomalous branches of nerve or the obturator vessels. Injury to the adductor longus tendon can lead to severe pain and immobility. Early detection before fibrosis is essential because it allows for complete removal.

Single incision mesh sling A single incision mesh sling requires only a vaginal incision and self-anchors to the obturator membrane (or endopelvic fascia in the direction of the retropubic space).

Pubovaginal sling This was the originally described "sling." It involves placing sling material, usually the patient's own autologous rectus fascia or fascia lata (alternatives include cadaveric, porcine, or mesh material) at the level of the bladder neck, traversing the retropubic space, and tying off-tension overlying the rectus fascia.

Readjustable sling The readjustable sling consists of an adjustable veritensor and polypropylene mesh and is typically used for refractory patients. The Prolene sutures on either side of this mesh sling (substitutable for biological material) are passed from the vaginal incision through the retropubic space and rectus fascia and are secured in the veritensor overlying the rectus fascia. The veritensor is adjusted once the patient is awake then the "key" is removed. It can also be reaccessed with a new key and adjusted at a time remote from the original procedure.[23]

PELVIC ORGAN PROLAPSE: NATIVE TISSUE AND MESH

Pelvic organ prolapse (POP) is the "descent of one or more of the anterior vaginal wall, posterior vaginal wall, the uterus (cervix), or the apex of the vagina (the vaginal vault or cuff scar after hysterectomy)."[1] It is further categorized by the prolapsing organ.

- Anterior compartment prolapse often involves the bladder and is known as a *cystocele.*
- Posterior compartment prolapse often involves the rectum and is referred to as a *rectocele.*
- Prolapse of bowel is called *enterocele.*
- Descent of the perineal body and levator plate is known as a *perineocele.*
- The involvement of all 3 compartments including the uterus is collectively known as *procidentia.*

POP can be completely asymptomatic. Symptoms occur most often once the prolapse passes the hymenal remnant. They may worsen as the prolapse advances, and include pelvic pressure, and sexual, defecatory, and urinary symptoms such as obstruction and urge urinary incontinence. Furthermore, severe consequences can result, such as urinary tract obstruction, urinary tract infections, or in cases of severe neglect ulceration with bowel evisceration (**Fig. 6**). Surgical options are considered if conservative measures are insufficient, if symptoms are a significant detriment to quality of life, or if there is a health consequence posed due to the POP.

Surgical correction of POP requires knowledge of the main supports available for a safe, durable repair. These supports include the arcus tendineus fascia pelvis, levator

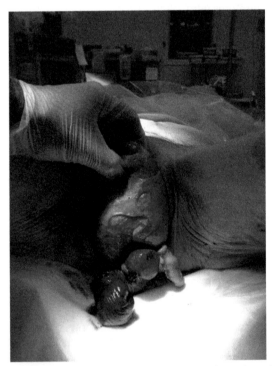

Fig. 6. Bowel evisceration via ulcerated procidencia in a neglected nursing home patient. (*Courtesy of* Brian Murray MD, Albany, NY.)

muscles, uterosacral ligaments, sacrospinous ligament, iliococcygeus muscle, rectus fascia, and the sacral promontory, which must be accessed without injuring the nerves, vessels, ureters, or adjacent organs within the pelvis. Assessment for involvement of each compartment is essential to completing the appropriate intervention. The vagina is "a house of cards," such that improving support to one compartment may increase strain on the others.

Treatment of POP has changed over time. In an effort to increase the durability of repairs, the use of mesh increased until 2008, at which point (and again in 2011) FDA warnings were published regarding mesh complications. Due to increased concerns over the use of transvaginal mesh, sacrocolpopexy placing mesh abdominally via minimally invasive techniques has increased.[24] Although vaginal mesh is still marketed, many companies have pulled their products from the market. Consequently, native tissue vaginal approaches have reemerged.

Due to the numerous repairs that have been available over time, it is important for the general surgeon to understand both current and historic approaches in the patient's surgical history, to plan further surgery or manage complications in a safe and effective manner.[25]

Vaginal Vault Suspension

For apical prolapse with or without the uterus present, there are 5 main options.

Vaginal approach

Sacrospinous ligament suspension Transvaginal suspension of the vaginal apex to the sacrospinous ligament undertakes both its dissection and suture placement in the extraperitoneal space.[26] Sutures are placed slightly caudad in the midportion of the sacrospinous ligament (**Figs. 7** and **8**). Injury can occur to the pudendal nerve and vessels laterally or the sciatic outflow more cephalad. There are many anatomic variations of the pudendal nerve. For example, the inferior rectal nerve (a branch) can penetrate directly through the sacrospinous ligament. Injury of this branch can lead to fecal incontinence. The sciatic nerve lies 2 cm from the sacrospinous ligament (**Fig. 9**).

Iliococcygeus suspension The iliococcygeus suspension uses similar principles to the sacrospinous ligament vault fixation, but in an effort to avoid the dangers surrounding the sacrospinous ligament, utilizes the iliococcygeus muscle.[27]

Vaginal uterosacral ligament suspension Intraperitoneal access is gained transvaginally via cuff dissection or at the time of hysterectomy. The vaginal apex is suspended to the uterosacral ligaments bilaterally (**Figs. 10–13**).[28] Due to the fact that the ureter is 1 cm from the uterosacral ligament on its cephalad end, ureteric injury rates are reported as high as 11%.[29] The majority of injuries are identified and addressed intraoperatively at the time with the administration of ureteric chromatic agents. It is debated whether to place ureteric stents before the procedure.

Mesh The most comprehensive pictorial for the mesh kits can be found in "Insertion and Removal of vaginal Mesh for Pelvic Organ Prolapse," by Muffly and Barber.[30] This article catalogs the products that were available in 2010, their routes of insertion, types of mesh, and sites of fixation. The mesh kits use the same points of fixation as native tissue surgery: the sacrospinous ligament, iliococcygeus muscle, arcus tendineus fascia pelvis, obturator fascia, and levator muscles. The route of trocar passage and type of mesh (open pore monofilament is preferable), as well as presence of infection will dictate the outcome and potential for complications (**Fig. 14**).

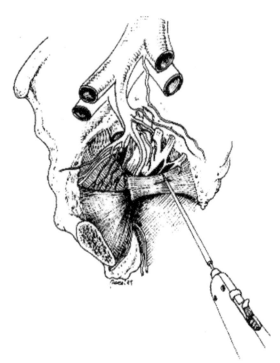

Fig. 7. Loaded inserter's shaft is pushed through the body of the coccygeus muscle and sacrospinous ligament, to the ischial spine to avoid the pudendal complex and sciatic nerve, found under the lateral third of the sacrospinous ligament. (*From* Giberti C. Transvaginal sacrospinous colpopexy by palpation-a new minimally invasive procedure using an anchoring system. Urology 2001;57(4):666–8; with permission.)

Abdominal approach

Abdominal sacrocolpopexy Abdominal sacrocolpopexy may be performed via an open, laparoscopic, or robotic-assisted approach. The peritoneum is dissected from the vagina, synthetic Y-mesh is tacked to the anterior and posterior aspect of the vagina, then sutured to the anterior longitudinal ligament at S1 and S2 (**Fig. 15**). Randomized studies have demonstrated that biological material is inferior and therefore synthetic mesh is uniformly used.[31] During dissection, injury to the ureter, bladder, rectum, hypogastric nerves, middle sacral vessels, or iliac vessels can occur. If the mesh is not reperitonealized, the patient is at risk of bowel obstruction due to adherence to the mesh. Rarely, sacral osteomyelitis or discitis can occur. Vaginal mesh erosion is a possibility, although of lower likelihood than with the vaginal approaches. The cervix is left in place due to high rates of erosion with concurrent trachelectomy.[32]

Cystocele Repair

Kelly Kennedy plication

Kelly Kennedy plication involves a midline plication of the pubocervical fascia (the circular muscular layers of the vagina) after dissecting under the vaginal mucosa (**Figs. 16** and **17**). Additional imbrication overlying the urethra is considered the Kelly plication with a 30% to 50% success rate for stress urinary incontinence.[33]

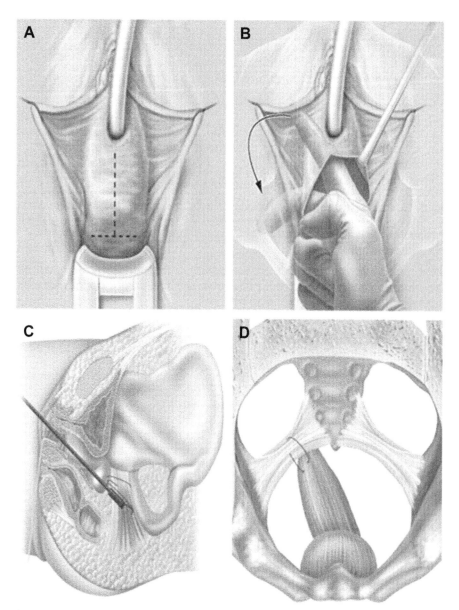

Fig. 8. Dissection for anterior sacrospinous vaginal vault suspension. (*A*) Incision (*dotted lines*). (*B*) Perforation into retropubic space through anterior vaginal wall incision and dissection. (*C*) Placement of suture in sacrospinous ligament with straight capiodevice. (*D*) Suspension of vaginal vault to sacrospinous ligament. (*From* Botros SM, Goldberg RP, Sand PK. Sacrospinous ligament suspension for vaginal vault prolapse. In: Raz S, Rodriguez L, editors. Female urology. Philadelphia: Saunders; 2008. p. 673–82; with permission.)

Site-specific graft augment

Site-specific graft augment may be undertaken with biological material (human cadaveric, porcine, bovine)[34] or mesh (**Fig. 18**). Currently, mesh is made of polypropylene monofilament but prior products included multifilament and small pore products

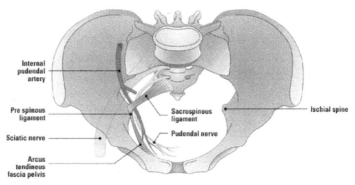

Fig. 9. Superior aspect of pelvis with sacrospinous ligament and iliococcygeus fascia and their relationship to major nerves and vessels. (*From* Maher CF. Iliococcygeus or sacrospinous fixation for vaginal vault prolapse. Obstet Gynecol 2001;98(1):40–4; with permission.)

with poor incorporation and tolerance. Site-specific grafts in cystocele repair are typically secured to the arcus tendineus fascia pelvis laterally (level II support), and/or the sacrospinous ligament (level I support) cephalad.

Lateral paravaginal repair (relatively historic)
The vagina is plicated in the midline and the lateral attachments are taken down and recreated with sutures to the lateral pelvic sidewall.[35] Although little is published on this technique, reports include relatively high transfusion rates.[36]

Anterior vaginal wall suspension
Anterior vaginal wall suspension is a needle suspension technique that involves helical sutures placed in a horizontal plane on each side of the vagina, as described regarding its application to stress urinary incontinence. The retroperitoneal space is entered bilaterally by taking down the endopelvic fascia. The surgeon's finger is passed up and under the anterior rectus sheath, protecting the bladder and other structures, such as ectopically positioned bowel. A small lower abdominal incision is created above the pubic symphysis and a dual pronged needle passer is passed to the

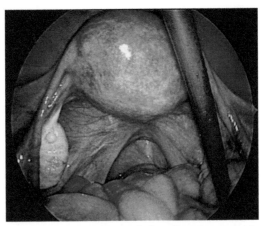

Fig. 10. Uterosacral ligaments are visible medially when the uterus is placed on tension (laparoscopic view).

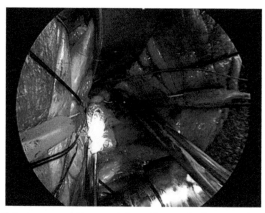

Fig. 11. Suture in the uterosacral ligament from the vaginal approach.

surgeon's finger bilaterally, then led into the vagina. The vaginal sutures are threaded into the passer and delivered from the vagina to the anterior abdominal wall, then tied overlying the rectus fascia off tension. Complications include hematoma and injury to the ilioinguinal nerve.[17]

Mesh kits

Mesh kits for anterior repair have been shown in randomized trials to decrease the incidence of reoperation for recurrence of prolapse but to increase the likelihood of reoperation for complications such as mesh erosion.[31] Mesh kits for support of the anterior vaginal wall can involve the following.[30]

- Trocar passage through the obturator membrane at 2 sites (closer to and farther from the pubic symphysis);

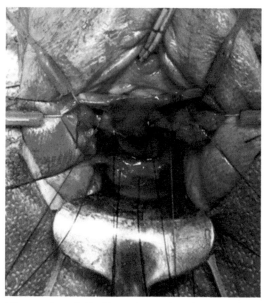

Fig. 12. Uterosacral ligament vault fixation sutures place in succession at the apex.

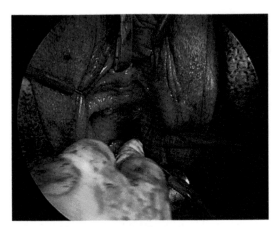

Fig. 13. Tying the uterosacral ligament suspension sutures.

- Fastening mechanisms from within the vaginal incision to the arcus tendineus fascia pelvis, levator muscles, or obturator foramen; or
- The addition of vault support fastening mechanisms including the sacrospinous ligaments bilaterally.

In general, the single-incision kits are easier to remove if needed, because the trocar-based mesh kits leave material adhered within planes of the bony and muscular pelvis.

Rectocele Repair

Rectocele repair can be achieved in many ways, and often includes a perineorrhaphy, reconstruction of the perineal body in the midline.

Posterior colporrhaphy

Mattress sutures plicate the rectovaginal muscularis across the midline similar to the midline Kelly Kennedy or rectovaginal fascial plication.[37]

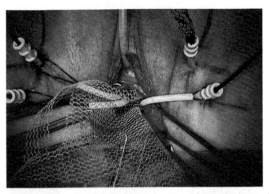

Fig. 14. After introducing the straps of the Gynecare Prolift mesh through the loops of the retrieval devices they are pulled sequentially through the cannulas. (*From* Reisenauer C. Anatomic conditions for pelvic floor reconstruction with polypropylene implant and its application for the treatment of vaginal prolapse. Eur J Obstet Gynecol Reprod Biol 2007;131(2):214–25; with permission.)

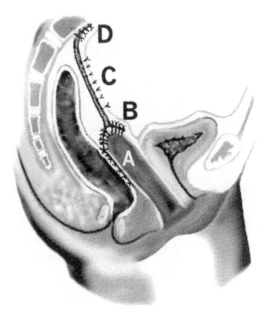

Fig. 15. Sagittal view of a completed abdominal sacrocolpopexy. Posterior wall enterocele repair (*A*) is shown with its attachment to the posterior limb of the mesh. The vagina is attached to the Y of the mesh (*B*), and the other end is attached to the anterior longitudinal ligament of the sacrum using multiple permanent sutures (*D*). The overlying peritoneum is then closed to completely cover the suspending mesh (*C*). (*From* Cespedes RD. Diagnosis and treatment of vaginal vault prolapse conditions. Urology 2002;60(1):8–15; with permission.)

Site-specific defect repair
Interrupted sutures reapproximate the detached edges of the rectovaginal fascia (the circular muscular layers of the vagina), correcting appreciable defects.[38] This method can be used in combination with the other techniques.

Site-specific graft augment
Site-specific graft augment with biological material (human cadaveric, porcine, bovine)[31,39] or synthetic graft.[40] When compared with traditional repair, this approach has poorer outcomes. However, the only high-quality data include porcine material,

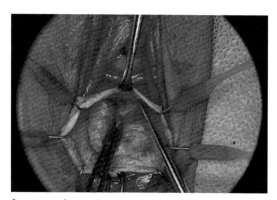

Fig. 16. Dissection for cystocele repair.

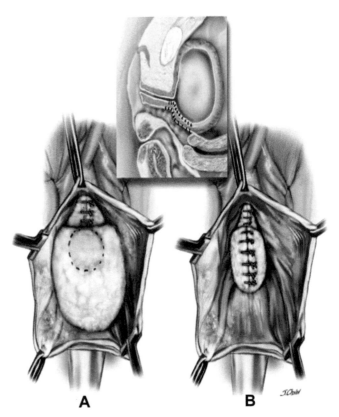

Fig. 17. Anterior colporrhaphy with Kelly–Kennedy plication. (*A*) The vaginal mucosa is opened and interrupted sutures are started under the urethra. (*B*) The completed colporrha-phy uses midline plication with interrupted sutures. Preferential support is provided to the proximal urethra over that provided to the bladder. (*From* Maher CF, Karram MM. Surgical management of anterior vaginal wall prolapse. In: Karram MM, Maher CF, editors. Surgical management of pelvic organ prolapse. Philadelphia: Saunders; 2013; with permission.)

which may be more immunogenic than human products. Mesh grafts overlying the rectum have led to rectovaginal fistula with significant difficulty in repair due to the dense adhesions of the surrounding tissue to the mesh and often overlying infection. Colostomy and removal of a significant margin of (if not all) the mesh, are fundamental to the operative plan (**Fig. 19**).[41]

Levator myorrhaphy
Levator myorrhaphy involves plicating the levator muscles in the midline as the foundation of the support for the rectal wall.[42] Pelvic pain and dyspareunia rates are high enough that this approach is not often used.

High midline levator myorrphaphy
High midline levator myorrphaphy typically involves opening the peritoneal cavity and fixing the vault of the vagina to a reconstructed shelf of levators high in the pelvis. This approach involves the closure of the enterocele inherent in an open peritoneal dissection. This approach reports lower rates of pain, perhaps due to the higher location on the levator muscles.[43]

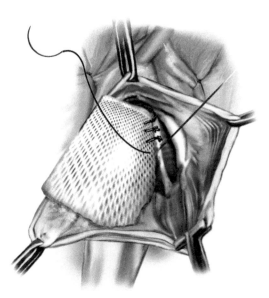

Fig. 18. Graft augmentation of lateral cystocele repair, suturing to the arcus tendineus fascia pelvis, the condensation of endopelvic fascia forming a fibrous band from the pubic symphysis to the ischial spine. (*From* Nitti VW, Karram M. Repair of anterior vaginal prolapse. In: Vaginal surgery for the urologist. Philadelphia: Saunders; 2012. p. 23–34; with permission.)

Mesh kits

As with the anterior repair, there are trocar-based kits and single incision site-specific kits. All involve mesh but as the kits evolved some reduced the volume of mesh or incorporated a biologic component. Most of these products have been removed from the market.

- Trocar routes typically traversed transgluteally and pararectally up through the iliococcygeus muscle or sacrospinous ligament.
- Single incision nontrocar fixation typically involves the sacrospinous ligament and the levator muscles.
- Depending on the mesh character and the plane of dissection, rectal perforation and erosion can be a serious consequence of this approach in addition to the typical risks of ureter, nerve and vascular injury. More subtle rectal findings could involve compression and kinking.

URGE URINARY INCONTINENCE

Urgency (urinary) incontinence is defined as "the complaint of involuntary loss of urine associated with urgency."[1] Treatments are typically behavioral and medical but for refractory cases the following options exist.

Onabotulinumtoxin A to Bladder Detrusor

Doses of 100 to 400 units are used, typically 100 units for those who void spontaneously and a starting dose of 200 units for those who self-catheterize. Urinary tract infection is the most common complication, followed by urinary retention requiring intermittent catheterization. Distant spread of toxin is a theoretic complication at these doses.

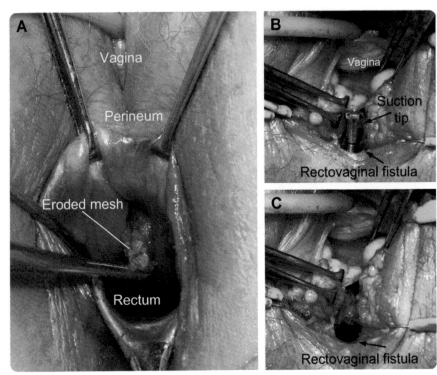

Fig. 19. Rectovaginal fistula. (*A*) Posterior mesh has eroded through the posterior vaginal wall and through the rectal wall, causing a rectovaginal fistula. (*B*) After removal of mesh, suction tip demonstrates rectovaginal fistula. (*C*) Vaginal side of fistulous tract is visible. (*From* Margulies RU, Lewicky-Gaupp C, Fenner DE, et al. Complications requiring reoperation following vaginal mesh kit procedures for prolapse. Am J Obstet Gynecol 2008;199(6):678.e1–4; with permission.)

Interstim Sacral Neuromodulation

Interstim sacral neuromodulation is an option for those with nonneurogenic overactive bladder. A lead is placed along the S3 nerve route and a low-grade vibration raises the threshold for neural communication in the pelvis.[44] Indications include not only urgency, frequency, and urge urinary incontinence, but also idiopathic urinary retention and fecal incontinence.[45]

Augmentation Cystoplasty

Augmentation cystoplasty involves augmentation of the bladder using ileum or other sections of bowel, described elsewhere in this issue (See Moritz Hansen, Matthew Hayn, Patrick Murray: The Use of Bowel in Urologic Reconstructive Surgery, in this issue). Electrolyte abnormalities, urinary retention, stones due to mucous build up, and perforation due to overdistension/delayed catheterization (a surgical emergency) are the most common complications.[46]

OBSTRUCTION
Urethral Diverticulum

Urethral diverticulum is an outpouching of the urethra that can be dissected and repaired to address its resultant urinary tract infections, postvoid dribbling, bladder outlet obstruction, and dyspareunia.[47] A Martius labial fat pad is often used for vascular interposition.

Urethral Stricture

Urethral stricture is rare in women. Urethral dilation is commonly used as first intervention. Maintenance of patency can be helped by periodic self-catheterization. Formal repair can be undertaken with urethral reconstruction.

Onabotulinumtoxin A to Sphincter or Bladder Neck

Onabotulinumtoxin A to sphincter or bladder neck can relax the internal or external urethral sphincter in a patient with primary (idiopathic) bladder neck obstruction or neurologic etiology for dyssynergia of either sphincter.

Incision of Bladder Neck

Incision of the bladder neck is used only rarely for women with primary bladder neck obstruction who are refractory to alpha blocker medical therapy and onabotulinumtoxin A. Stress urinary incontinence is a predictable risk and self-catheterization may be a preferred mode of therapy.

Levator Dysfunction

For levator dysfunction and behavioral dysfunction of the external urethral sphincter, pelvic floor physical therapy is an extremely useful intervention for incomplete emptying, urinary urgency frequency, incontinence, dyspareunia, and defecatory dysfunction related to a dysfunctional pelvic floor.[48] Onabotulinumtoxin A can be injected directly into the external urethral sphincter and levator muscles in cases refractory to physical therapy and oral muscle relaxants.[49]

Prolapse of the anterior vaginal wall can lead to obstruction, as discussed.

SUMMARY

Surgery for female voiding dysfunction is varied and depends on the clinical picture at presentation. Review of the prior operative note, and a general understanding of the type of procedures performed, will typically shed light on the organs affected by complications or future surgical planning.

ACKNOWLEDGMENTS

The authors thank John Harmon for his expertise in the written language and contribution to this work.

REFERENCES

1. Haylen BT, de Ridder D, Freeman RM, et al. An International Urogynecological Association (IUGA)/International Continence Society (ICS) joint report on the terminology for female pelvic floor dysfunction. Neurourol Urodyn 2010;29(1):4–20.
2. Walsh LP, Zimmern PE, Pope N, et al, Urinary Incontinence Treatment Network. Comparison of the Q-tip test and voiding cystourethrogram to assess urethral hypermobility among women enrolled in a randomized clinical trial of surgery for stress urinary incontinence. J Urol 2006;176(2):646–9 [discussion: 650].
3. DeLancey JO. Structural support of the urethra as it relates to stress urinary incontinence: the hammock hypothesis. Am J Obstet Gynecol 1994;170(6):1713–20 [discussion: 1720–3].

4. Sand PK, Bowen LW, Panganiban R, et al. The low pressure urethra as a factor in failed retropubic urethropexy. Obstet Gynecol 1987;69(3 Pt 1):399–402.

5. Dobberfuhl AD, De EJ. Female stress urinary incontinence and the mid-urethral sling: is obstruction necessary to achieve dryness? World J Urol 2015;33(9): 1243–50.

6. Klarskov N, Lose G. Urethral injection therapy: what is the mechanism of action? Neurourol Urodyn 2008;27(8):789–92.

7. Corcos J, Collet JP, Shapiro S, et al. Multicenter randomized clinical trial comparing surgery and collagen injections for treatment of female stress urinary incontinence. Urology 2005;65(5):898–904.

8. Mayer RD, Dmochowski RR, Appell RA, et al. Multicenter prospective randomized 52-week trial of calcium hydroxylapatite versus bovine dermal collagen for treatment of stress urinary incontinence. Urology 2007;69(5):876–80.

9. Ghoniem G, Corcos J, Comiter C, et al. Cross-linked polydimethylsiloxane injection for female stress urinary incontinence: results of a multicenter, randomized, controlled, single-blind study. J Urol 2009;181(1):204–10.

10. Keegan PE, Atiemo K, Cody J, et al. Periurethral injection therapy for urinary incontinence in women. Cochrane Database Syst Rev 2007;(3):CD003881.

11. Dmochowski RR, Blaivas JM, Gormley EA, et al. Update of AUA guideline on the surgical management of female stress urinary incontinence. J Urol 2010;183(5): 1906–14.

12. Marshall VF, Marchetti AA, Krantz KE. The correction of stress incontinence by simple vesicourethral suspension. Surg Gynecol Obstet 1949;88(4):509–18.

13. Kammerer-Doak DN, Cornella JL, Magrina JF, et al. Osteitis pubis after Marshall-Marchetti-Krantz urethropexy: a pubic osteomyelitis. Am J Obstet Gynecol 1998; 179(3 Pt 1):586–90.

14. Burch JC. Urethrovaginal fixation to Cooper's ligament for correction of stress incontinence, cystocele, and prolapse. Am J Obstet Gynecol 1961;81:281–90.

15. Takacs EZ, Philippe E. Role of needle suspensions. In: Raz S, Rodriguez LV, editors. Female urology. New York: Elsevier; 2008. p. 362–74.

16. Raz S, Klutke CG, Golomb J. Four-corner bladder and urethral suspension for moderate cystocele. J Urol 1989;142(3):712–5.

17. Coskun B, Lavelle RS, Alhalabi F, et al. Anterior vaginal wall suspension procedure for moderate bladder and uterine prolapse as a method of uterine preservation. J Urol 2014;192(5):1461–7.

18. Pereyra AJ. A simplified surgical procedure for the correction of stress incontinence in women. West J Surg Obstet Gynecol 1959;67(4):223–6.

19. Raz S. Modified bladder neck suspension for female stress incontinence. Urology 1981;17(1):82–5.

20. Schaeffer AJ, Stamey TA. Endoscopic suspension of vesical neck for urinary incontinence. Urology 1984;23(5):484–94.

21. Gittes RF, Loughlin KR. No-incision pubovaginal suspension for stress incontinence. J Urol 1987;138(3):568–70.

22. Nager C, Tulikangas P, Miller D, et al. Position statement on mesh midurethral slings for stress urinary incontinence. Female Pelvic Med Reconstr Surg 2014; 20(3):123–5.

23. Errando C, Rodriguez-Escovar F, Gutierrez C, et al. A re-adjustable sling for female recurrent stress incontinence and sphincteric deficiency: outcomes and complications in 125 patients using the Remeex sling system. Neurourol Urodyn 2010;29(8):1429–32.

24. Wang LC, Awamlh BA, Hu JC, et al. Trends in mesh use for pelvic organ prolapse repair from the Medicare database. Urology 2015;86:885–91.

25. Maher C, Baessler K. Surgical management of anterior vaginal wall prolapse: an evidence-based literature review. Int Urogynecol J Pelvic Floor Dysfunct 2006; 17(2):195–201.

26. Morley GW, DeLancey JO. Sacrospinous ligament fixation for eversion of the vagina. Am J Obstet Gynecol 1988;158(4):872–81.

27. Medina CA, Croce C, Candiotti K, et al. Comparison of vaginal length after iliococcygeus fixation and sacrospinous ligament fixation. Int J Gynaecol Obstet 2008;100(3):267–70.

28. Shull BL, Bachofen C, Coates KW, et al. A transvaginal approach to repair of apical and other associated sites of pelvic organ prolapse with uterosacral ligaments. Am J Obstet Gynecol 2000;183(6):1365–73 [discussion: 1373–4].

29. Barber MD, Visco AG, Weidner AC, et al. Bilateral uterosacral ligament vaginal vault suspension with site-specific endopelvic fascia defect repair for treatment of pelvic organ prolapse. Am J Obstet Gynecol 2000;183(6):1402–10 [discussion: 1410–1].

30. M Muffly T, Barber MD. Insertion and removal of vaginal mesh for pelvic organ prolapse. Clin Obstet Gynecol 2010;53(1):99–114.

31. Maher C, Feiner B, Baessler K, et al. Surgical management of pelvic organ prolapse in women. Cochrane Database Syst Rev 2013;(4):CD004014.

32. Tan-Kim J, Menefee SA, Luber KM, et al. Prevalence and risk factors for mesh erosion after laparoscopic-assisted sacrocolpopexy. Int Urogynecol J 2011; 22(2):205–12.

33. Kelly HA, Dumm WM. Urinary incontinence in women, without manifest injury to the bladder. 1914. Int Urogynecol J Pelvic Floor Dysfunct 1998;9(3):158–64.

34. Cormio L, Mancini V, Liuzzi G, et al. Cystocele repair by autologous rectus fascia graft: the pubovaginal cystocele sling. J Urol 2015;194(3):721–7.

35. Young SB, Daman JJ, Bony LG. Vaginal paravaginal repair: one-year outcomes. Am J Obstet Gynecol 2001;185(6):1360–6 [discussion: 1366–7].

36. Scotti RJ, Garely AD, Greston WM, et al. Paravaginal repair of lateral vaginal wall defects by fixation to the ischial periosteum and obturator membrane. Am J Obstet Gynecol 1998;179(6 Pt 1):1436–45.

37. Maher CF, Qatawneh AM, Baessler K, et al. Midline rectovaginal fascial plication for repair of rectocele and obstructed defecation. Obstet Gynecol 2004;104(4): 685–9.

38. Cundiff GW, Weidner AC, Visco AG, et al. An anatomic and functional assessment of the discrete defect rectocele repair. Am J Obstet Gynecol 1998; 179(6 Pt 1):1451–6 [discussion: 1456–7].

39. Grimes CL, Tan-Kim J, Whitcomb EL, et al. Long-term outcomes after native tissue vs. biological graft-augmented repair in the posterior compartment. Int Urogynecol J 2012;23(5):597–604.

40. Paraiso MF, Barber MD, Muir TW, et al. Rectocele repair: a randomized trial of three surgical techniques including graft augmentation. Am J Obstet Gynecol 2006;195(6):1762–71.

41. Yamada BS, Govier FE, Stefanovic KB, et al. Vesicovaginal fistula and mesh erosion after Perigee (transobturator polypropylene mesh anterior repair). Urology 2006;68(5):1121.e5–7.

42. Natale F, La Penna C, Padoa A, et al. High levator myorrhaphy for transvaginal suspension of the vaginal apex: long-term results. J Urol 2008;180(5):2047–52 [discussion: 2052].

43. Natale F, La Penna C, Padoa A, et al. High levator myorraphy versus uterosacral ligament suspension for vaginal vault fixation: a prospective, randomized study. Int Urogynecol J 2010;21(5):515–22.

44. Noblett K, Siegel S, Mangel J, et al. Results of a prospective, multicenter study evaluating quality of life, safety, and efficacy of sacral neuromodulation at twelve months in subjects with symptoms of overactive bladder. Neurourol Urodyn 2016; 35(2):246–51.

45. Wexner SD, Coller JA, Devroede G, et al. Sacral nerve stimulation for fecal incontinence: results of a 120-patient prospective multicenter study. Ann Surg 2010; 251(3):441–9.

46. Greenwell TJ, Venn SN, Mundy AR. Augmentation cystoplasty. BJU Int 2001; 88(6):511–25.

47. Crescenze IM, Goldman HB. Female urethral diverticulum: current diagnosis and management. Curr Urol Rep 2015;16(10):540.

48. Fitzgerald MP, Anderson RU, Potts J, et al. Randomized multicenter feasibility trial of myofascial physical therapy for the treatment of urological chronic pelvic pain syndromes. J Urol 2013;189(1 Suppl):S75–85.

49. Adelowo A, Hacker MR, Shapiro A, et al. Botulinum toxin type A (BOTOX) for refractory myofascial pelvic pain. Female Pelvic Med Reconstr Surg 2013; 19(5):288–92.

Surgical Management of Male Voiding Dysfunction

Jessica Mandeville, MD*, Arthur Mourtzinos, MD, MBA

KEYWORDS

- Benign prostatic hypertophy • Lower urinary tract symptoms
- Transurethral resection of the prostate • Holmium laser enucleation of the prostate
- Photoselective vaporization of the prostate • Open simple prostatectomy

KEY POINTS

- BPH is a common, surgically correctable cause of voiding dysfunction and troublesome lower urinary tract symptoms in males.
- Indications for surgical intervention in the management of BPH include urinary retention, recurrent urinary tract infections, bladder stone formation, upper urinary tract deterioration, and failure of medical management.
- Numerous surgical interventions are available for the management of BPH. The procedure of choice is determined by patient and surgeon preference, desired outcome, prostate size, and other patient-related factors (ie, anticoagulation use).

 Video content accompanies this article at http://www.surgical.theclinics.com

INTRODUCTION

Male voiding dysfunction is associated with various genitourinary conditions including urethral stricture, idiopathic detrusor overactivity, neurogenic bladder (ie, from spinal cord injury), neurologic disorders (ie, stroke, parkinsonism), poorly controlled diabetes, and benign prostatic hyperplasia (BPH). All of these conditions are associated with troubling lower urinary tract symptoms (LUTS), which can have a negative impact on quality of life. This article focuses on the management of male voiding dysfunction and LUTS related to BPH.

Disclosure Statement: J. Mandeville has provided educational lectures for Lumenis, but has no financial relationship with the company. A. Mourtzinos has nothing to disclose.
Department of Urology, Lahey Hospital and Medical Center, 41 Mall Road, Burlington, MA 01805, USA
* Corresponding author.
E-mail address: jessica.a.mandeville@lahey.org

Surg Clin N Am 96 (2016) 491–501
http://dx.doi.org/10.1016/j.suc.2016.02.006
0039-6109/16/$ – see front matter © 2016 Elsevier Inc. All rights reserved.

ETIOLOGY AND EPIDEMIOLOGY OF BENIGN PROSTATIC HYPERPLASIA AND LOWER URINARY TRACT SYMPTOMS

BPH is a histologic diagnosis characterized by enlargement of the prostate gland from a nonmalignant proliferation of glandular and stromal elements in the transition zone of the prostate.[1] Development of BPH in males is an age-related process. Histologic evidence of BPH is identified in approximately 10% of men in their 30s, in 50% to 60% of men in their 60s, and in up to 90% of men in their 70s and 80s.[1,2]

BPH may be entirely asymptomatic or associated with a wide variety of LUTS. The LUTS develop as a result of bladder outlet obstruction from the enlarged prostate. LUTS is separated into voiding-related symptoms or storage-related symptoms (**Box 1**).[2,3] Numerous self-completed, validated questionnaires exist for the assessment of LUTS related to BPH and the most commonly used tool is the International Prostate Symptoms Score. Symptoms are considered mild if the score is seven or less, moderate if the score is 8 to 19, and severe if the score is 20 to 35. The quality of life question response ranges from zero to six, with a score of zero indicating the patient is "delighted" with their symptoms and a score of six indicating the symptoms are "terrible." Severity of symptoms is not well correlated with prostate size or patient age. However, the risk for developing urinary retention does increase with increasing symptom score and higher preoperative symptoms scores are associated with successful postoperative outcomes in patients undergoing surgery for BPH/LUTS.[1,2] The International Prostate Symptoms Score is also useful for assessing treatment success (medical or surgical).

MANAGEMENT OF BENIGN PROSTATIC HYPERPLASIA AND LOWER URINARY TRACT SYMPTOMS

A wide variety of treatments are available for the management of BPH/LUTS. The most commonly used initial measures are conservative (watchful waiting, behavioral modification, oral fluid management, or medical therapy with α-blockers and/or 5α-reductase inhibitors). However, these management options are outside of the scope of this review.

Surgical intervention is often necessary for patients with complications related to BPH including urinary retention, development of bladder calculi, recurrent urinary tract infections, recurrent prostatic bleeding, or impairment of renal function related to upper urinary tract obstruction. Additional indications for surgical intervention are severe symptoms, failure of medical therapy, intolerance of medical therapy, or patient preference to avoid medications.

Currently, urologic surgeons and their patients have a wide variety of surgical treatment options available for management of BPH/LUTS. These treatments include

---

Box 1
Lower urinary tract symptoms that may be associated with BPH

Voiding symptoms
- Slowing urinary stream
- Hesitancy in initiating urinary stream
- Straining to initiate urinary stream
- Sensation of incomplete bladder emptying
- Postvoid dribbling of urine

Storage symptoms
- Increased daytime urinary frequency (>7 voids per day)
- Nocturia (waking to void at night)
- Urgency of urination
- Urgency-related incontinence of urine

office-based procedures, operating room–based transurethral surgeries, and open or laparoscopic surgeries (**Box 2**). The treatment of choice depends on patient and surgeon preference, expected outcomes, prostate size, and other patient-related factors (ie, surgical risk, anticoagulation, anatomic abnormalities).

PREOPERATIVE EVALUATION

Preoperatively, digital rectal examination and prostate-specific antigen are assessed to evaluate for the presence of underlying prostate cancer (although prostate-specific antigen can often be elevated simply from prostatic enlargement). Urine culture should routinely be obtained before surgery and any infection treated with culture-specific antibiotics. In patients with hematuria or a history suggesting causes of LUTS other than BPH (ie, history of stricture), cystoscopy should be carried out before surgery. Transrectal ultrasound sizing of the prostate is optional and is helpful in determining the most appropriate surgical approach and planning operative times.

OFFICE-BASED PROCEDURES
Transurethral Microwave Therapy

With the development of new technologies and changes in reimbursement schedules, some treatments for BPH have moved into the office environment. Typically these procedures are performed in patients with small glands or in patients who cannot tolerate an anesthetic. Transurethral microwave therapy (TUMT) is a heat-based therapy considered an alternative office-based treatment to transurethral resection of the prostate (TURP) in patients who have LUTS. Because of its ease of administration and minimal discomfort, it has become an attractive option for many patients. TUMT treatment is based on increasing intraprostatic temperatures greater than 45°C, which cause coagulation necrosis in the targeted periurethral glandular tissue of the transition zone.[4] The heat is delivered through a catheter with a microwave antenna to carefully selected sections of the prostate gland. Several devices are available commercially; the main differences between the various systems are the degree of energy delivered, the design of the antenna, and the cooling system.

TUMT is performed in an outpatient setting without the need for an anesthesiologist.[5] Local anesthesia is administered with intraurethral 2% lidocaine jelly

---

Box 2
Surgical management options for BPH/LUTS

Office-based procedures
- Transurethral microwave therapy
- Transurethral needle ablation

Transurethral electrosurgical procedures
- Transurethral resection of the prostate
- Bipolar transurethral vaporization of the prostate

Transurethral laser procedures
- Holmium laser ablation of the prostate
- Holmium laser enucleation of the prostate
- Photoselective vaporization of the prostate (green light)

Open surgical procedures
- Open simple prostatectomy (transvesical or retropubic)

Laparoscopic/robotic procedures
- Robotic-assisted laparoscopic simple prostatectomy

approximately 10 to 15 minutes before the procedure. The bladder is subsequently emptied with straight catheterization and 50 mL of 2% lidocaine solution is instilled into the bladder for 10 minutes. With the assistance of a transrectal ultrasound, the TUMT catheter is placed into the bladder and the balloon is inflated. The rectal probe for temperature assessment is inserted and treatment is begun. The most common complications are prolonged postoperative catheterization times; urinary tract infections; and irritative voiding symptoms, such as dysuria and urinary frequency.[6]

Transurethral Needle Ablation

Transurethral needle ablation (TUNA) of the prostate is another temperature-based minimally invasive alternative in men with LUTS resulting from prostatic hypertrophy. TUNA uses the thermal properties of radiofrequencies.[7] The TUNA catheter is fitted with two deployable needles angled 40° from each other. The needles deliver thermal energy from an automated generator that maintains a target temperature of more than 45°C at the periphery and approximately 100°C at the center.[8] Coagulation necrosis is achieved at a mean of 3 mm from the tip of the needles through agitation of water molecules causing friction and subsequent heat. Depth of penetration of the needles is based on prostate volume assessment and urethral length measurements. Protective shields are deployed 5 to 6 mm over the shaft of the needle to protect the urethra. This is considered one of the major advantages of the TUNA technique because it protects the integrity of the urothelium and theoretically allows the performance of the procedure with minimal discomfort to the patient.[9] At the end of the procedure, the instrument is removed and the bladder is emptied. A catheter may or may not be placed at the end of the procedure. Patients reportedly tolerate the procedure well with minimal discomfort and significant symptom score improvement.[10]

SURGICAL PROCEDURES
Monopolar Transurethral Resection of the Prostate

Monopolar TURP is the historical gold standard therapy for LUTS secondary to obstruction from BPH (small to medium sized glands). In the 1980s, TURP was the most common operation in the Medicare population after cataract surgery.[11] Over the past 20 years, there has been a progressive decrease in the number of TURP procedures. This is caused by an increased use of medical therapies and minimally invasive surgical procedures (ie, TUMT, TUNA, laser, and vaporization techniques). Multiple factors have driven this trend, including reimbursement changes, but there has been no clear evidence that these new techniques are more efficacious or cost-effective than traditional TURP.[12]

The standard technique of the procedure has not changed. The patient is placed in the dorsal lithotomy position and the urethra is dilated to accommodate the resectoscope sheath (typically 26F catheter). The scope is then passed through the anterior and posterior urethra into the bladder under direct vision to prevent any urethral false passages. The resection technique varies according to the size of the prostate and user preference; however, it should be performed in an orderly fashion. A trough should be resected that identifies the capsule (typically between the 5- and 7-o'clock positions from the bladder neck to the verumontanum, encompassing the median lobe/median bar tissue) and resection of the lateral lobes is then continued down to the same plane (starting at the bladder neck and carried distally to the apex of each lateral lobe). Surgeons should take caution not to undermine the bladder neck and should avoid resection distal to the verumontanum (to prevent injury to the external urethral sphincter). In addition, the ureteral orifices should be identified and not violated.

Typically, most urologists use nonhemolytic irrigating solutions, such as 1.5% glycine, 3% sorbitol, or 3% mannitol, because of the inherent danger of using water where absorption can cause hemolysis and shock. The other solutions listed are not isotonic and can also cause serious side effects if excessive amounts are absorbed, specifically TURP syndrome. TURP syndrome is characterized by hypertension, bradycardia, visual disturbances, mental confusion, and nausea caused by a dilutional hyponatremia. Cerebral or bronchial edema can result if left untreated. Serum sodium levels should be monitored frequently and corrected with judicious infusion of intravenous hypertonic sodium chloride and furosemide. Procedures are typically performed under spinal anesthesia to monitor patients for TURP syndrome. Several attempts have been made to improve the modern TURP by altering instrumentation focused on mainly improving hemostasis and safety. Nonetheless, regardless of the configuration of TURP loops, hemostasis is determined by the balance of wattage, power, voltage, surface contact, and exposure time to tissue.[13,14]

TURP has durable very long-term follow-up results documented in urology literature, with follow-up ranging from 8 to 22 years.[15] The data from most recent cohort studies do suggest that patient morbidity decreases with increased urologist caseload volume. Overall morbidity rates can range from 11% to 30% with urinary retention and urinary tract infections most commonly seen.[16] Transfusion rates have been seen up to 20% in early studies; although more recent studies have shown rates as low as 2% to 4%.[17] It is extremely important to alert any patient undergoing a bladder outlet procedure, especially TURP, of the high risk of retrograde ejaculation and the consequences for fertility and sexual functioning. Although most studies demonstrate objective long-term efficacy of TURP, quality of life and patient satisfaction measures are rare.

Bipolar Transurethral Resection of the Prostate

Bipolar TURP was developed to allow the operation to be performed in a normal saline environment and theoretically allow for longer and safer resection.[14] The traditional monopolar TURP uses an active electrode to transmit energy into tissue and a return electrode at the skin to complete the circuit.[11] Bipolar technology allows high initializing voltage to establish a voltage gradient in the gap between two electrodes. The active and return poles are thus incorporated into the electrode design.[18] This energy converts the saline into a plasma field of highly ionized particles disrupting the molecular bonds between the tissues. The high-temperature loop provides rapid vaporization and desiccation of prostate tissue and results in a "cut and seal" effect.[19] Because these charge ions have only a short penetration of 50 to 100 μm, there should be less collateral thermal damage to the surrounding tissue and less tissue char.[15] Bipolar TURP is performed in the exact same manner as monopolar TURP.

Several types of bipolar resection devices are available. In addition, surgeons are now performing bipolar transurethral vaporization of the prostate procedures. In these procedures, a bipolar button is used in a similar fashion as a bipolar loop with the intent of vaporizing the tissue instead of cutting the tissue. The vaporization procedure is carried out in essentially the same fashion as a TURP procedure (Video 1). Bipolar TURP allows for longer resection times without the risk of hyponatremia and TURP syndrome. Some have proposed that the slower pace of resection is also more comfortable for the resident in training and only enhances resident training in the future.[14] To date, no case reports have documented any case of clinically significant TURP syndrome with saline bipolar TURP.

Laser Therapy for Benign Prostatic Hyperplasia

The development of laser-based surgical techniques has challenged the idea that TURP and open simple prostatectomy should remain the gold standards for the management of BPH/bladder outlet obstruction. Traditionally, TURP has been considered the surgery of choice for managing small-to-moderate-sized glands (up to 60–80 g), whereas open simple prostatectomy has been considered the optimal treatment of larger glands (>80). With the advent of laser-based procedures that are less invasive and associated with fewer complications, these techniques have gained widespread acceptance among urologists and have begun to rapidly supplant more traditional surgical therapies.

Although numerous lasers suitable for the management of BPH exist, those most commonly used are the holmium:yttrium-aluminum-garnet (Ho:YAG) laser and the KTP ("green light") laser. Additional laser therapies that are currently less commonly used include diode lasers and thulium lasers. The focus here is on Ho:YAG and KTP applications for BPH management.

Holmium laser physics

The Ho:YAG laser is a pulsed, solid-state laser that emits a wavelength of 2140 nm (infrared). It is rapidly absorbed by water and the depth of penetration is 0.5 mm. Therefore, when the laser fiber is more than 0.5 mm from the target tissue (ie, prostate) the energy is dissipated in water and no detrimental effects on the tissue occur. Because of the high water content of the prostate, the holmium wavelength is well absorbed allowing for either laser ablation or resection/enucleation of prostate tissue. The Ho:YAG laser energy is delivered through small (typically 550–1000 μm), flexible fibers that are precisely controlled by the surgeon. The energy is delivered in a saline milieu, removing the risk of developing hyponatremia and TURP syndrome, which is seen when prostate resections are done with hypotonic irrigants.[20,21] An additional benefit of the Ho:YAG laser is its excellent hemostatic effects, which allows the surgeon to perform resection or ablation in the setting of antiplatelet or anticoagulation therapy when absolutely necessary (although cessation of antiplatelets and anticoagulants is typically preferred whenever possible). Finally, in patients with concomitant bladder stones, the stones are treated simultaneously using the Ho:YAG laser.

Holmium laser ablation of the prostate

Holmium laser ablation of the prostate (HoLAP) is typically carried out using a 26F catheter resectoscope with laser bridge and continuous-flow normal saline irrigation. The laser bridge steadies the fiber within the scope to allow for better control of the laser fiber. A 550-μm side-firing laser fiber is used to deliver the Ho:YAG laser energy. A Ho:YAG laser capable of generating a power of 80 W or higher is required.

Various HoLAP techniques have been described. One of the most commonly used techniques includes the creation of troughs at the 5- and 7-o'clock positions from the bladder neck to a point proximal to the verumontanum. The troughs are deepened until capsule is identified (a fibrous, shiny, white surface with delicate vessels). Next, the tissue between the 5- and 7-o'clock troughs (median lobe tissue) is ablated until capsule is identified. Ablation is carried out by positioning the laser fiber close to, but not touching the prostate tissue. The tissue is slowly ablated by rotating the side-firing laser fiber. After the median lobe tissue is ablated, the lateral lobes are ablated in a similar fashion starting at the bladder neck and moving distally toward the apex. Once capsule is identified throughout, the procedure is completed and typically, a catheter is left in place overnight.[6]

Before the development of high powered Ho:YAG lasers, HoLAP had limited utility in the management of BPH because of slow ablation times and inefficient tissue removal. However, with the advent of higher powered Ho:YAG lasers (80–120 W), HoLAP has re-emerged as a treatment option for small-to-moderate-sized glands, particularly because this procedure is simpler to perform than holmium laser enucleation of the prostate (HoLEP; discussed next).[20]

Holmium laser enucleation of the prostate

Gilling and colleagues[22] first described HoLEP in the mid-1990s. Over the past two decades, the HoLEP technique has been found to be an excellent option for the surgical management of prostates of all sizes, including extremely large glands, which previously would have been treated only with open simple prostatectomy. The procedure has evolved to become a minimally invasive, endoscopic equivalent to open simple prostatectomy, with significantly less morbidity (ie, less blood loss, significantly lower risk of blood transfusion, shorter hospital stay, and shorter length of catheterization).[20]

HoLEP is also performed using a 26F catheter resectoscope with laser bridge and continuous-flow normal saline irrigation. A 550-μm end-firing laser fiber is used to deliver the laser energy. A Ho:YAG laser capable of generating a power of 100 to 120 W is used. A morcellator device with 5-mm reciprocating blades controlled by foot pedal is also required to remove the enucleated tissue.

The procedure as described by Gilling[23] has been well documented. It begins with creating bilateral incisions extending from the bladder neck (5 and 7 o'clock) to the verumontanum. The incisions are deepened until capsule is identified (in instances where no median lobe is present, a single incision is made at the 6-o'clock position). After completion of the bladder neck incisions, the median lobe tissue is enucleated starting at the verumontanum. The fibers connecting the median lobe tissue to the capsule are divided, working side-to-side between the bladder neck incisions. The resectoscope beak is used to elevate the median lobe off of the capsule and create counter-traction during enucleation. The median lobe is pushed up through the bladder neck and the remaining fibers are divided to completely free the median lobe tissue. The lateral lobes can then be enucleated. The distal aspect of the bladder neck incision of each lateral lobe is extended inferolaterally and underneath the apex of the lobe. The apex is then lifted off of the capsule using the beak of the resectosope. The apical incision is then carried up to the 2-o'clock position (left lobe) or 11-o'clock position (right lobe). Then, the bladder neck is incised at the 12-o'clock position (anterior commissure) to release the anterior aspect of both lobes. This incision is then carried distally and laterally toward the verumontanum. The anterior incision and the bladder neck incisions are joined along the plane of the capsule. The dissection is continued until each lobe is freed entirely and pushed into the bladder. After achieving excellent hemostasis in the prostatic bed, the tissue is morcellated in the bladder. A long rigid nephroscope (typically used for percutaneous kidney surgery) is used for morcellation. The bladder must remain fully distended throughout morcellation and contact between adenoma and morcellator blades must be carefully maintained at all times to prevent bladder injury.[23] After all tissue is morcellated, a catheter is left in place overnight.

The technique has been modified by Lingeman and colleagues[24] and is the preferred technique of the authors of this article. In this modification, one initial bladder neck incision is made and the median lobe dissection is incorporated into the dissection of one of the lateral lobes. Additionally, the dissection of the lateral lobe is continued across the entire anterior surface of the gland to open a space between capsule and anterior commissure before division of the anterior commissure. Finally, the apical mucosal strips are divided by encircling the lateral lobes with the resectoscope and placing the tissue on stretch away from the sphincter.[24] (See videos at http://www.urologybook.com/holmium-laser-enucleation-of-the-prostate-holep/).[25]

Photoselective Vaporization of the Prostate Physics

Photoselective vaporization of the prostate (PVP) is performed using a 532-nm laser. The laser was initially developed by doubling the frequency of a pulsed neodymium:YAG laser with a KTP crystal. This generates a visible green wavelength (532 nm) and thus the laser is referred to as a "green light" laser. This wavelength is rapidly absorbed by hemoglobin within the prostate tissue. This in turn allows for rapid photoselective vaporization secondary to rapid photothermal vaporization of heated intracellular water. The depth of penetration is 0.8 mm and the coagulation zone is 1 to 2 mm. These properties of the 532-nm wavelength laser allow PVP procedures to be performed in the setting of active antiplatelet or anticoagulant therapy when absolutely necessary. PVP procedures are performed using a variety of different laser systems with powers ranging from 60 to 180 W. The higher power systems allow for more rapid vaporization of prostate tissue.[20,26]

Photoselective Vaporization of the Prostate Procedure

The goal of a PVP procedure is to create a defect similar to that created by standard TURP. The laser fiber is used at "near-contact" mode (0.5 mm distance between the fiber and the prostate tissue) to achieve maximal energy delivery. The formation of bubbles on the surface of the prostate tissue is a surrogate for efficient vaporization, whereas bubble diminishment is considered a sign of proximity to the capsule, where vaporization efficiency decreases secondary to decreased vascularity of the fibrous capsule. Various techniques for tissue removal exist. These including side-to-side sweeping from the bladder neck to the apex in a clockwise-counterclockwise fashion; the "spiral technique" where the middle lobe and lateral lobes are ablated in separate sections; and the vaporization-incision technique, which incorporates some aspect of HoLEP (bladder neck incision, apical incisions, high lateral lobe incisions) followed by ablation of the median lobe, lateral lobes, and apices. Placement of a catheter at the end of the procedure is done at the discretion of the surgeon, but is not mandatory.[27]

OPEN SIMPLE PROSTATECTOMY

With the advent of laser technologies and laparoscopic and robotic systems, use of open simple prostatectomy for the management of BPH is on the decline. However, for patients with very large prostates, patients with concomitant bladder stones or large bladder diverticuli, or patients with a urethral abnormality (ie, stricture) the procedure remains an effective and viable option, especially when laser and robotic platforms are not readily available.

Open simple prostatectomy is performed in a retropubic (incision directly through prostatic capsule) or transvesical fashion. The transvesical approach is preferred in the setting of concomitant bladder stones and/or bladder diverticula and is the most commonly used approach. In the transvesical approach, a midline incision from below the umbilicus to the pubic bone is typically used. The extraperitoneal prevesical space is then bluntly developed and self-retaining retractors are placed. The bladder is distended with saline through a 22F three-way Foley catheter placed in a sterile fashion before starting the procedure. A midline cystotomy is created and the retractors are positioned such that the dome of the bladder can be retracted to aid exposure to the prostate. If necessary, 5F ureteral catheters are placed to help identify the ureteral orifices. Then, a circumferential incision is made around the prostate, distal to the trigone, and a plane between adenoma and prostatic capsule is sharply developed. Blunt finger dissection is then used to enucleate the adenoma. Finally, the apical prostatic urethra is transected by placing a finger at the apex of the prostate and pulling posteriorly. Hemostasis is achieved in the prostatic fossa using electrocautery and/or absorbable sutures. Vicryl sutures are then placed at the 5- and 7-o'clock positions to advance the bladder mucosa to the prostatic urethra. The bladder is then closed in two layers with Vicryl sutures. The 22F three-way Foley catheter is left in place.[28] A suprapubic tube can also be left in place at the surgeon's discretion but is often unnecessary. Typically a catheter is left in place for about 1 week and is removed after a postoperative cystogram reveals no leak.

ROBOTIC SIMPLE PROSTATECTOMY

Robotic simple prostatectomy is yet another option for the management of large prostatic adenomas. Bladder stones and bladder diverticuli can also be treated simultaneously with this approach.

At the author's institution, robotic simple prostatectomy is performed via a transperitoneal approach. The patient is positioned in the same fashion as used for a robotic radical prostatectomy and the same port configuration is used.[29] The procedure is carried out in a transvesical fashion in the same manner as an open simple prostatectomy. In this case, however, finger dissection is replaced by dissection using monopolar robotic scissors. Hemostasis in the prostatic fossa is achieved with electrocautery and suture ligation if needed. The bladder is closed and a Foley catheter is left in place (18–22F catheter). A Jackson Pratt drain can be left in place at the discretion of the surgeon. As with open simple prostatectomy, a catheter is left in place for a week and is removed after a cystogram reveals no leak.

COMPLICATIONS OF BENIGN PROSTATIC HYPERPLASIA SURGERY

Complications of all transurethral BPH surgeries include bleeding, need for blood transfusion, urinary tract infection, retrograde ejaculation (usually permanent), temporary or permanent urinary incontinence, painful urination, urethral stricture, bladder neck contracture, or bladder or ureteral injury. The incidence of each complication depends on the surgery performed and the experience of the surgeon. Additional complications of open or robotic simple prostatectomy include injury to surrounding organs (ie, bowel) or vascular structures, wound infection, surgical site hernia, and bladder leak. All potential complications should be extensively reviewed with the patient before proceeding with surgery.

SUMMARY

BPH is a common medical condition in aging males, which can lead to bothersome LUTS that can negatively impact quality of life. Fortunately, when symptoms are severe or BPH-related complications occur, such as urinary retention, recurrent urinary tract infections, recurrent hematuria, or upper tract deterioration, numerous interventions are available for surgical management. The appropriate technique depends on multiple factors including prostate size, anesthetic risk, need for uninterrupted anticoagulation, the presence of concomitant disease (ie, bladder stones or diverticula), available technology, and surgeon experience.

SUPPLEMENTARY DATA

Supplementary data related to this article can be found at http://dx.doi.org/10.1016/j.suc.2016.02.006.

REFERENCES

1. Bushman W. Etiology, epidemiology and natural history. Urol Clin North Am 2009; 36:403–15.
2. Thorpe A, Neal D. Benign prostatic hyperplasia. Lancet 2003;361:1359–67.
3. Abrams P, Cardozo L, Fall M, et al. The standardization of terminology of lower urinary tract function: report from the Standardization Subcommittee of the International Continence Society. Neurourol Urodyn 2002;21:167–78.
4. Roehrborn CG, Preminger G, Newhall P, et al. Microwave thermotherapy for benign prostatic hyperplasia with the Dornier urowave: results of a randomized, double-blind, multicenter, sham-controlled trial. Urology 1998;51:19–28.
5. Larson TR, Blute ML, Bruskewitz RC, et al. A high efficiency microwave thermoablation system in the treatment of benign prostatic hyperplasia: results of a randomized, double-blind, multicenter clinical trial. Urology 1998;51:731–42.
6. Walmsley K, Kaplan SA. Transurethral microwave thermotherapy for benign prostate hyperplasia: separating truth from marketing hype. J Urol 2004;172: 1249–55.
7. Chapple CR, Issa MM, Woo H. Transurethral needle ablation. A critical review of radiofrequency thermal therapy in the management of benign prostatic hyperplasia. Eur Urol 1999;35:119–28.
8. Minardi D, Garofalo F, Yehia M, et al. Pressure-flow studies in men with benign prostatic hypertrophy before and after treatment with transurethral needle ablation. Urol Int 2001;66:89–93.
9. Namiki K, Shiozawa H, Tsuzuki M, et al. Efficacy of transurethral needle ablation of the prostate for the treatment of benign prostatic hyperplasia. Int J Urol 1999;6: 341–5.
10. Schulman CC, Zlotta AR. Transurethral needle ablation: histopathological, radiological and clinical studies of a new office procedure for treatment of benign prostatic hyperplasia. Prog Clin Biol Res 1994;386:479–86.
11. Wei JT, Calhoun E, Jacobsen SJ. Urologic diseases in America project: benign prostatic hyperplasia. J Urol 2005;173:1256–61.
12. Yu X, Elliott SP, Wilt TJ, et al. Practice patterns in benign prostatic hyperplasia surgical therapy: the dramatic increase in minimally invasive technologies. J Urol 2008;180:241–5.
13. Nudell DM, Cattolica EV. Transurethral prostatectomy: an update. Linthicum (MD): American Urological Association. AUA update series, vol. XIX. 2000. Lesson 5.
14. Issa MM. Technological advances in transurethral resection of the prostate: bipolar versus monopolar TURP. J Endourol 2008;22(8):1587–95.
15. Reich O, Gratzke C, Stief CG. Techniques and long-term results of surgical procedures for BPH. Eur Urol 2006;49:970–8.
16. Reich O, Gratzke C, Bachman A, et al. Morbidity, mortality and early outcome of transurethral resection of the prostate: a prospective multicenter evaluation of 10,654 patients. J Urol 2008;180:246–9.
17. Wendt-Nordahl G, Bucher B, Hacker A, et al. Improvement in mortality and morbidity in transurethral resection of the prostate over 17 years in a single center. J Endourol 2007;21(9):1081–7.

18. Smith D, Khoubehi B, Patel A. Bipolar electrosurgery for benign prostatic hyperplasia: transurethral electrovaporization and resection of the prostate. Curr Opin Urol 2005;15:95–100.
19. Ho HS, Cheng CW. Bipolar transurethral resection of prostate: a new reference standard? Curr Opin Urol 2008;18:50–5.
20. Mandeville JA, Gnessin E, Lingeman JE. New advances in benign prostatic hyperplasia: laser therapy. Curr Urol Rep 2011;12:56–61.
21. Lerner LB, Tyson MD. Holmium laser applications of the prostate. Urol Clin North Am 2009;4:485–95.
22. Gilling PJ, Kennett K, Das Ak, et al. Holmium Laser Enucleation of the Prostate (HoLEP) with transurethral tissue morcellation: an update on the early clinical experience. J Endourol 1998;12:457–9.
23. Gilling P. Surgical atlas: holmium laser enucleation of the prostate (HoLEP). BJU Int 2008;101:131–42.
24. Dusing MW, Krambeck AE, Terry C, et al. Holmium laser enucleation of the prostate: efficiency gained by experience and operative technique. J Urol 2010;184: 635–40.
25. Mandeville JA. Holmium laser enucleation of the prostate (HoLEP). UrologyBook. N.p., 2012. Available at: http://www.urologybook.com/. Accessed September 28, 2015.
26. Rieken M, Bachmann A. Laser treatment of benign prostate enlargement – which laser for which prostate? Nat Rev Urol 2014;11:142–52.
27. Sountoulides P, de la Rosette J. Update on photoselective vaporization of the prostate. Curr Urol Rep 2008;9:106–12.
28. Thiel DD, Petrou SP. Electroresection and open surgery. Urol Clin North Am 2009; 36:461–70.
29. Leslie S, de Castro Abreu AL, Chopra S, et al. Transvesical robotic simple prostatectomy: initial clinical experience. Eur Urol 2014;66:321–9.

Diagnosis and Management of Hematuria

Gabriella J. Avellino, MD, Sanchita Bose, MD, David S. Wang, MD*

KEYWORDS

- Hematuria • Trauma • Malignancy • Infection • Urolithiasis • Workup
- Clot retention • CBI

KEY POINTS

- Hematuria can be caused by a variety of etiologies, found along the entire genitourinary tract, including urolithiasis, urinary tract infection, malignancy, iatrogenic causes and trauma.
- The most important aspects of triaging and initial management of a patient with hematuria are assessing hemodynamic stability, determining the underlying cause of hematuria, and ensuring urinary tract drainage.
- Hematuria workup should be pursued in all patients presenting with hematuria in whom benign causes of bleeding have been ruled out.

INTRODUCTION

Hematuria is a complex condition with a multitude of causes and treatments. It can be a daunting situation when an otherwise nonurologic surgical patient has this condition. This article provides an overview of the many aspects of this condition and provides guidelines for treatment. In general, collaboration with the urology, and occasionally nephrology, services is recommended in treating the general surgery patient with hematuria. After reading this article, the reader will gain knowledge on common etiologies, diagnosis, treatment, outcomes, and follow-up of the surgical patient with hematuria to provide the best possible patient care.

Hematuria is commonly encountered in the inpatient setting where it accounts for 4% to 20% of inpatient urology consults and hospitalizations.[1] *Hematuria* is the presence of blood cells in the urine. Gross hematuria is when blood is visible in the urine. Microscopic hematuria is defined as 3 or more red blood cells per high-powered field in a properly collected urine sample.

The initial evaluation of patients presenting with gross hematuria is 3-fold: assess hemodynamic stability, determine the underlying cause of hematuria, and ensure urinary drainage. The most important consideration in the initial evaluation of a patient

Disclosures: The authors have nothing to disclose.
Department of Urology, Boston Medical Center, Boston University School of Medicine, 725 Albany Street, Suite 3B, Boston, MA 02118, USA
* Corresponding author.
E-mail address: DavidS.Wang@bmc.org

with hematuria is hemodynamic stability with assessment of vital signs, physical examination, and hemoglobin/hematocrit, because an unstable patient must be treated emergently. Examples of etiologies of hematuria that may cause emergent bleeding include, but are not limited to, trauma such as intraperitoneal bladder rupture, ureteroarterial fistula, and hemorrhagic cystitis. By contrast, painless gross hematuria without hemodynamic compromise is a condition that is generally worked up on an outpatient basis. For this reason, it is extremely important to ensure that these patients have outpatient urologic follow-up scheduled.

The best approach to treating a patient with hematuria is to identify the underlying cause of hematuria, because the etiologies are diverse and often have very different treatments. Common etiologies of hematuria in the surgical inpatient include urinary tract infection (UTI), urolithiasis, malignancy, and trauma or iatrogenic causes (eg, traumatic urethral catheter placement or anticoagulation).

There are several medications (such as phenazopyridine, nitrofurantoin, phenytoin, and warfarin) that can cause or give the appearance of hematuria. Thus, inpatient medications should be evaluated. Additionally, patients may be anticoagulated, which may cause hematuria from a variety of sources such as benign prostatic hyperplasia (BPH) or undiagnosed urinary tract malignancies.

Gross hematuria should always be considered significant, because it is a sign of malignancy until proven otherwise. Roughly 4% of patients with microscopic hematuria and up to 40% of patients with gross hematuria could be harboring a malignancy.[2]

RELEVANT ANATOMY AND PATHOPHYSIOLOGY

The etiology of hematuria can originate from anywhere along the urinary tract, including the kidneys, ureters, bladder, prostate, and urethra (**Table 1**).

Kidney and Ureter

Specifically from the kidney, hematuria can be of glomerular origin, including medical renal disease, and nonglomerular origin, which includes urologic disorders. Urologic sources of hematuria from the kidney and ureter may include masses, both benign and malignant, infection, urolithiasis, arteriovenous malformation, and trauma.

Kidney masses may represent metastasis or be primary renal tumors. Although infrequent, the most common malignancies to metastasize to the kidneys include lung, colorectal, head and neck, breast, and gastrointestinal tumors.[3] Renal tumors can be intraparenchymal or urothelial. Upper tract urothelial tumors can be found anywhere along the ureters and in the renal pelvis.

Table 1 Relevant anatomy and anatomic contributors to hematuria			
Kidney/Ureter	**Bladder**	**Prostate**	**Urethra**
• Glomerular	• Uncomplicated cystitis	• BPH	• Urethritis
• Tumor	• Radiation/hemorrhagic cystitis	• Prostate cancer	• Trauma
◦ Parenchymal		• Prostatitis	◦ Disruption
◦ Urothelial	• Tumor		◦ Traumatic Foley removal/placement
• Infection	• Trauma/rupture		• Urethral mass
◦ Pyelonephritis			• Urethral caruncle
◦ Calculi			• Urethral stricture
• Trauma			
• Ureteraoarterial fistula			

Abbreviation: BPH, benign prostatic hyperplasia.

Infection of the kidney, or pyelonephritis, may cause microscopic or gross hematuria. Pyelonephritis often results from ascending infection from the bladder (cystitis) and can lead to high fevers and lateralizing flank pain. These symptoms can also be present in patients with renal or ureteral calculi. Thus, if the suspicion is high (known history of nephrolithiasis, chronically bed bound patient, strong family history of kidney stone formation), there should be a low threshold to image the patient with noncontrast computed tomography (CT).

Blunt, penetrating, or iatrogenic trauma can lead to hematuria from anywhere along the urinary tract. The kidneys are the most frequently injured genitourinary organ, in up to 5% of civilian traumas and 24% of traumatic abdominal solid organ injuries. The kidneys are especially at risk of deceleration injuries owing to their relatively fixed position by the renal pelvis and vascular pedicles in the retroperitoneum.[4] Accounting for only 1% of urologic injuries, ureteral injuries are infrequent. Iatrogenic ureteral injury during gynecologic, urologic or colorectal surgeries accounts for 80% of ureteral injuries.[5]

Bladder

Bladder sources of hematuria include trauma, infection, hemorrhagic cystitis (from radiation and/or chemotherapy exposure), and tumors. Bladder ruptures are categorized as intraperitoneal, about 30% of the time, extraperitoneal 60%, and both in the remaining 10%.[6] Although more than 85% of blunt bladder injuries are associated with pelvic fractures, less than 10% of blunt pelvic fracture patients are found to have bladder injuries.[5] They occur rarely in blunt abdominal trauma owing to the location of the bladder in a relatively protected position in the pelvis. The typical site of intraperitoneal rupture is at the dome of the bladder, often in setting of a full bladder. Extraperitoneal bladder ruptures often occur at the bladder neck or the base of the bladder. Blood at meatus in the setting of trauma and pelvic fractures should make the clinician suspicious of urethral or bladder injury.

Cystitis refers to any inflammation of the bladder, whether infectious or noninfectious in origin. Infectious causes can be bacterial, viral, and fungal. Uropathogenic *Escherichia coli* is the most common cause of UTIs. These bacteria have unique properties that allow them to bind to the outermost layer of the urothelium, enter the cells, replicate, and eventually lead to cell lysis. Less common, viral cystitis is typically seen in immunosuppressed patients owing to adenovirus and BK virus.

Noninfectious etiologies of cystitis include radiation and chemical cystitis, which can lead to hemorrhagic cystitis. Radiation-induced cystitis can be seen at any time after treatment, and there are no known risk factors for who will develop this complication. Radiation cystitis leads to damage of urothelium via apoptosis initiated by DNA damage and can also affect the muscular layers of the bladder as well as the vasculature. Chemical cystitis can be from various medications, for example, cyclophosphamide and/or ifosfamide chemotherapy. These medications are metabolized by the liver, resulting in the formation of a harmful metabolite acrolein, which is filtered into the urine, inducing urothelial damage.[7]

Bladder tumors are a common cause of gross and microscopic hematuria; approximately 80% to 90% of patients with bladder cancer present with painless gross hematuria. Transitional cell carcinoma (or urothelial carcinoma) accounts for 90% of bladder cancers and develops in the inner layer (urothelium) of the bladder. It is described as a field change defect, meaning that it can affect the entire urothelium, with significant potential for recurrence owing to highly malignant tumor biology. The remaining 10% of bladder cancers include but are not limited to squamous cell, adenocarcinoma, and small cell. Risk factors for developing bladder cancer are outlined in **Box 1**.

> **Box 1**
> **Risk factors for urologic malignancy**
>
> - Smoking history
> - Advanced age
> - Male gender
> - History of pelvic irradiation or certain chemotherapeutics (eg, cyclophosphamide)
> - Chronic bladder inflammation (indwelling catheter, chronic urinary tract infections)
> - Occupational exposures (eg, aromatic amines, aniline dyes, benzene)

Prostate

Prostatic causes of hematuria can largely be attributed to prostatic hyperplasia. The prostatic hyperplastic process is owing to an imbalance between cell death and cell proliferation, which eventually leads to cell accumulation.[8] In this process, there is also expression of vascular endothelial growth factor, which makes the prostate an extremely vascular organ prone to bleeding. Prostatic malignancy and infection of the prostate, or prostatitis, are other contributors to hematuria of prostatic source. Bacterial prostatitis is the result of focal uropathogenic bacteria residing in the prostate gland. The most common cause of bacterial prostatitis, both acute and chronic, is the Enterobacteriaceae family of Gram-negative bacteria.[9] Locally advanced prostate cancer may also cause hematuria.

Urethra

Urethral causes of hematuria include infection (urethritis), urethral masses, and trauma. Urethritis is inflammation of the urethra, and is usually infectious in origin. As with any infection, a urinalysis and culture as well as testing for *Neisseria gonorrhea* and chlamydia are useful. An uncommon cause of emergent urethral bleeding is in the setting of traumatic Foley catheter manipulation or removal (eg, by a demented or delirious patient or during transfers). After traumatic catheter removal, reinsertion of the catheter is recommended.[1] If resistance is met on reinsertion, there should be further evaluation of urethral integrity, either with bedside cystoscopy or retrograde urethrogram.

CLINICAL PRESENTATION AND EXAMINATION

Patients with gross hematuria have a wide range of presentations (**Table 2**). As mentioned, the first and most important part of evaluation of a patient with hematuria is hemodynamic stability. Patients with hypotension, tachycardia, and low hemoglobin/hematocrit may require emergent intervention. This can involve surgical intervention (ie, fulguration of prostatic bleeding, angioembolization by interventional radiology) as well as resuscitation.

Obtaining a thorough history is essential in evaluating patients with hematuria because the history often provides clues for diagnosis of underlying etiology (eg, a strong family history of prostate cancer or a long history of smoking provides further evidence of likely urologic malignancy). Although patients with hematuria may be asymptomatic, common presenting symptoms include dysuria, urinary frequency and/or urgency, and abdominal and/or flank pain.

In the physical examination of the patient with hematuria, it is important to perform a focused examination of the abdomen, flanks, pelvic examination in women, digital

Table 2
Clinical presentations by etiology

Urinary Tract Infection	Urolithiasis	Malignancy	Prostate	Hemorrhagic Cystitis	Trauma
• Dysuria • Hematuria • Frequency/urgency • Incontinence • Small volume voids • Foul-smelling, cloudy urine • Suprapubic pain	• Symptoms of urinary tract infection • Lateralizing flank pain • Fevers	• Often painless • Irritative voiding symptoms (frequency, urgency, dysuria)	• Enlarged prostate on digital rectal examination • Clot retention • Range of symptoms (frequency, urgency, decreased stream, nocturia)	• Persistent bleeding from bladder • Urgency • Frequency • Bladder pain	• Hematuria • Blood at meatus • Clinical correlation • Inability to void

rectal examination in men, and external genitourinary examination. Pain on digital rectal examination can clue the clinician into a diagnosis of prostatitis, and a nodule on digital rectal examination raises the concern for prostatic malignancy. Flank or costovertebral angle tenderness may signal a diagnosis of pyelonephritis or urolithiasis. Pain from obstructing ureteral calculi can often radiate to the lower abdomen or scrotum.

In addition to a focused physical examination, as discussed, the urine must also be examined. The color and viscosity of the urine often provides valuable clinical information. As with bleeding in other areas of the body, dark red/brown urine often signifies the presence of old blood, whereas bright red blood likely signifies active, new bleeding. Increased viscosity of urine as well as the presence of clots in voided urine is concerning because this may signal that a patient may develop clot retention. Clot retention is defined as blood clots within the bladder that obstruct the flow of urine causing symptomatic urinary retention.

Urinary Tract Infection

UTIs can occur in any part of the genitourinary tract (cystitis, urethritis, prostatitis, pyelonephritis, epididymitis). Although patients with a UTI can be asymptomatic, common symptoms associated with cystitis include dysuria, hematuria, urinary frequency and/or urgency, incontinence of urine, small volume voids, foul-smelling urine, and suprapubic pain. An indurated and tender epididymis in addition to the above symptoms is an easily localizable feature of epididymitis. Symptoms associated with upper UTIs, namely pyelonephritis, include these symptoms with the addition of fevers, rigors, flank pain, nausea, and vomiting. Although symptoms are very helpful in the diagnosis of UTI, they do not accurately localize the infection within the genitourinary tract.[10] UTI in the setting of obstructive uropathy or stones is a urologic emergency.

Patients with urolithiasis often present with dysuria and hematuria along with intense lateralizing flank pain. When the suspicion is high, CT abdomen/pelvis without contrast in the prone position is the modality that often diagnoses ureteral and renal stones. It is important to understand the indications for urgent intervention (ie, placement of ureteral stent or nephrostomy tube) for obstructing stones, which include fever, uncontrollable pain despite treatment with narcotics, solitary kidney, renal dysfunction, bilateral ureteral stones, and hemodynamic instability.

Urologic Malignancy

Patients with occult urologic malignancy often present with painless gross hematuria, which may be the only abnormality on presentation. Irritative voiding symptoms (frequency, urgency, dysuria) can also be symptoms of malignancy, particularly carcinoma in situ of the bladder. Roughly 80% of patients with bladder carcinoma in situ present with irritative voiding symptoms, and the presence of these symptoms doubles the risk of harboring carcinoma in situ in patients with hematuria (from 5% to 10%).[11] However, the symptom combination of hematuria and voiding dysfunction is quite common in a variety of urologic pathology including UTI, prostatic hypertrophy, and urolithiasis, which makes diagnosis quite complex.

Hemorrhagic Cystitis

A particularly difficult to manage etiology of gross hematuria is hemorrhagic cystitis. This condition is characterized by diffuse, persistent bleeding from the bladder mucosa. The severity of bleeding can range from mild bleeding managed conservatively to life-threatening bleeding requiring blood transfusion, bladder irrigation, and/or operative intervention. Hemorrhagic cystitis can be associated with irritative symptoms, including urinary urgency, frequency, and bladder pain.[12] Typically hemorrhagic cystitis is only seen in patients with known risk factors, such as prior pelvic radiation and cyclophosphamide chemotherapy. Reports indicate that up to 5% of patients who receive pelvic radiation will experience moderate or severe persistent gross hematuria.[13]

Trauma

Trauma patients often present with multiple injuries and hematuria as a result of urinary tract injury. Although patients with renal and bladder injuries often present with gross hematuria, a patient with urethral disruption/injury may present with inability to void and blood at urethral meatus. In ureteral trauma, gross hematuria is unfortunately not a reliable indicator of injury, and these injuries are often diagnosed in a delayed fashion. Suspicion for ureteral injury should arise in patients with bowel, bladder, or retroperitoneal injuries or in patients with high velocity pelvic or vertebral fractures.[14]

Prostatic Enlargement

Prostatic enlargement may cause hematuria in men in a variety of scenarios, including BPH, prostatitis, and advanced prostate cancer. The prostate can bleed owing to a variety of aggravators (including Foley catheterization, infection, and anticoagulation). Localization of hematuria to the prostate should be determined after a complete evaluation of the hematuria is completed; other etiologies for the hematuria must be excluded.[1] Hematuria from prostatic enlargement has a range of presentations from mild bleeding to recalcitrant bleeding with clots and thus has a variety of treatments.

Ureteroarterial Fistula

Ureteroarterial fistula is an infrequent but very serious cause of gross hematuria. It can be life threatening. This diagnosis requires a high degree of suspicion. Patients may present with gross hematuria, symptomatic anemia, and lateralizing flank pain. Risk factors include chronic indwelling stents, previous pelvic radiation, pelvic or vascular surgery, and vascular disease.[15]

DIAGNOSTIC PROCEDURES AND DIAGNOSIS

After excluding benign causes, the presence of hematuria should precipitate a urologic evaluation. The workup for hematuria includes history, examination, laboratory studies, cystoscopy, and upper tract imaging (with CT urogram, which is the standard, or MR urogram vs renal ultrasound with retrograde pyelography for patients with renal dysfunction; **Table 3**). The initial step in diagnosis is to obtain a properly collected, midstream clean catch urinary specimen and identify 3 or more red blood cells per high-power field. A dipstick test is not adequate to identify microhematuria because it can result positive in the setting of oxidation or myoglobinuria. This must be confirmed by a microscopic urinalysis. This analysis will also allow the identification of red blood cell casts, proteins, and dysmorphic red blood cells, which can indicate a medical renal source for hematuria. A urine culture should also be sent to assess for infection. If the workup is unremarkable but microscopic hematuria persists, a urologic evaluation can be repeated in 3 to 5 years.

In the history, in addition to assessing risk factors for urologic malignancy, the provider should inquire about medical renal disease, UTI, trauma, and menstruation. Physical examination should include a thorough abdominal and genital examination and blood pressure reading.

Laboratory tests should include the estimated glomerular filtration rate, creatinine, and blood urea nitrogen to evaluate renal function. Renal function can determine eligibility for further diagnostic testing. Although once considered a mandatory part of the workup, urine cytology has limited use and should not be part of the initial workup for asymptomatic microscopic hematuria.[16]

Cystoscopy, which involves direct visualization of the urethra and bladder by camera, should be performed for all patients older than 35 years of age. Cystoscopy should be done at the discretion of the physician for any patients younger than 35 years, such as if there is concern for malignancy owing to exposures or irritative voiding symptoms. This can be done in the office setting for the appropriately selected patient. Cystoscopy allows identification of urethral lesions, strictures, and false passages, bladder lesions or masses, and lateralizing hematuria from a ureteral orifice. Additionally, retrograde radiographic studies can be done if fluoroscopy is available.

The gold standard for imaging in hematuria workup is multi-phasic CT urography. This includes 3 phases with and without contrast: a noncontrast phase for identification of stones, a nephrogenic phase for evaluation of renal masses, and an excretory phase for assessment of filling defects in the collecting system (ureters and bladder). Another option is MR urography. If CT or MRI are unavailable or patient is ineligible owing to pregnancy, iodinated contrast allergy, or renal insufficiency, renal and bladder ultrasound examination with retrograde pyelogram is an option.

In settings of traumatic hematuria, if stable enough for imaging, the patient should undergo intravenous contrast-enhanced CT of the abdomen and pelvis with delayed images to evaluate the collecting system. If the patient is too unstable and proceeds directly to operating room without imaging, an intravenous pyelogram can be obtained and should be performed if nephrectomy is being considered to confirm presence of contralateral kidney.

Table 3 Hematuria workup		
Cystoscopy	**Urine Cytology**	**Upper Tract Imaging**
• Evaluates urethral and bladder mucosa for masses	• Examines urine for cancer cells • Not recommended in asymptomatic microhematuria • Consider in high-risk patients	• CT urogram gold standard • Renal ultrasound with retrograde pyelogram vs MR urogram in renal insufficiency

If bladder rupture is suspected, a CT or plain film cystogram can elucidate extravasation. A cystogram involves images captured after filling the bladder and then after emptying to identify any extravasated contrast concealed by the distended bladder.[5] Contrast outlining bowel supports an intraperitoneal rupture. Contrast localized in the pelvis supports an extraperitoneal rupture. If there is concern of urethral injury, a retrograde urethrogram should be done before Foley catheter placement and will show extravasation of contrast outside the urethra.

If the source of hematuria has not yet been clarified by imaging methods already mentioned or if the patient is hemodynamically unstable, percutaneous angioembolization can be diagnostic and therapeutic as an alternative to surgical exploration.[5]

INTERVENTIONS AND TREATMENT

Management and treatment can vary depending on the etiology of hematuria.

Urinary Tract Infections

Infections of the urinary tract (pyelonephritis, cystitis, prostatitis, epididymitis, and urethritis) are common and treatable causes of hematuria. In terms of management of these patients, all patients should have urine culture performed before initiation of antibiotics. Antibiotic selection should focus on coverage of uropathogens (Gram-negative and Gram-positive bacteria). Antibiotic coverage should be broad when initiated, and eventually narrowed based on culture data. A hospital's antibiograms should be used in antibiotic selection. Consider consultation with the infectious disease service in patients with complex infections to further aid in antibiotic selection and duration of therapy.

Urolithiasis

With kidney stone disease affecting 1 in 11 people in the United States, it is a very common and important entity for clinicians to learn to diagnose and manage.[17] Unlike cholelithiasis, appendicitis, and other surgical conditions, surgical treatment of stones is not the endpoint in stone therapy, because patients have a high incidence of recurrence of disease. In terms of stone management, it is important to recognize which patients can be managed non-operatively with medical expulsive therapy and which patients will require urgent surgical intervention with ureteral stenting or percutaneous nephrostomy tube placement.

There are several indications for the urgent surgical management of ureteral stones. These indications include intractable pain, solitary kidney, bilateral ureteral stones with obstruction, high-grade unilateral obstruction, renal dysfunction, abnormal ureteral anatomy, infection (which can manifest with fever, sepsis, and positive urinalysis and urine culture), hemodynamic compromise, and stones that are unlikely to pass spontaneously.[18]

If the patient is hemodynamically compromised or septic, it is prudent to proceed with percutaneous nephrostomy decompression, because this procedure requires less manipulation of the urinary tract. Although the general surgery patient may have nonurologic causes for being hemodynamically compromised, a concurrent obstructing stone must be addressed.

Medical expulsive therapy is a non-invasive and viable approach to managing the patient with uncomplicated urolithiasis (ie, in the absence of factors requiring urgent intervention). The ideal candidate for medical expulsive therapy is a patient with a stone but without signs of hemodynamic compromise, infection, or obstruction. It should be noted that the size and location of the ureteral stone are extremely important. The rate of spontaneous passage is much greater for distal ureteral stones (71%)

than for proximal ureteral stones (22%).[19] Medical expulsive therapy includes high-rate intravenous fluids, adequate pain control with narcotics, and alpha-1 antagonist therapy, most commonly tamsulosin, although there is a debate in current literature on the utility of tamsulosin.[20]

Urologic Malignancy

Gross hematuria should always be taken seriously as a "red flag" for urologic malignancy. Should painless gross hematuria be present in the general surgery patient in the absence of other etiologies of hematuria (trauma, infection, urolithiasis, etc), urologic malignancy should be high on the differential. In addition to referral to urology, the general surgeon can begin the process of working up gross hematuria by ordering laboratory and imaging studies. Urology completes the evaluation with cystoscopy, as an outpatient in the majority of cases, to rule out urethral and bladder mucosal pathology.

Clot Retention

The initial management of hematuria is resuscitation and bladder drainage. It is also important to identify risk factors and reversible causes for severe hematuria. In terms of catheter selection, large-bore catheters are preferable to ease passage of clots. Urinary catheters are sized in the French system, where 1 French equals 0.33 cm in circumference (not luminal diameter). In patients with severe hematuria and passage of clots, the best catheters to choose are large bore ($\geq$22 French) with 3 channels to allow for the possibility of manual and continuous bladder irrigation (CBI).[1] After the catheter is in place, manual irrigation with normal saline using catheter-tipped syringes should be performed to clear any clots from the bladder. Should the urine clear after adequate manual irrigation, the focus should be on conservative management with hydration and resuscitation. Should severe hematuria and clots persist despite adequate manual irrigation, then CBI may be used. In CBI, irrigation fluid continuously flows into a patient's bladder via a third port on the 3-way urethral catheter and is drained out via the exit port. Although CBI is an excellent treatment for severe hematuria, patients must be monitored for catheter obstruction during CBI, which raises the risk of bladder perforation. If bleeding persists despite this treatment, the clinician should consider intravesical therapy, cystoscopy with fulguration, or embolization (**Box 2**).

Box 2
Clot Retention

Assess hemodynamic stability/resuscitate

Identify etiology

Place large catheter ($\geq$22 French), manually irrigate

Urine clears

  Hydration

  Resuscitation

  Hematuria workup

Urine does not clear

  Imaging to evaluate clot burden

  Start continuous bladder irrigation

  Assess for reversible causes of hematuria (such as anticoagulation status)

  Consider operative intervention or intravesical therapy

Prostatic Hematuria

Prostate-related gross hematuria can be due to prostatitis, BPH, or advanced prostate cancer. The initial management of these patients is the same as with any patient with severe hematuria (bladder drainage, resuscitation, treatment of reversible causes).

In patients with acute prostatic bleeding owing to BPH, use of 5-alpha reductase inhibitor (finasteride) should be considered. Finasteride is associated with decreased prostatic blood flow by inhibition of vascular endothelial growth factor expression.[21] Finasteride is dosed 5 mg once daily and is associated with sexual side effects (decreased libido and trouble with erections and ejaculation).

Patients with advanced prostate cancer may also present with hematuria. If stable, the patient may be considered for surgical treatment (limited transurethral resection of prostate), radiation therapy, or androgen deprivation for control of hematuria. Androgen deprivation decreases prostate tissue vascularity and can control refractory bleeding from the prostate.[1] Should hematuria from BPH or prostate cancer persist despite conservative therapies, operative intervention should be considered (cystoscopy with fulguration and clot evacuation, embolization).

Hemorrhagic Cystitis

Hemorrhagic cystitis presents with severe hematuria due to diffuse bladder mucosal bleeding. The patient may even present with clot retention. Often the patient endorses a history of passing significant clot burden and has known risk factors (ie, history of pelvic radiation, cyclophosphamide chemotherapy). If a patient is scheduled to receive cyclophosphamide, the administration of 2-mercaptoethane sulfonate sodium (Mesna) can be bladder protective by neutralizing the harmful metabolite acrolein. These patients should also undergo a full hematuria workup to rule out other causes of hematuria, namely active urologic malignancy. The acute management of these patients remains the same as discussed. There are additional treatments that can be used for these patients such as intravesical agents (alum, aminocaproic acid, etc), fulguration with electrocautery, and hyperbaric oxygen. If still unable to control, urinary diversion (cystectomy, bilateral percutaneous nephrostomy) is an option.

Urotrauma

Traumatic injury to the urinary tract often results in gross hematuria. Patients with urinary tract trauma frequently present in the setting of multiple organ injuries. Trauma is the cause of 150,000 deaths per year in the United States and is the leading cause of death in adults under 45 years of age.[22] Treatment of urinary tract trauma is complex and is based on the organ that is injured. Intraperitoneal bladder rupture usually requires operative management, whereas extraperitoneal rupture can be managed nonoperatively with catheterization. Urethral injury may be managed with Foley catheter alone or may require urinary diversion, repair, or ureteral stenting. Urethral injury may require diversion with suprapubic tube and delayed repair.

Traumatic urethral catheterization and removal can also cause hematuria. Urethral catheter trauma may be remedied simply with replacement or manipulation of the catheter; however, about 30% may require prolonged catheterization, CBI, cystoscopy, or suprapubic tube placement. Urethral catheter placement can cause traumatic hematuria, especially in men with BPH or on anticoagulation.

Ureteroarterial Fistulae

Although it is an uncommon cause of hematuria, ureteroarterial fistula is a life-threatening condition. The general surgeon should have a high degree of suspicion

---

Box 3
Hematuria: pearls and pitfalls

- To limit urethral catheter trauma in men, inflate the Foley catheter balloon only if:
  - Catheter is completely hubbed at urethral meatus at junction with the balloon port.
  - There is return of urine.
- Make sure the patient's catheter is not obstructed while he or she is on continuous bladder irrigation, particularly if complaining of abdominal pain.
- A large-bore catheter ($\geq$22 French) should be used for bladder lavage/continuous bladder irrigation
- All patients with gross hematuria warrant a hematuria workup.
- Obtain urinalysis and urine culture on all patients with hematuria.

---

of this condition in patients presenting with hematuria, lateralizing flank pain, down-trending blood counts, and risk factors (chronic indwelling ureteral stents, history of pelvic irradiation or pelvic and/or vascular surgery). Immediate involvement of vascular surgery or endovascular treatment by interventional radiology is essential.

SUMMARY

Hematuria in the general surgery patient is a unique and complex situation that warrants close investigation. After careful evaluation of history and physical examination, laboratory tests, and indicated imaging, the source may remain elusive. In a study screening patients with hematuria on initial microscopic urinalysis, 2% were found to have bladder cancer, 22% infection, 10% BPH, and 65% remained of unknown cause.[23]

The general surgeon should take into consideration the circumstances under which new-onset gross hematuria develops. For example, if in the postoperative period, consider the operation, anticoagulation status, and whether the patient had a urethral catheter placed. Iatrogenic hematuria can be owing to unidentified intraoperative complications, such as laceration or thermal injury to ureter or bladder, or inflation of urethral catheter balloon in urethra.[24] Certain medications can alter the urine color to give the appearance of hematuria; thus, the medication list should be reviewed.

Gross hematuria can occasionally lead to a symptomatic reduction in hematocrit requiring transfusion, which can occur in cases related to trauma, ureteroarterial fistula, and hemorrhagic cystitis. Thus, these etiologies should be dealt with emergently.

In this article, we have outlined some of the most common causes of hematuria that a general surgeon may encounter, such as UTIs, urolithiasis, urologic malignancy, urinary tract arterial fistulae, prostatic bleeding, hemorrhagic cystitis, and trauma, as well as the clinical scenario of clot retention. Pearls and pitfalls of addressing hematuria are provided to the reader in **Box 3**. We hope that reading this article provides the general surgeon with an armamentarium of knowledge to properly triage and initiate diagnosis and treatment of the complex general surgery patient with hematuria.

REFERENCES

1. Linder BJ, Boorjian SA. Management of emergency bleeding, recalcitrant clots and hemorrhagic cystitis. AUA Update Series. Maryland: American Urological Association Education and Research, Inc; 2015; 34 (lesson 3).
2. Grossfeld GD, Litwin MS, Wolf JS Jr, et al. Evaluation of asymptomatic microscopic hematuria in adults: an American Urologic Association best practice policy – part I: definition, detection, prevalence, and etiology. Urology 2001;57(4):599–603.

3. Zhou C, Urbauer DL, Fellman BM, et al. Metastases to the kidney: a comprehensive analysis of 151 patients from a tertiary referral centre. BJU Int 2015 [Epub ahead of print] Available at: www.bjui.org.

4. Morey AF, Brandes S, Dugi DD, et al. Urotrauma: AUA guideline. J Urol 2014; 192(2):327–35.

5. Gross JA, Lehnert BE, Linnau KF, et al. Imaging of urinary system trauma. Radiol Clin North Am 2015;53(4):773–88.

6. Morey AF, Iverson AJ, Swan A, et al. Bladder rupture after blunt trauma: guidelines for diagnostic imaging. J Trauma 2001;51:683.

7. Haldar S, Dru C, Bhowmick NA. Mechanisms of hemorrhagic cystitis. Am J Clin Exp Urol 2014;2(3):199–208.

8. Roehrborn C. Chapter 91: Benign prostatic hyperplasia. In: Wein AJ, Kavoussi LR, Novick AC, et al, editors. Campbell-Walsh urology. 10th edition. Philadelphia: Saunders; 2011. p. 2570–610.

9. Nickel J. Chapter 11: Prostatitis and related conditions, orchitis and epididymitis. In: Wein AJ, Kavoussi LR, Novick AC, et al, editors. Campbell-Walsh urology. 10th edition. Philadelphia: Saunders; 2011. p. 327–56.

10. Nguyn H. Chapter 13. Bacterial infections of the urinary tract. In: Tanagho EA, McAninch JW, editors. Smith's General Urology. 16th edition. New York: McGraw-Hill Companies Inc; 2004. p. 203–27.

11. Zincke H, Utz DC, Farrow GM. Review of Mayo Clinic experience with carcinoma in situ. Urology 1985;26(4 Suppl):39–46.

12. Liem X, Saad F, Delouya G. A practical approach to the management of radiation-induced hemorrhagic cystitis. Drugs 2015;75(13):1471–82.

13. Linder BJ, Tarrell RF, Boorjian SA. Cystectomy for Refractory Hemorrhagic Cystitis: Contemporary Etiology, Presentation and Outcomes. The Journal of Urology 2014;192(6):1687–92.

14. Elliott SP, McAninch JW. Ureteral injuries from external violence: the 25-year experience at San Francisco General Hospital. J Urol 2003;170:1213.

15. Krambeck AE, DiMarco DS, Gettman MT, et al. Ureteroiliac artery fistula: diagnosis and treatment algorithm. Urology 2005;66(5):990–4.

16. Cargan J, Kavoussi LR. Chapter 3: Lack of utility of routine urine cytology as part of hematuria workups. In: Wein AJ, Kavoussi LR, Novick AC, et al, editors. Campbell-Walsh urology. 10th edition. Philadelphia: Saunders; 2014.

17. Pearle MS, Goldfarb DS, Assimos DG, et al. Medical management of kidney stones: AUA guideline, American Urological Association; 2014. Maryland: American Urological Association Education and Research Inc. Available at: https://www.auanet.org/education/guidelines/management-kidney-stones.cfm. Accessed August 30, 2015.

18. Matlaga BR, Lingeman JE. Chapter 48: Surgical management of upper urinary tract calculi. In: Wein AJ, Kavoussi LR, Novick AC, et al, editors. Campbell-Walsh urology. 10th edition. Philadelphia: Saunders; 2011. p. 1357–410.

19. Morse RM, Resnick MI. Ureteral calculi: natural history and treatment in an era of advanced technology. J Urol 1991;145:263–5.

20. Pickard R, Starr K, MacLennan G, et al. Medical expulsive therapy in adults with ureteric colic: a multicentre, randomised, placebo-controlled trial. Lancet 2015; 386:341–9.

21. Rastinehad AR, Ost MC, VanderBrink BA, et al. Persistent prostatic hematuria. Nat Clin Pract Urol 2008;5:159.

22. Centers for disease control and prevention: injury prevention & control: data & statistics (WISQARSTM). Available at: http://www.cdc.gov/injury/wisqars/LeadingCauses.html. Accessed September 27, 2015.

23. Elias K, Svatek RS, Gupta S, et al. High risk patients with hematuria are not evaluated according to guideline recommendations. Cancer 2010;116(12):2954-9.

24. Leuck AM, Wright D, Ellingson L, et al. Complications of Foley catheters—is infection the greatest risk? J Urol 2012;187(5):1662-6.

Diagnosis and Management of Nephrolithiasis

Johann P. Ingimarsson, MD[a], Amy E. Krambeck, MD[a],
Vernon M. Pais Jr, MD[b,c],*

KEYWORDS

- Nephrolithiasis • Urolithiasis • Management • Diagnosis

KEY POINTS

- Nephrolithiasis can be caused by general surgical conditions, including malabsorption in Crohn's disease, ulcerative colitis, and pancreatitis and can occur in patients after bariatric surgery.
- Removal of a parathyroid adenoma can significantly decrease stone formation in patients with hyperparathyroidism.
- Low-dose unenhanced computed tomography scan has emerged as the gold standard imaging modality in the acute setting, whereas retroperitoneal ultrasound scan is a common option in the nonacute setting.
- Interventions include shock wave lithotripsy, ureteroscopy, percutaneous nephrolithotomy, and, rarely, open or laparoscopic surgery.
- These options vary in likelihood of rendering the patient stone free and in respective contraindications, risks, side effects, and need for additional procedures.

INTRODUCTION
Prevalence

Nephrolithiasis is a common reason for urgent patient presentation for medical or surgical evaluation. The incidence and prevalence of kidney stones has increased in the last decades among adults, adolescents and children. In their lifetime, 7% of females and 11% of males in the United States will be affected by kidney stones.[1]

Disclosure Statement: The authors have nothing to disclose.
[a] Department of Urology, Mayo Clinic, 200 First Street Southwest, Rochester, MN 55905, USA; [b] Section of Urology, Department of Surgery, Geisel School of Medicine at Dartmouth, Hanover, NH, USA; [c] Section of Urology, Dartmouth Hitchcock Medical Center, Lebanon, NH 03756, USA
* Corresponding author. Section of Urology, Dartmouth Hitchcock Medical Center, Lebanon, NH 03756.
E-mail address: Vernon.m.pais@dartmouth.edu

Surg Clin N Am 96 (2016) 517–532
http://dx.doi.org/10.1016/j.suc.2016.02.008
0039-6109/16/$ – see front matter © 2016 Elsevier Inc. All rights reserved.

Extent and Cost

Nephrolithiasis results in at least 1.2 million emergency department visits in the United States annually and 41,000 surgical interventions.[2,3] The estimated cost of kidney stones in 2007 was $3.8 billion with a projected further increase in cost of $1.2 billion by 2030.[4]

Morbidity and Prognosis

The most common morbidity of a kidney stone is renal colic, a condition resulting in pain, often acute, with need for acute medical and surgical intervention. More severe sequelae include sepsis from an obstructed infected stone and deterioration in renal function. Furthermore, ureteral stones, if left impacted for prolonged periods, can result in ureteral scar and stricture.[5]

Kidney stone recurrence rates vary by the underlying metabolic cause, but on average, after a stone event, 31% recur with another symptomatic kidney stone within 10 years.[6]

Risk Factors

Risk factors for kidney stone formation include increasing age, male sex, race (highest among whites), lower socioeconomic status, obesity, diabetes, and gout disease.[1] Additionally, dietary and endocrine factors are also known to greatly affect risk of kidney stones.[7]

Relevance to the General Surgeon

Likely the most common way for a kidney stone to come to the attention of a general surgeon is as a differential diagnosis for acute abdomen.

Outside of the acute setting, of particular relevance to the general surgeon, is the knowledge that malabsorptive intestinal diseases and conditions, such as Crohn's disease, ulcerative colitis, pancreatitis, and short gut syndrome increase risk of stone formation. The same is true for surgical interventions, such as bariatric surgery, colectomy, and any surgery leading to less absorptive physiology or decreased small bowel length.

Further, hyperparathyroidism, although uncommon (comprising <5%) is an important modifiable cause of renal stones.[8] The general surgeon can substantially decrease the risk of or completely prevent stone formation via surgical removal of an active parathyroid adenoma.

Finally, knowledge of the procedures performed to remove stones is useful for the general surgeon, as there is a known risk of injury to the adjacent structures, including pleura and colon for which intraoperative assistance of the general surgeon may be requested.

RELEVANT ANATOMY AND PATHOPHYSIOLOGY
Anatomy

Anatomically the kidneys are retroperitoneal organs in close proximity to liver, spleen, colon, duodenum, adrenals, diaphragm, and the lowest ribs.[9] This anatomy is relevant when stones are removed percutaneously, as there is potential injury to these organs when a percutaneous needle is introduced and an access tract, often up to 1 cm in diameter, is developed with dilators.

Should a kidney stone move and progress down the ureter, it will encounter 3 classically described areas of decreased luminal diameter. The first is at the ureteropelvic junction, the second occurs where the ureter crosses over the iliac vessels (external compression), and the third occurs where the ureter passes through the muscle layers of the bladder wall to emerge at the ureteral orifice. These areas of narrowing are the most common sites at which a ureteral stone is likely to become impacted and result in up-stream obstruction.[9]

Pathophysiology

When a solute is added to a solution (such as urine), it dissolves until its saturation point. Because of the presence of crystallization inhibitors, the concentration of clinically relevant crystals such as calcium oxalate can exceed their saturation point, existing in a metastable supersaturated state. From this state, stones may form in urine.[10,11]

In urine, the aforementioned inhibitors include molecules such as citrate, glycoproteins, and magnesium, whereas other factors, such as epithelial cells, urinary casts, red blood cells and even other crystals, can act as nucleating centers in urine, promoting stone formation. The pH can also affect the solubility of solutes in urine.[10]

Alternatively, severe enough super saturation can result in spontaneous crystallization and stone formation in the urine of the renal pelvis (homogenous nucleation).[11]

Given the above, kidney stones can be either intraparenchymal, calyceal, in the pelvis, or in the ureter upon diagnosis.

The size and the location of a kidney stone will affect its natural history and its management. A small renal pelvis or upper pole stone is likely to travel down the ureter and pass spontaneously with or without symptoms, whereas a larger stone or a stone in the dependent lower pole is less likely to do so. Success rates of treatments are also associated with stone location, size, number, and complexity.[12]

Renal stones can have numerous chemical compositions. Calcium-based stones are by far the most common. Frequently, renal stones show a mixture of more than one of the below-mentioned crystals.

Calcium oxalate accounts for 60% to 65% of stones in North America and as high as 90% in India. These findings may result from a combination of decreased fluid intake or relative dehydration, high dietary sodium, conditions that lead to high urinary excretion of calcium, and abnormalities in oxalate handling.[13] These risk factors, as they relate to general surgical conditions, are discussed below.

Calcium phosphate accounts for 10% to 20% of stones in western countries. Calcium phosphate stones may result from states of hypercalciuria (either primary or secondary to hypercalcemia) and disorders of urinary acidification, as calcium phosphate is poorly soluble in alkaline urine.[14] Urinary alkalization occurs in states such as renal tubular acidosis but may also be iatrogenically induced by medications including carbonic anhydrase inhibitors and topiramate.[15]

Uric acid stones account for 5% to 10% of stones. They may be associated with excessive protein intake or abnormalities in protein and uric acid metabolism but form frequently in the absence of either, as the supersaturation of uric acid rapidly increases in the setting of low urine volume or low urine pH. Opposite to calcium phosphate stones, they are poorly soluble in acidic urine and cannot form in alkaline urine.[16]

Ammonium acid urate stones are rare (0.2%–3%) but warrant special mention to the general surgeon. It has been theorized that they form in the setting of gastrointestinal loss of water and electrolytes that cause a volume-depleted state with intracellular acidosis. This state results in elevated urinary ammonia excretion in high enough concentrations to crystalize with urate.[17] In North America these stones are associated with a history of inflammatory bowel diseases or ileostomy diversion, laxative abuse, and morbid obesity.[18]

Other stones include struvite, an ammonium stone composition primarily caused by chronic urinary infection with urease-positive bacteria converting urea to ammonium (1%–14%); cystine stones, caused by a genetic disorder causing an impairment of transport of the amino acid cystine (1%–4%); and other rarer stones (0%–4%).[19]

Stone composition affects surgical treatment and likelihood of recurrence. As an example, harder stones, such as cystine and some calcium phosphate stones, are resistant to shock wave lithotripsy.[20] Struvite stones typically harbor bacteria; if they are infected, they must be completely eradicated.[21] Pure uric acid stones may potentially be resolved by altering urine pH.[22] Finally, the chemical composition affects post-surgical dietary and medical management with regard to decreasing risk of recurrence.

Pathophysiology of General Surgery Conditions Resulting in Stone Formation

Certain gastrointestinal conditions and disease states increase the risk of kidney stone formation. The primary variables that can be altered are elevated urinary excretion of oxalate (stone promoter), decreased urine citrate (stone inhibitor), urine acidification (promotes some stones) and decreased urine volume (less dilution, thus, more super-saturated urine).[23]

The increased urinary excretion of oxalate is thought primarily to be caused by increased enteric uptake, primarily in the setting of fat malabsorption, thus, known as *enteric hyperoxaluria*. As fat is malabsorbed, calcium ions are saponified in it and lost via steatorrhea. Under normal circumstances, the calcium binds to oxalate to form calcium oxalate crystals, which are not absorbed by the intestine and excreted fecally. In the absence of free luminal calcium, however, there is excess free oxalate, which is absorbed by the intestine.[23] At the same time, unconjugated bile salts and long-chain fatty acids have been found to increase oxalate permeability in the intestine, further increasing the uptake of oxalate.[24,25] Additionally, in disease states in which vitamin B6 is malabsorbed, the liver is induced to produce endogenous oxalate.[25] Finally, loss of oxalate degrading bowel flora such as *Oxalobacter formigenes*, either caused by inflammatory bowel conditions or antibiotic use, will increase availability of intestinal oxalate to be absorbed. Because oxalate is predominantly eliminated by renal excretion, increased oxalate uptake leads to increased urinary oxalate and calcium oxalate stone formation.[26,27] In addition to kidney stone formation, enteric hyperoxaluria can lead to renal insufficiency and ultimately end-stage renal disease. The true incidence of end-stage renal disease remains unreported, and most of our current knowledge comes from case series.[28] In one study, 8 of 11 patients presenting with nephropathy secondary hyperoxaluria eventually had end-stage renal failure, emphasizing the gravity of this condition and need for awareness of it in patients with fat malabsorptive conditions.[29]

Citrate is a potent inhibitor of stone formation. Its urinary levels are primarily controlled by acid-base status, as acidosis results in increased citrate utilization by mitochondria; thus, less free citrate is available for urinary excretion.[30] Therefore, any state resulting in chronic subclinical metabolic acidosis can result in low urinary citrate.

Acidosis can also result in excess net renal excretion of acids as a compensation mechanism, lowering the urinary pH and therefore increasing the risk of uric acid and ammonium acid urate stones.

Any state resulting in excessive gastrointestinal fluid losses will result in decreased urine volume and, thus, higher supersaturation of urine crystals and stone formation.[10]

Examples of disorders with increased risk of stone formation

Patients with ileostomy tend to lose excessive fluids. This loss results in more concentrated urine with higher likelihood of solutes being supersaturated. The most common stones, calcium oxalate, become more common. Additionally, loss of bicarbonate leads to a lower urinary pH, increasing the risk of urine acid and ammonium acid urate stones.[31]

Inflammatory bowel diseases Patients with Crohn's disease and ulcerative colitis are found to have an increased incidence in calcium oxalate stones compared with a healthy population. This increased incidence is thought to be primarily associated with fat malabsorption and resulting enteric hyperoxaluria[32]

Chronic pancreatitis Pancreatic insufficiency often leads to fat malabsorption, resulting in hyperoxaluria and oxalate stone formation.[33]

Bariatric surgery Growing evidence in the literature shows a higher kidney stone rate among patients having undergone bariatric surgery. With increasing postoperative malabsorption, the likelihood of symptomatic stone events increases. Thus, gastric banding and sleeve gastrectomy have stone rates similar to obese controls, whereas the adjusted hazard ratio of a symptomatic stone event was 2.5 patients having undergone Roux-en-Y gastric bypass and 5.2 for the more malabsorptive procedures, such as very long limb Roux-en-Y gastric bypass and biliopancreatic diversion/duodenal switch. The most predominant stone type is calcium oxalate stones.[34]

Hyperparathyroidism Although surgical intervention (such as aforementioned gastric bypass) may lead to kidney stone formation, surgery can also cure the underlying pathology that leads to stone formation. This is exemplified with primary hyperparathyroidism.[35]

Although the reason for stone formation is somewhat uncertain, it is known that parathyroid hormone (PTH) stimulates formation of active 1,25 vitamin D, with stimulation of bone resorption to release calcium and gastrointestinal absorption of calcium, leading to hypercalcemia. Although PTH does increase tubular reabsorption of calcium, net renal calcium excretion increases in part because the filtered load of calcium increases. As a result, kidney stones develop in about 20% of patients with hyperparathyroidism.[36,37]

Parathyroidectomy of a hyperactive adenoma results in a significant decrease in stone formation. Although for the first few years it remains higher, at 10 years it is the same as in the general population.[35]

With this in mind, the International Workshop on the Management of Asymptomatic primary hyperparathyroidism recommends that imaging indicating calcium-containing stones in a primary hyperparathyroidism patient warrants parathyroidectomy.[38]

Similarly, in a stone patient with hypercalcemia, PTH levels should be checked.[7]

PATHOPHYSIOLOGY OF RENAL COLIC AND STONE PASSAGE

Obstruction of urinary flow leads to increased upstream intraluminal pressure. This pressure leads to hydronephrosis, causing stretch and stimulation of nerve endings in the urothelium, resulting in colicky pain. Additionally, the smooth muscle in the ureteral wall contracts in an attempt to expel the stone and can go into spasm.[39]

The afferent nerves of the kidney and ureter enter the spinal cord at the T11 to L1 levels, en route to the central nervous system. These pathways are not specific to the kidney and ureter but are shared with afferent nerves from the gastrointestinal organs, other urinary organs, and genitalia. As such, pain can be perceived by the patient as rising from these organs, making for a presentation of an acute abdomen.[39] Nausea and vomiting may be caused by the common innervation pathway of the renal pelvis, stomach, and intestines through the celiac axis and vagal nerve afferents.[39]

Hematuria, although not always present, is caused by the rough surface of the stone injuring superficial blood vessels in its path.[40]

CLINICAL PRESENTATION AND EXAMINATION
Symptoms

The most common presentations of kidney stone are pain, hematuria, nausea, vomiting, and urinary tract infection (**Box 2**).

The location and nature of the pain can change based on stone location, although there is not a reliable correlation between pain location and stone location. This finding is particularly true in the elderly.[41] Intermittent pain indicates incomplete or intermittent obstruction, whereas constant pain indicates complete obstruction.[42] As mentioned earlier, because of the shared innervation of the ureter with adjacent organs, the pain can be perceived as coming from intestine, groin, bladder, and internal or external genitalia. In particular, ipsilateral testicular, labial, or groin areas are common sites of referred pain from distal ureteral calculi. Although it is classically described that a patient with renal colic is writhing, unable to find a comfortable position, this is not universal finding.[39,41]

Because obstruction is the mechanism by which stones cause pain, nonobstructing stones are not believed to be able to cause pain. Thus, in a patient with acute abdomen or flank or back pain and an imaging finding of a nonobstructing stone or an intraparenchymal stone, an alternate cause for the pain needs to be sought.

Hematuria may be macroscopic but more often is microscopic. The absence of hematuria does not exclude stone. The accuracy of hematuria for predicting stone has been reported as only 62%.[40]

Urgency, frequency, dysuria, and pain at meatus are common findings, as the stone traverses the transluminal bladder wall, thus, irritating the bladder urothelium. The condition can easily be mistaken for cystitis. If a stone passes into the bladder, it often becomes asymptomatic. Because the urethra has a larger diameter then the ureter, the actual passage of stones through the urethra is often less symptomatic and may be fully asymptomatic.[43]

Nausea and vomiting are present in about half of acute cases, making distinction from a gastrointestinal etiology more challenging.[43]

Of particular concern is a kidney stone presentation associated with fevers, chills, and rigors, as upper tract urinary tract infection that is not draining because of an obstructive stone carries a high risk of systemic inflammatory response syndrome and severe sepsis development. In addition to cultures and antibiotics, urinary drainage, in the form of a ureteral stent or a nephrostomy tube, must be performed.[12,42]

Physical Examination

General

In classical descriptions, a patient with renal colic is writhing, unable to find a comfortable position. This is a common finding but not universal.

Vital signs

Renal colic can induce tachycardia and hypertension. Renal colic generally does not cause fevers unless associated with urinary tract infection.[42]

Abdominal and flank examination

Costovertebral angle percussion tenderness is frequently found and is often quite severe. Given the retroperitoneal location of the kidney and the ureter, the abdomen is usually soft, nontender, nondistended, and without signs of peritoneal irritations. Examination findings of the genitalia and groin are normal.[42]

Laboratory Work

Serum chemistry results are most often within normal range. Elevation of creatine can be seen in a solitary kidney or in patients with a baseline decrease in renal function. Creatine elevation may also result from dehydration as a result of colic-related nausea and emesis.[40]

An increase in neutrophils and white blood cells may be noted as stress response or if there is an associated urinary tract infection.[42]

On a urinalysis, microscopic hematuria is common.[40] Although urinary crystals may be noted, crystalluria is a common finding in normal controls and is not diagnostic of urolithiasis.[44] The presence of white cells, leukocyte esterase, and nitrites should raise the suspicion of an underlying infection.[4]

Imaging

Noncontrast computed tomography

Noncontrast, low-dose (or ultra–low-dose) computed tomography (CT) scans have become the gold standard for diagnosis of urolithiasis and has replaced intravenous pyelography (IVP) as such. This type of CT offers high sensitivity (>95%) and specificity (98%) for the detection of stones.[45] This type of CT offers more anatomic stone and renal detail, which is especially relevant when mapping out large branched stones or complex collecting system anatomy. In addition, it offers anatomic information of surrounding organs.[46]

Noncontrast CT avoids the intravenous contrast need for an IVP and allows for better quality imaging in the obese compared with ultrasound scan and in many institutions is often more accessible than ultrasonography.[46]

The main drawback of noncontrast CT is the amount of ionizing radiation, which is of particular concern in frequent stone formers and young patients. The average stone protocol CT scan in North America results in 11 mSv, but ultra–low-dose protocols are available with 1 mSv are available.[47,48]

Retroperitoneal ultrasound scan

Retroperitoneal ultrasound scan offers moderate sensitivity (45%) and specificity (88%–94%), albeit lower than CT scan.[49] Retroperitoneal ultrasound is less expensive than CT; however, it is operator dependent, and there is risk of over- and undercalling stone size.[47] Because there is no radiation, retroperitoneal ultrasound is a reasonable study for the nonacute setting, in follow-up, and in children and pregnant women. The European Association of Urology Guidelines recommends this method as the primary imaging modality, although a CT scan should be obtained for acute flank pain.[12]

Plain radiograph of abdomen and pelvis

Radiograph of the kidney, ureter, and bladder offers lower radiation dose than CT (0.6–1 mSv), with lower sensitivity and specificity. It is easily available and can be routinely use for follow-up if the primary stone is radio-opaque but should not be a primary study in acute circumstances.[12,50,51]

Intravenous pyelogram

Previously the gold standard for kidney stone detection, IVP has essentially been replaced by CT. Low-dose CT scans can now be performed with a similar or less amount of radiation without the need for intravenous contrast. CT can be done in a faster manner, as IVP often requires delayed imaging to allow contrast excretion into a partially obstructed collecting system. IVP still has a role in discerning ureteral stones from phleboliths.

Nuclear functional renal scan

Nuclear functional renal scans have a limited role in renal stone diagnosis and are occasionally used to confirm obstruction when there is doubt. The scans also have a role in assessing differential renal function, as a patient may be best served with observation or nephrectomy in the setting of a stone in a poorly functioning kidney as opposed to complex stone-removing procedures.[52]

MANAGEMENT AND AVAILABLE PROCEDURES
Observation

Small nonobstructing and intraparenchymal stones may potentially neither grow nor move down the ureter and, thus, not cause symptoms. By 3 years, 22% will grow significantly, 28% will cause colic, and another 2% will cause silent obstruction.[53] Observation, with serial imaging to assess for interval growth, is a reasonable alternative in these cases, at least in the short term, as the risk of complications of intervention may not outweigh the benefit.[12]

Medical Expulsive Therapy

Should a small stone (<10 mm) travel down the ureter and cause renal colic, it may pass spontaneously. Success rates are higher and passage time shorter the smaller the stone is and the further it is down the ureter at the time of presentation. Thus, a 1-mm stone has about an 87% chance of passage; a 2- to 4-mm stone, 76%; 5 to 7 mm, 60%; 8 to 9 mm, 48%; and 10 mm or larger, 25%. Similarly, a proximal stone has a 48% chance of passage; a midureteral stone, a 60% chance of passage; and a distal stone, a 75% to 79% chance of spontaneous passage.[54] The smaller and further distal the stone is, the shorter the time of passage, although this may vary from hours to 30 days.

The use of medication to affect ureteral passage rates is known as *medical expulsive therapy* (MET). Alpha blockers inhibit ureteral smooth muscle contraction and peristalsis with decrease basal tone. Calcium channel blockers inhibit calcium influx and prostaglandins, thus, decreasing contractions in the ureter.[55]

MET is found to increase successful passage of a ureteral stone by 44% to 66%.[55] It also decreases pain and number of colic episodes (**Table 1**).[56]

This therapy is a recommended treatment option for the informed patient, both by the American Urology Association and the European Association of Urology.[12,57] Should medical expulsive therapies fail, either because of intractable pain, prolonged course, or sequelae, such as infection or worsening renal function, then surgical intervention is indicated.[12]

Table 1
Medical expulsive therapy versus no medical expulsive therapy

	MET	Controls	Difference
Time of passage (d)	4–30	8–31	3.6[a]
Colic events	23%	40%	17%
Need for auxiliary procedures	12%	33%	11%

[a] weighted mean in meta-analysis.
Data from Fan B, Yang D, Wang J, et al. Can tamsulosin facilitate expulsion of ureteral stones? A meta-analysis of randomized controlled trials. Int J Urol 2013;20:818–30.

AVAILABLE SURGICAL PROCEDURES

- Temporizing drainage
- Shock wave lithotripsy

- Ureteroscopy
- Percutaneous nephrostomy
- Open or laparoscopic stone surgery

PROCEDURE TECHNIQUE

In certain acute settings, such as where a stone is believed to cause an obstructed urinary tract infection or acute deterioration in renal function, urgent decompression of the renal pelvis is needed. This decompression can be done either by placing a percutaneous nephrostomy tube or a ureteral stent cystoscopically.[12]

Shock Wave Lithotripsy

The basis of shock wave lithotripsy (SWL) is to fracture stones using focused shock waves into smaller fragments, which can then be passed spontaneously. Numerous versions of SWL devices (lithotripters) are available, with different means of generating the shock wave. These include electrohydraulic (spark gap), electromagnetic, and piezoelectric shock waves. The shock wave is generated inside the lithotripter and then it is focused to an external point with parabolic reflectors or acoustic lenses. The patient is positioned in such a way that the focal point is on the stone in question. To ensure correct position of the patient and stone, fluoroscopic or ultrasound guidance is used and the patient or lithotripter moved until the stone is in the focal point. Because sound and shock waves are best conducted in liquid, the treatment head of the lithotripter is pushed against the patient's body with water or aqueous gel in between as the medium.[58]

The primary benefit of SWL is that it does not require instrumentation of the patient's urinary tract or placement of a ureteral stent. Many patients poorly tolerate stent because of bladder spams and flank discomfort. However, SWL for many stone locations has a lower likelihood of rendering the patient stone free, as it may be difficult to verify that the stone was fractured into small enough pieces to pass down the ureter spontaneously. Therefore, the need for additional treatments is higher (**Table 2**).[12,57]

SWL does not have a high success rate for very large stones (2 cm or higher) or in certain hard stones, such as cysteine, and certain calcium phosphate stones.

SWL is contraindicated in the setting of obstruction distal to the stone, in patients on anticoagulation, in pregnant patients, and in patients with a known urinary tract infection. Complications include blockage of ureter from fragments (<4%), sepsis (1%), clinically significant bleeding (0.6%), and injury to gastrointestinal organs (1.8%). Long-term effects on hypertension, renal function, and diabetes have also been reported but remain debated.[59]

Table 2
Stone-free rates: SWL versus ureteroscopy from American Urology Association guidelines

Location	SWL (%)	URS (%)
Distal ureter	74	94
Mid ureter	73	86
Proximal ureter	82	81

Ureteroscopy

The basis of ureteroscopy is to advance a small diameter scope (most often 2–3 mm in diameter) in a retrograde manner up the urethra and bladder to the ureter and kidney and fracture the stone(s) with laser energy via a laser fiber through the scope. The fragments can either be broken down into smaller fragments that can then be extracted with a wire basket or further fractured to submillimeter fragments (dusting) with the plan of having them pass spontaneously.[60]

This method can be achieved either with a semirigid scope in the distal ureter, allowing for better irritant flow and visibility, or a flexible ureteroscope in the more proximal ureter and kidney, allowing for complete inspection of the urinary collecting system.

Ureteroscopy offers superior stone-free rates to those of SWL in most clinical scenarios and, thus, fewer secondary procedures for residual stones.[12,57]

Because ureteroscopy may induce inflammation in the ureter initially after surgery, a ureteral stent is often needed to ensure drainage and prevent colic from temporary obstruction. As mentioned earlier, stent discomfort is common in the form of bladder spasm and flank pain.[60]

There are few contraindications to ureteroscopy other than untreated urinary tract infection. Complications other than stent discomfort are rare, but these included ureteral stricture (1%–2%), ureteral injury (3%–6%), urinary tract infection (2%–4%), and sepsis (2%).[57]

Percutaneous Nephrolithotomy

Both SWL and ureteroscopy are limited by the size of stones that can be treated successfully. In percutaneous nephrolithotomy (PCNL), a percutaneous access tract up to 1 cm in diameter is created through the kidney and allows access to the largest renal stones, which can be fractured accordingly and then removed.

Percutaneous nephrolithotomy allows for the insertion of larger-diameter rigid scopes directly into the renal pelvis. Through these, both suction and more potent energy sources, such as ultrasound and pneumatic lithotripsy, can be applied, greatly facilitating stone fracturing and clearance. In addition, larger flexible scopes can be introduced via the ureter, with improved visibility and working capacity.[61]

The access is obtained under fluoroscopic or ultrasound guidance, either preoperatively by an interventional radiologist or during surgery by the urologist. A posterior approach is typically used to avoid the anterior surrounding organ and to take advantage of the relatively less vascularized watershed area between the anterior and posterior branches of the renal artery.[62–64]

The primary appeal of PCNL is superior stone-free rates compared with SWL and ureteroscopy in large and complex stones (**Table 3**).[12]

Because it involves establishing and dilating a tract through the renal parenchyma, PCNL does carry the risk of bleeding, which may need transfusion (7%) or angioembolization (0.5%). PCNL is, therefore, contraindicated in patients on anticoagulation. Because of posterior access and the low-lying posterior aspect of the pleural sulcus, there is a risk of hydro-, hemo- and pneumothorax (1.5%). The risk is higher if the access is obtained between the ribs, which may be needed in certain circumstances.[12] Treatment of these conditions may require a chest tube as with other causes of these conditions.

Table 3 Ureteroscopy versus PCNL		
	PCNL (%)	Ureteroscopy (%)
Stone free	95	84
Complication rate	16	13

Data from De S, Autorino R, Kim FJ, et al. Percutaneous nephrolithotomy versus retrograde intrarenal surgery: a systematic review and meta-analysis. Eur Urol 2015;67:125–37.

Table 4
Ureteral stone management based on American Urology Association guidelines

Stone Size	Primary Option	Secondary Option
<10 mm	Offer MET in a patient informed of the expected course, benefits, and risks, with scheduled follow-up and imaging, proceeding to intervention if MET fails	Either SWL or ureteroscopy
>10 mm	Either SWL or ureteroscopy	—

Data from Preminger GM, Tiselius HG, Assimos DG, et al; EAU/AUA Nephrolithiasis Guideline Panel. 2007 guideline for the management of ureteral calculi. J Urol 2007;178:2418–34.

Although much less frequent (cumulative average in reported series is 0.4%), injuries to surrounding organ, such as the retro-renal colon, duodenum, spleen, or liver are known complications.[12] Colonic injuries have been successfully managed by pulling the nephrostomy tube into the colonic lumen and leaving it to drain. At the same time, a retrograde ureteral stent is placed. This placement diverts the fecal and urinary streams and allows for successful outcomes. However, the need for colectomy and bowel diversion may be required based on the clinical scenario.[63] Successful conservative management of duodenal injury has been described with nasogastric tube decompression, fasting, and parental feeding, but explorative surgery remains the classical approach to any duodenal trauma.[64] In either setting, should the patient develop peritonitis, an explorative laparotomy is mandatory. Splenic injuries secondary to PCNL abide by the general trauma surgery principles and can be treated with observation, angioembolization, or laparotomy, based on the severity of the injury.[65] Liver injury during PCNL is rare and can most often be managed conservatively.[66]

Open or Laparoscopic Surgery for Stone Disease

Surgeries for stone disease include anatrophic nephrolithotomy and pyelolithotomy but are rarely used, given higher morbidity and complication rates, so are thus generally reserved for select cases. These techniques may be considered in rare cases in which SWL, ureteroscopy, and percutaneous nephrolithotomy fail or are unlikely to be successful.[12]

Table 5
Renal stone management based on the European Association of Urology guidelines

Stone Size/Location	Primary Option	Secondary Option
>20 mm	PCNL	Ureteroscopy or SWL
10–20 mm, located in lower pole of kidney	If unfavorable for shockwave: ureteroscopy or PCNL	—
	If favorable[a] for shockwave: ureteroscopy or PCNL	SWL
10–20 mm elsewhere in kidney	Ureteroscopy or SWL or PCNL	—
<10 mm	Ureteroscopy or SWL	PCNL

[a] None of the following: Shockwave-resistant stones, steep infundibular-pelvic angle, long lower pole calyx, or narrow infundibulum.

Data from Türk C, Petřík A, Sarica K, et al. EAU guidelines on interventional treatment for urolithiasis. Eur Urol 2016;69(3):475–82.

Box 1
Overview of diseases seen by the general surgeon that increase risk of kidney stones

Disease/Condition	Metabolic Abnormality	Resulting Stone Type

Colectomy/ileostomy
Chronic diarrhea
Laxative abuse
	1. Dehydration
	
	2. Loss of bicarbonate – renal
	   retention of acid – increased
	   urine pH
		1. All types
		
		2. Uric acid stones
		   Ammonium acid urate

Fat malabsorption • Inflammatory bowel disease • Pancreatitis • Bariatric surgery	Saponification of calcium resulting in excess enteric oxalate. Increased per ability to oxalate	Calcium oxalate stones
Altered bowel flora	Loss of oxalate consuming bacteria	Calcium oxalate stone
Hyperparathyroidism	PTH-induced increase in enteric calcium absorption— compensatory hypercalciuria	Any calcium stones

SELECTION OF PROCEDURE

For many ureteral and renal stones, more than one option for surgical treatment may be available. Choices may vary with patient factors, patient preference, and urologist expertise. The American Urology Association and the European Association of Urology have published thorough reviews of outcomes and complications, which are offered in **Tables 1–5** and **Boxes 1–3** regarding the management of ureteral and renal stones.

Box 2
Signs and symptoms of renal colic

- Sudden onset—brought by sudden obstruction to outflow

- Intermittent versus constant
  - Intermittent suggestive of incomplete obstruction
  - Constant suggestive complete obstruction
  - If chronically obstructed may become painless

- Location of pain
  - Flank, lower abdomen, genitalia, groin

- Nausea vomiting
  - Present in about 50% of cases

- Hematuria
  - Present in 64% of cases

- Fever
  - Sign of a confined, nondraining upper tract infection. Must be surgically drained.

- Costovertebral angle tenderness to percussion

- Abdominal and genitalia examination findings often benign

- Laboratory values most often normal. Elevated creatinine and microscopic hematuria common.

- Significantly elevated white count should raise concern of nondraining urinary tract infection

Box 3		
Comparison of treatment options		
Procedure	**Pro**	**Con**
SWL	Avoids instrumentation of the patient	Lower stone-free rates
	Avoids the need of stent placement	More often requires secondary procedures
		Patient must pass stone fragments, which can block the ureter
Ureteroscopy	Higher stone-free rates	Commonly requires stent placement
	Can be performed on an anticoagulant end patient	Low risk of ureteral injuries
	Can be performed on pregnant patients	
PCNL	Highest stone-free rates	Highest bleeding risk
		Low, but real risk of injury to adjacent organs
Open or laparoscopic surgery	May be of benefit in rare cases of complex stones in complex anatomy	Most invasive

REFERENCES

1. Scales CD Jr, Smith AC, Hanley JM, et al. Urologi diseases in America project, prevalence of kidney stones in the United States. Eur Urol 2012;62:160–5.

2. Eaton SH, Cashy J, Pearl JA, et al. Admission rates and costs associated with emergency presentation of urolithiasis: analysis of the nationwide emergency department sample 2006-2009. J Endourol 2013;27:1535–8.

3. Table 9-19 and 9-20 Urinary tract stones. In: Litwin MS, Saigal CS, editors. Urologic diseases in America. US department of health and human services, public health service, National Institutes of Health, National Institute of Diabetes and Digestive and Kidney Diseases. Washington, DC: US Government Printing Office; 2012. p. 331–2. NIH Publication No. 12-7865.

4. Antonelli JA, Maalouf NM, Pearle MS, et al. Use of the national health and nutrition examination survey to calculate the impact of obesityand diabetes on cost and prevalence of urolithasis in 2030. Eur Urol 2014;66:724–9.

5. Mugiya S, Ito T, Maruyama S, et al. Endoscopic features of impacted ureteral stones. J Urol 2004;171:89–91.

6. Rule AD, Lieske JC, Li X, et al. The ROKS nomogram for predicting a second symptomatic stone episode. J Am Soc Nephrol 2014;25:2878–86.

7. Pearle MS, Goldfarb DS, Assimos DG, et al, American Urological Assocation. Medical management of kidney stones: AUA guideline. J Urol 2014;192:316–24.

8. Heath H 3rd, Hodgson SF, Kennedy MA. Primary hyperparathyroidism. Incidence, morbidity, and potential economic impact in a community. N Engl J Med 1980;24(302):189–93.

9. Anderson JK, Caddedu JA. Surgical antomy of the retroperitoneum, adrenals, kidney and ureters. In: Wein AJ, Kavoussi LT, editors. Campbell-Walsh Urology. Elsevier; 2012. p. 3–32.

10. Aggarwal KP, Narula S, Kakkar M, et al. Nephrolithiasis: molecular mechanism of renal stone formation and the critical role played by modulators. Biomed Res Int 2013;2013:292–5.

11. Smith LH. Renal stones. Solutions and solute. Endocrinol Metab Clin North Am 1990;19:767–72.
12. Türk C, Petřík A, Sarica K, et al. EAU guidelines on interventional treatment for urolithiasis. Eur Urol 2016;69(3):475–82.
13. Matlaga BR, Williams JC Jr, Kim SC, et al. Endoscopic evidence of calculus attachment to Randall's plaque. J Urol 2006;175:1720–4.
14. Tiselius HG. A hypothesis of calcium stone formation: an interpretation of stone research during the past decades. Urol Res 2011;39:231–43.
15. Kaplon DM, Penniston KL, Nakada SY. Patients with and without prior urolithiasis have hypocitraturia and incident kidney stones while on topiramate. Urology 2011;77:295–8.
16. Mehta TH, Goldfarb DS. Uric acid stones and hyperuricosuria. Adv Chronic Kidney Dis 2012;19:413–8.
17. Dick WH, Lingeman JE, Preminger GM, et al. Laxative abuse as a cause for ammonium urate renal calculi. J Urol 1990;143:244–7.
18. Soble JJ, Hamilton BD, Streen SB. Ammonium acid urate calculi: a reevaluation of risk factors. J Urol 1999;161:869–73.
19. Pearle MS, Lotan Y. Urinary lithiasis. In: Wein AJ, Kavoussi LT, editors. Cambpellwalsh urology. Elsevier; 2012. p. 1257–86.
20. Dretler SP. Stone fragility—a new therapeutic distinction. J Urol 1988;139: 1124–7.
21. Teichman JM, Long RD, Hulbert JC. Long-term renal fate and prognosis after staghorn calculus management. J Urol 1995;153:1403–7.
22. Rodman JS. Intermittent versus continuous alkaline therapy for uric acid stones and ureteral stones of uncertain composition. Urology 2002;60:378.
23. Dobbins JW, Binder HJ. Importance of the colon in enteric hyperoxaluria. N Engl J Med 1977;296:298–301.
24. Caspary WF, Tonissen J, Lankisch PG. 'Enteral' hyperoxaluria. Effect ofcholestyramine, calcium, neomycin, and bile acids on intestinal oxalate absorption in man. Acta Hepatogastroenterol 1977;24:193–200.
25. Hoyer-Kuhn H, Kohbrok S, Volland R, et al. Vitamin B6 in primary hyperoxaluria I: first prospective trial after 40 years of practice. Clin J Am Soc Nephrol 2014;9: 468–77.
26. Kumar R, Ghoshal UC, Singh G, et al. Infrequency of colonization with oxalobacter formigenes in inflammatory bowel disease: possible role in renal stone formation. J Gastroenterol Hepatol 2004;19:1403–9.
27. Kharlamb V, Schelker J, Francois F, et al. Oral antibiotic treatment of Helicobacter pylori leads to persistently reduced intestinal colonization rates with Oxalobacter formigenes. J Endourol 2011;25:1781–5.
28. Nazzal L, Puri S, Goldfarb DS. Enteric hyperoxaluria: an importnant cause of ESKD. Nephrol Dial Transplant 2016;31(3):375–82.
29. Nasr SH, D'Agati VD, Said SM, et al. Oxalate nephropathy complicating Roux-en-Y gastric bypass: an underrecognized cause of irreversible renal failure. Clin J Am Soc Nephrol 2008;3:1676–83.
30. Hamm LL, Hering-Smith KS. Pathophysiology of hypocitraturic nephrolithiasis. Endocrinol Metab Clin North Am 2002;31:885–93, viii.
31. Evan AP, Lingeman JE, Coe FL, et al. Intra-tubular deposits, urine and stone composition are divergent in patients with ileostomy. Kidney Int 2009;76:1081–8.
32. Hylander E, Jarnum S, Jensen HJ, et al. Enteric hyperoxaluria: dependence on small intestinal resection, colectomy, and steatorrhoea in chronic inflammatory bowel disease. Scand J Gastroenterol 1978;13:577–88.

33. Cartery C, Faguer S, Karras A, et al. Oxalate nephropathy associated with chronic pancreatitis. Clin J Am Soc Nephrol 2011;6:1895–902.

34. Lieske JC, Mehta RA, Milliner DS, et al. Kidney stones are common after bariatric surgery. Kidney Int 2015;87:839–45.

35. Mollerup CL, Vestergaard P, Frøkjaer VG, et al. Risk of renal stone events in primary hyperparathyroidism before and after parathyroid surgery: controlled retrospective follow up study. BMJ 2002;325:807–10.

36. Kumar R, Thompson JR. The regulation of parathyroid hormone secretion and synthesis. J Am Soc Nephrol 2011;22:216–24.

37. Parks JH, Coe FL, Evan AP, et al. Clinical and laboratory characteristics of calcium stone-formers with and without primary hyperparathyroidism. BJU Int 2009;103:670–8.

38. Bilezikian JP, Brandi ML, Eastell R, et al. Guidelines for the management of asymptomatic primary hyperparathyroidism: summary statement from the fourth international workshop. J Clin Endocrinol Metab 2014;99:3561–9.

39. Shokeir AA. Renal colic: new concepts related to pathophysiology, diagnosis and treatment. Curr Opin Urol 2002;12:263–9.

40. Safriel Y, Malhotra A, Sclafani SJ, et al. Hematuria as an indicator for the presence or absence of urinary calculi. Am J Emerg Med 2003;21:492–3.

41. Krambeck AE, Lieske JC, Li X, et al. Effect of age on the clinical presentation of incident symptomatic urolithiasis in the general population. J Urol 2013;189:158–64.

42. Gulmi FA, Felsen D. Pathophysiolgy of urinary tract obstruction. In: Smith AD, Badlani GH, editors. Smith's textbook of endourology. West Sussex (United Kingdom): Wiley-Blackwell; 2012. p. 95–119.

43. Carter MR, Green BR. Renal calculi: emergency department diagnosis and treatment. Emerg Med Pract 2011;13:1–17.

44. Robert M, Boularan AM, Delbos O. Evaluation of the risk of stone formation: study on crystalluria in patients with recurrent calcium oxalate Urolithiasis. Eur Urol 1996;29:456–61.

45. Dalrymple NC, Verga M, Anderson KR, et al. The value of unenhanced helical computerized tomography in the management of acute flank pain. J Urol 1998;159:735.

46. Viprakasit DP, Sawyer MD, Herrell SD, et al. Limitations of ultrasonography in the evaluation of urolithiasis: a correlation with computed tomography. J Endourol 2012;26:209.

47. Lukasiewicz A, Bhargavan-Chatfield M, Coombs L, et al. Radiation dose index of renal colic protocol CT studies in the United States: a report from the American College of Radiology National Radiology Data Registry. Radiology 2014;271:445–51.

48. Sagara Y, Hara AK, Pavlicek W, et al. Abdominal CT: comparison of low-dose CT with adaptive statistical iterative reconstruction and routine-dose CT with filtered back projection in 53 patients. AJR Am J Roentgenol 2010;195:713.

49. Ray AA, Ghiculete D, Pace KT, et al. Limitations to ultrasound in the detection and measurement of urinary tract calculi. Urology 2010;76:295.

50. Astroza GM, Neisius A, Wang AJ, et al. Radiation exposure in the follow-up of patients with urolithiasis comparing digital tomosynthesis, non-contrast CT, standard KUB, and IVU. J Endourol 2013;27:1187.

51. Chen TT, Wang C, Ferrandino MN, et al. Radiation exposure during the evaluation and management of nephrolithiasis. J Urol 2015;194:878–85.

52. Bird VG, Gomez-Marin O, Leveillee RJ, et al. A comparison of unenhanced helical computerized tomography findings and renal obstruction determined by furosemide 99m technetium mercaptoacetyltriglycine diuretic scintirenography for patients with acute renal colic. J Urol 2002;16:1597–603.

53. Dropkin BM, Moses RA, Sharma D, et al. The natural history of nonobstructing asymptomatic renal stones managed with active surveillance. J Urol 2015;193:1265–9.

54. Coll DM, Varanelli MJ, Smith RC. Relationship of spontaneous passage of ureteral calculi to stone size and location as revealed by unenhanced helical CT. AJR Am J Roentgenol 2002;178:101–3.

55. Seitz C, Liatsikos E, Porpiglia F, et al. Medical therapy to facilitate the passage of stones: what is the evidence? Eur Urol 2009;56:455–71.

56. Hollingsworth JM, Rogers MA, Kaufman SR, et al. Medical therapy to facilitate urinary stone passage: a meta-analysis. Lancet 2006;368:1171–9.

57. Preminger GM, Tiselius HG, Assimos DG, et al. EAU/AUA nephrolithiasis guideline panel. 2007 guideline for the management of ureteral calculi. J Urol 2007;178:2418–34.

58. Cleveland RO, McAteer JA. Physics of shock wave lithotripsy. In: Smith AD, Badlani GH, editors. Smith's textbook of endourology. West Sussex (United Kingdom): Wiley-Blackwell; 2012. p. 529–53.

59. Lee FJ, Tan YH. Complications of shock wave lithotripsy. In: Smith AD, Badlani GH, editors. Smith's textbook of endourology. West Sussex (United Kingdom): Wiley-Blackwell; 2012. p. 529–53.

60. Lahme S. Ureteroscopic management of renal calculi. In: Smith AD, Badlani GH, editors. Smith's textbook of endourology. West Sussex (United Kingdom): Wiley-Blackwell; 2012. p. 529–53.

61. Lasser MS, Pareek G. Percutaneos lithotripsy and stone extraction. In: Smith AD, Badlani GH, editors. Smith's textbook of endourology. West Sussex (United Kingdom): Wiley-Blackwell; 2012. p. 529–53.

62. Wolf JS. Percutaneous approaches to the upper urinary tract system. In: Wein AJ, Kavoussi LT, editors. Cambpell-walsh urology. Elsevier; 2012. p. 1324–59.

63. Gerspach JM, Bellman GC, Stoller ML, et al. Conservative management of colon injury following percutaneous renal surgery. Urology 1997;49:831–6.

64. Culkin DJ, Wheeler JS Jr, Canning JR. Nephroduodenal fistula. A complication of percutaneous nephrolithotomy. J Urol 1985;134:528–30.

65. Dent D. Splenic injury: angio vs operation. J Trauma 2007;62:s26.

66. El-Nahas AR, Mansour AM, Ellaithy R, et al. Case report: conservative treatment of liver injury during percutaneous nephrolithotomy. J Enduorl 2008;22:1649–52.

Genitourinary Prosthetics

A Primer for the Non-urologic Surgeon

Garjae Lavien, MD*, Uwais Zaid, MD, Andrew C. Peterson, MD

KEYWORDS

- Artificial urinary sphincter • Penile prosthesis • Testicular prosthesis
- Perioperative management • Erectile dysfunction • Urinary incontinence

KEY POINTS

- There are several implanted urologic devices that may affect surgical care by the general surgeon in the future.
- Given the numbers of penile prostheses and anti-incontinence procedures being performed, all surgeons must evaluate for the presence of urologic prosthetics in patients undergoing nonurologic surgery.
- Patients with artificial urinary sphincters must have their devices deactivated in the open position before any attempt at urethral instrumentation and catheterization.
- Injury to device components of urologic prosthetics in a sterile operative field can be managed with immediate or delayed revision.
- Injury to device components in the setting of an infected operative field can be managed with immediate removal of components and replacement at a later operative session.

INTRODUCTION

Genitourinary prosthetics are used in the management of a variety of urologic conditions with the goal of restoring function and improving the quality of lives of affected patients. Urologic prosthetics may be encountered by general surgeons during clinical assessments when evaluating patients for a multitude of nonurologic surgeries.

Erectile dysfunction (ED) is estimated to affect up to 30 million men in the United States.[1] It can have a devastating impact on both the physical and the psychological aspects of men's health and is frequently attributable to a progressive decline in neurologic, hormonal, and vascular function. More than 50% of men between the ages of 40 and 70 experience some level of ED.[2] Despite the increasing role of phosphodiesterase type 5 inhibitors, such as sildenafil (Viagra), tadalafil (Cialis), vardenafil (Levitra HCl), and avanafil (Stendra) in the management of ED, the penile prostheses

Disclosure Statement: The authors have nothing to disclose.
Genitourinary Survivorship Program, Division of Urology, Duke University Medical Center, DUMC 3146, Durham, NC 27710, USA
* Corresponding author.
E-mail address: garjae.lavien@duke.edu

Surg Clin N Am 96 (2016) 533–543
http://dx.doi.org/10.1016/j.suc.2016.02.009
0039-6109/16/$ – see front matter © 2016 Elsevier Inc. All rights reserved.

remain a standard treatment option, with excellent durability and patient/partner satisfaction. This satisfaction is reflected by the number of annual penile prosthesis implantations performed in the United States, increasing from 17,540 cases in 2000, to 22,420 in 2009, to approximately 30,000 in the present day.[3] Penile prostheses have also been used in the treatment of refractory ischemic priapism[4,5] and to facilitate condom catheter usage in spinal cord patients.[6]

Similar to ED, urinary incontinence is a condition that carries a significant economic and health burden with a prevalence of 11.2% in men age 45 to 64 years to 31% in men older than 65 years old.[7,8] The most common cause of stress incontinence in men include the various treatments for prostate cancer: radiation therapy, brachytherapy, and surgical removal of the prostate. Stress urinary incontinence, which is defined as the involuntary leakage of urine with effort or exertion, or with coughing or sneezing, is managed in men surgically when conservative treatment modalities are unsuccessful. With the surge in the number of anti-incontinence procedures and devices available within the armamentarium of urologists, there has been a subsequent increase in the number of anti-incontinence procedures being performed, as reflected in case logs of certifying and recertifying urologists from 2004 to 2010 showing an increase from 1936 to 3366 treatments per year.[9]

Given these findings, it is very likely that surgeons in other disciplines will encounter patients who present with existing genitourinary prosthetics during workup for nonurologic surgery. In this article, an overview is presented of the 3 most common types of urologic prosthetics non-urologic surgeons may encounter: the testicular prosthesis, the penile prosthesis, and the artificial urinary sphincter (AUS).

TYPES OF GENITOURINARY PROSTHESIS
Testicular Prosthesis

Testicular prostheses (**Fig. 1**) are used in cases of anorchism or monorchism, which can occur as a complication of testicular torsion, scrotal trauma, radical orchiectomy for testicular cancer, and sexual reassignment surgery. Patient acceptance and satisfaction rates are high.[10,11] These devices consist of a silicone elastomer filled with saline and are designed to mimic the natural testicle in size and consistency. Placement is performed through an inguinal incision or high scrotal incision, and these can be fixed in place with a nonabsorbable suture to the dartos of the scrotum to prevent migration. Varying sizes allow surgeons to place prostheses that account for the volume of the scrotal sac, the

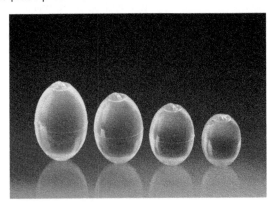

Fig. 1. Torosa saline-filled testicular prosthesis. (© Coloplast Corp. REPRINTED WITH PERMISSION-ALL RIGHTS RESERVED. Coloplast® and Torosa Testicular Prosthesis® are registered trademarks of Coloplast A/S.)

size of the contralateral testes, as well as the patient's wishes. General surgeons may be consulted about patients with scrotal masses and should consider this in their differential when faced with a scrotal ultrasound that is abnormal. A urologic history and physical examination may prevent unnecessary exploration in these patients.

Semirigid Penile Prostheses

Semirigid penile prostheses (**Fig. 2**) are solid implants placed into each corpus cavernosum. These devices consist of a silicone cylinder containing a central malleable core consisting of articulating titanium and polyethylene segments. The design allows a patient to bend their penis as required for sexual intercourse and permits downward deflection for concealment when not in use. This type of prosthesis is advantageous in patients with poor manual dexterity. It also carries a decreased risk of infection and mechanical failure compared with the inflatable penile prosthesis but does have higher rates of extrusion to the skin and erosion into the urethra.[12]

Inflatable Penile Prostheses

Inflatable penile prostheses consist of "2-piece" and "3-piece" inflatable penile prostheses. The 2-piece inflatable penile prosthesis (**Fig. 3**) consists of paired intracorporeal cylinders and a scrotal pump. When a patient activates the pump, fluid within the cylinders is transferred from the proximal part of the cylinders to the distal portion of cylinders, providing the necessary rigidity to facilitate sexual intercourse. Two-piece inflatable penile prostheses facilitate implantation in select cases whereby placement of a retroperitoneal reservoir may be challenging, such as in patients with prior pelvic surgery, renal transplant, or pancreas transplant patients with exocrine drainage via the bladder.[12,13] Three-piece inflatable penile prostheses (**Fig. 4**) consist of paired cylinders, a scrotal pump, and a fluid reservoir, which is placed in the space of Retzius or between transversalis fascia and the rectus abdominis. The scrotal pump allows fluid to be transferred from the reservoirs to the cylinder via tubing connections, thus providing patients with an on-demand artificial erection while providing improved cosmesis in the flaccid state compared with the semirigid prosthesis. Some advocate avoiding 3-piece inflatable penile prosthesis placement in select populations, such as those at risk for subsequent abdominal and pelvic operations. For instance, Cuellar and Sklar[13] noted a high rate of device malfunction in renal transplant patients related

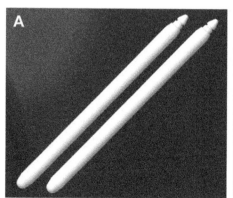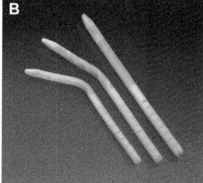

Fig. 2. (*A*) AMS spectra. (*B*) Coloplast Genesis. ([*A*] Image provided courtesy of Boston Scientific. © 2016 Boston Scientific Corporation or its affiliates. All rights reserved.; and [*B*] © Coloplast Corp. REPRINTED WITH PERMISSION-ALL RIGHTS RESERVED. Genesis® Malleable Penile Prosthesis is a registered trademark of Coloplast A/S.)

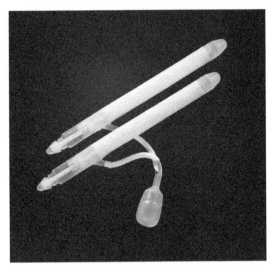

Fig. 3. AMS Ambicor inflatable penile prosthesis. (Image provided courtesy of Boston Scientific. © 2016 Boston Scientific Corporation or its affiliates. All rights reserved.)

to complications from the extraperitoneal location of the reservoir. In patients undergoing kidney transplant, the investigators noted an 8.7% rate of iatrogenic injury to these reservoirs and proposed that this may stem from the unfamiliarity of the reservoir size and location during extraperitoneal exploration by transplant surgeons.

Artificial Urinary Sphincter

Since its introduction in 1972,[14] the AUS remains a standard option for treatment of male stress urinary incontinence. Although other urinary sphincter models do exist on the market outside of the United States,[15] the AMS 800 (American Medical Systems, Minnetonka, MN, USA) remains the only US Food and Drug Administration–approved urinary sphincter in the United States.[16] Approximately 5000 devices are placed worldwide annually with multiple studies demonstrating high satisfaction rates and

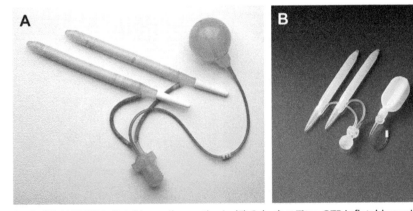

Fig. 4. (A) AMS 700 inflatable penile prosthesis. (B) Coloplast Titan OTR inflatable penile prosthesis. ([A] Image provided courtesy of Boston Scientific. © 2016 Boston Scientific Corporation or its affiliates. All rights reserved.; and [B] © Coloplast Corp. REPRINTED WITH PERMISSION- ALL RIGHTS RESERVED. Titan® Touch Penile Implant is a registered trademark of Coloplast A/S.)

improvement in the quality of lives of affected men.[17-19] Major indications for place-ment of the AUS include stress urinary incontinence secondary to treatment of prostate cancer through either surgical removal of the prostate gland or pelvic radiation. Benign indications also include urinary incontinence from transurethral prostatectomy, pelvic trauma, urethral surgery, or neurogenic causes. Patients must have the manual dexter-ity as well as the mental capacity to safely operate the sphincter multiple times a day.

The AUS consists of 3 components: a control pump, a pressure-regulating balloon, and a fluid-filled cuff. The control pump is placed in a sub-dartos pouch in the anterior scrotum, while the pressure-regulating balloon is placed in the preperitoneal space be-ing inserted either with a lower abdominal incision or through the inguinal canal.[20] A deactivation button is located on the upper portion of the control pump. When pressed, this prevents fluid from being transferred between the components. Cuff sizes range from 3.5 cm to 11 cm, and the size of the cuff is determined by the surgeon intra-operatively. The pressure-regulating balloon is available in 3 preset pressures (51–60, 61–70, 71–80 cm H_2O), which is transmitted through the entire device. The fluid-filled cuff is placed around the urethra, although variations in placement such as the trans-corporal approach have been used by urologists for revision surgery.[21] The cuff is placed through a perineal incision or high scrotal incision, while the scrotal pump and pressure-regulating balloon are placed through a lower abdominal incision below the rectus fascia or pushed through the inguinal canal using the same incision that was used for the cuff. The fluid consists of normal saline or contrast medium, which can facilitate identification of device and allows for troubleshooting postoperatively (**Fig. 5**).

When activated, the sphincter provides continuous continence by occlusion of the urethra with the cuff filled with fluid. To urinate, the patient squeezes the pump in his scrotum 1 to 4 times, which cycles fluid from the pump to the pressure-regulating balloon (**Fig. 6**). This process allows the same volume of fluid to drain from the cuff

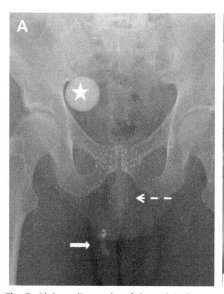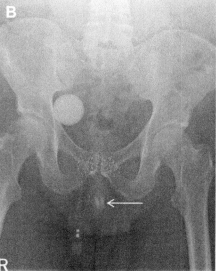

Fig. 5. Plain radiographs of the pelvis demonstrating the components of a contrast filled AUS in a deactivated state. In (*A*), the scrotal pump (*filled arrow*), urethral cuff (*dashed arrow*), and pressure-regulating balloon (*star*) are noted. In (*B*), increased uptake in the urethral cuff is noted (*thin arrow*), demonstrating activation of the device. Multiple seeds from his prior brachytherapy treatment of his prostate cancer are noted.

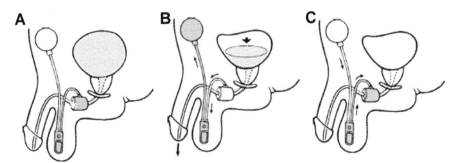

Fig. 6. With an AUS, (A) the urethral cuff (*asterisk*) provides continuous occlusion when activated. Squeezing of the control pump (*B*) transmits fluid in the scrotal pump to the reservoir to allow fluid to exit the urethral cuff and permit voiding. After 3 minutes have passed to allow for volitional voiding, the cuff automatically refills (*C*).

into the pump in a unidirectional fashion, allowing the patient to void volitionally. A delay-fill resistor in the device slows down urethral cuff refilling, allowing a patient 2 to 4 minutes to void before automatic urethral occlusion returns.

PERIOPERATIVE CONSIDERATIONS FOR GENITOURINARY PROSTHESES
Antibiotic Coverage for Nonurologic Surgery

Preoperative antibiotic prophylaxis is used by many surgical subspecialties for prevention of surgical site infection.[22] Surgeons may proceed with antibiotic prophylaxis at their discretion when proceeding with a nonurologic surgical intervention on patients with a urologic prosthetic. When planning for surgical exploration in the patient with an AUS or penile prosthesis, surgeons must assess the risk of exposing the device during surgery. Preoperative planning may be warranted in conjunction with a urologic surgeon as determined by the clinical picture. In cases with high risk of exposure, the authors recommend a preoperative urinalysis and culture to ensure sterility of the urine as well as preoperative antibiotic coverage to protect the urologic device. The American Urologic Association guidelines on antimicrobial prophylaxis recommend use of an aminoglycoside (5 mg/kg) and a first- or second-generation cephalosporin or vancomycin for operative cases involving implantation of a prosthetic device.[23]

Urethral Catheterization with an Artificial Urinary Sphincter or Penile Prosthesis

The authors recommend placement of urethral catheters in these patients only when absolutely necessary! Before urethral catheter placement, it is essential that the AUS be deactivated. Placement of a urethral catheter in the setting of an activated AUS will lead to mucosal trauma and ischemia of the urethra with possible subsequent erosion of the cuff into the urethral lumen.[24–26] This complication may be devastating and ultimately requires removal of the entire device relegating the patient to a state of debilitating incontinence for many months before repeat implantation. Inappropriate urethral catheterization is also a common reason for subsequent litigation.[27] The deactivation button can be located by palpating the upper portion of the control pump in the scrotum. Deactivation is carried out by pressing the scrotal pump to allow emptying of the urethral cuff. Once the scrotal pump partially fills (after a wait of 30–60 seconds), the deactivation button is pushed before complete filling. A slight palpable dimple that remains on the scrotal pump indicates the device is appropriately deactivated. Patients are instructed to carry identification cards, which not only has the name of surgeon who implanted the device but also explains the deactivation process to health care providers that are unfamiliar with the patient's history. Medical identification bracelets have also been recently developed to provide notice in events where patients are unable to communicate this pertinent history to medical providers. Deactivation may be done by the patient, although urologic consultation is warranted if it is not clear that the device is deactivated.

In cases whereby intraoperative urethral catheter drainage is absolutely required, it is imperative to ensure proper management. Many surgical cases may only require opening of the device and deactivating it, thus allowing collection of urine through a condom catheter or into pads because the patient is typically already incontinent (thus the reason for placement of the device in the first place). If a catheter is absolutely required for surgery (for temperature monitoring, strict fluid output assessment, and so on), the authors recommend placement of the smallest possible (10–12 French) urethral catheter to facilitate bladder drainage during an operation. Whenever feasible, the catheter should be removed within 72 hours; this will help minimize injury to the cuff as well as urethral erosion. In cases of prolonged urinary retention where a patient is unable to void or leak sufficiently in the setting of a deactivated device, the authors recommend suprapubic catheter placement.

Management of Traumatic Urethral Catheterization

Suspicion of a traumatic urethral catheterization in the setting of an activated AUS should be considered in cases whereby clinicians note significant difficulty with catheterization or new-onset hematuria. Urology consultation is warranted in these cases. It is the authors' practice to perform immediate urethroscopy for assessment of the urethra to evaluate for cuff erosion. In cases whereby erosion of the cuff into the urethra is identified, explantation of the device is performed with removal of all components. Urethral repair should be performed at the time of removal, which may reduce the likelihood of development of a urethral stricture.[28] In cases whereby mucosal trauma is identified without obvious urethral cuff erosion, the device is deactivated, and further urethral instrumentation is avoided to facilitate urethral rest. Repeat urethroscopy is performed 2 weeks from the inciting event for repeat assessment of the cuff; the device is then activated under direct vision to ensure that an occult urethral injury is not missed with the AUS in an activated state.

GENERAL SURGICAL CONSIDERATIONS
Inguinal Hernias

The development of inguinal hernias after AUS or penile prosthesis has been described.[29] This development of inguinal hernias is thought to be due to weakening of the posterior wall of the inguinal canal because of incision of the transversalis fascia when placing the balloon in a preperitoneal fashion. However, the prevalence of inguinal hernias after AUS placement is not well defined. Leroy and colleagues[30] described using a laparoscopic transabdominal preperitoneal approach for correction of hernias in patients with an existing AUS, which allows early identification of the reservoir, to minimize the risk of inadvertent injury that may be encountered through a traditional anterior inguinal approach.

Small Bowel Obstruction

Literature surrounding small bowel obstruction due to a reservoir from either an AUS or penile prosthesis when those parts are placed intraperitoneal is limited to case reports.[31,32] These cases may stem from inadvertent blind placement of the reservoir through the peritoneum, which can be related to scarring in the space of Retzius. These cases have been managed successfully with exploratory laparotomy and removal of the offending reservoir.

Vascular Complications

Vascular complications related to AUSs and inflatable penile prosthesis are rare; when they do occur, comanagement with vascular surgery is advised. Deep venous thrombosis has been described after 3-piece inflatable penile prosthesis placement.[33,34] Deep venous thrombosis has been attributed to mechanical compression of the pelvic veins by the reservoir leading to stasis and thrombus formation; this is managed by repositioning of the reservoir along with simultaneous anticoagulation. One case was also managed with venous thrombectomy.[34] Arterial insufficiency leading to critical limb ischemia has also been described and presents with acute right lower extremity edema and pain in the immediate postoperative period.[35] This arterial insufficiency was treated with repositioning of the reservoir from outside the space of Retzius to an ectopic position along with use of a smaller volume reservoir.

Managing Iatrogenic Injuries to the Device During Nonurologic Surgery

Literature regarding management of intraoperative injury to AUSs and penile prosthesis in nonurologic surgery is sparse. The authors' experience for intraoperative management of genitourinary prostheses in nonurologic surgery is based on the approach to retained urologic devices and sterile erosions described in the urologic literature. Cefalu and colleagues[36] demonstrated in their retrospective review that intentionally draining and leaving existing reservoirs from inflatable penile prostheses and AUSs in situ during noninfected reoperative surgery does not increase infection rates compared with cases when all components are removed. Boateng and colleagues[37] managed tubing erosion of AUS with antibiotic irrigation and reinsertion with no postoperative infectious complications. Singla and Singla[38] showed that in very select cases eroded components from an AUS can be managed nonsurgically long term, although the authors prefer to proceed with device removal in these types of cases.

At the authors' institution, injuries to urologic prostheses within a grossly contaminated operative field (ie, fecal spillage, abscess, or infected body fluids) are managed with immediate explantation of all components. However, if the pseudocapsule of the device is not opened or in cases whereby the operative field is sterile, and the clinical situation is deemed not appropriate for immediate repair of the device (ie, unstable patient, unavailable device components), nonabsorbable sutures are tied to the tubing to enable identifying components at a later operative session and to prevent seepage of body fluid into the device itself. This course of action can be followed by delayed revision of the device. When urologic consultation is available intraoperatively and the urologic surgeon has experience with prosthetic surgery, a device that is damaged during surgical exploration may be immediately repaired in specific cases. This immediate repair requires the facility to have on hand the components needed to repair the device, a sterile field, and an operative team familiar with exploration and revision of the device. Device exploration when no injury to a component is suspected must be avoided because this may lead to unnecessary damage and incision into the pseudocapsule, thus exposing the device to further infection.

SUMMARY

ED and urinary incontinence are 2 conditions that carry a significant burden to the quality of lives of those that are affected. The use of genitourinary prosthetics, such as the penile prosthesis and AUS, are used effectively in men with these conditions. With the increase in utilization of penile prosthesis and AUSs, it is important for all surgeons irrespective of their specialty to recognize preoperatively whether their patients have genitourinary prosthetics to facilitate preoperative planning. The need for deactivation of AUS before urethral catheterization cannot be understated in order to minimize unnecessary morbidity of urethral injury and erosion. The length of urethral catheterization in patients with either type of device should be limited given the risk of infection to the device. Communication with a urologist before nonurologic surgery can help mitigate the potential consequences.

REFERENCES

1. Wessells H, Joyce G, Wise M, et al. Erectile dysfunction. J Urol 2007;177(5): 1675–81.
2. Selvin E, Burnett A, Platz E. Prevalence and risk factors for erectile dysfunction in the US. Am J Med 2007;120(2):151–7.
3. Montague DK. Penile prosthesis implantation in the era of medical treatment for erectile dysfunction. Urol Clin North Am 2011;38(2):217–25.
4. Ralph DJ, Garaffa G, Muneer A, et al. The immediate insertion of a penile prosthesis for acute ischaemic priapism. Eur Urol 2009;56(6):1033–8.
5. Tausch TJ, Mauck R, Zhao LC, et al. Penile prosthesis insertion for acute priapism. Urol Clin North Am 2013;40(3):421–5.
6. Perkash I, Kabalin JN, Lennon S, et al. Use of penile prostheses to maintain external condom catheter drainage in spinal cord injury patients. Paraplegia 1992;30(5):327–32.
7. Tikkinen KA, Agarwal A, Griebling TL. Epidemiology of male urinary incontinence. Curr Opin Urol 2013;23(6):502–8.
8. Shamliyan TA, Wyman JF, Ping R, et al. Male urinary incontinence: prevalence, risk factors, and preventive interventions. Rev Urol 2009;11(3):145–65.
9. Poon SA, Silberstein JL, Savage C, et al. Surgical practice patterns for male urinary incontinence: analysis of case logs from certifying American urologists. J Urol 2012;188(1):205–10.
10. Yossepowitch O, Aviv D, Wainchwaig L, et al. Testicular prostheses for testis cancer survivors: patient perspectives and predictors of long-term satisfaction. J Urol 2011;186(6):2249–52.
11. Zilberman D, Winkler H, Kleinmann N, et al. Testicular prosthesis insertion following testicular loss or atrophy during early childhood—technical aspects and evaluation of patient satisfaction. J Pediatr Urol 2007;3(6):461–5.
12. Sadeghi-Nejad H, Fam M. Penile prosthesis surgery in the management of erectile dysfunction. Arab J Urol 2013;11(3):245–53.
13. Cuellar DC, Sklar GN. Penile prosthesis in the organ transplant recipient. Urology 2001;57(1):138–41.
14. Scott FB, Bradley WE, Timm GW. Treatment of urinary incontinence by an implantable prosthetic urinary sphincter. J Urol 1974;112(1):75–80.
15. Vakalopoulos I, Kampantais S, Laskaridis L, et al. New artificial urinary sphincter devices in the treatment of male iatrogenic incontinence. Adv Urol 2012;2012:439372.
16. U.S. Food and Drug Administration. AMS sphincter 800™ urinary prosthesis— P000053. 2001. Available at: http://www.accessdata.fda.gov/scripts/cdrh/cfdocs/cftopic/pma/pma.cfm?num=p000053. Accessed August 7, 2015.
17. Peterson AC, Webster GD. Artificial urinary sphincter: lessons learned. Urol Clin North Am 2011;38(1):83–8.
18. Van der Aa F, Drake MJ, Kasyan GR, et al. The artificial urinary sphincter after a quarter of a century: a critical systematic review of its use in male non-neurogenic incontinence. Eur Urol 2013;63(4):681–9.

19. Ratan HL, Summerton DJ, Wilson SK, et al. Development and current status of the AMS 800 artificial urinary sphincter. EAU-EBU Update Series 2006;4(3):117–28.

20. Chung PH, Morey AF, Tausch TJ, et al. High submuscular placement of urologic prosthetic balloons and reservoirs: 2-year experience and patient-reported outcomes. Urology 2014;84(6):1535–40.

21. Guralnick ML, Miiler E, Toh KL, et al. Transcorporal artificial urinary sphincter cuff placement in cases requiring revision for erosion and urethral atrophy. J Urol 2002;167(5):2075–9.

22. Bratzler DW, Houck PM, Surgical Infection Prevention Guidelines Writers Workgroup, et al. Antimicrobial prophylaxis for surgery: an advisory statement from the National Surgical Infection Prevention Project. Clin Infect Dis 2004;38(12):1706–15.

23. Wolf J, Bennett C, Dmochowski R, et al. Best practice policy statement on urologic surgery antimicrobial prophylaxis. 2014. Available at: https://www.auanet.org/education/guidelines/antimicrobial-prophylaxis.cfm. Accessed September 6, 2015.

24. Seideman CA, Zhao LC, Hudak SJ, et al. Is prolonged catheterization a risk factor for artificial urinary sphincter cuff erosion? Urology 2013;82(4):943–6.

25. Khoury JM, Webster GD, Perez LM. Urethral cuff erosion as a result of urinary catheterization in patients with an artificial urinary sphincter. N C Med J 1994;55(5):162–4.

26. Steidle CP, Mulcahy JJ. Erosion of penile prostheses: a complication of urethral catheterization. J Urol 1989;142(3):736–9.

27. Osman NI, Collins GN. Urological litigation in the UK National Health Service (NHS): an analysis of 14 years of successful claims. BJU Int 2011;108(2):162–5.

28. Rozanski AT, Tausch TJ, Ramirez D, et al. Immediate urethral repair during explantation prevents stricture formation after artificial urinary sphincter cuff erosion. J Urol 2014;192(2):442–6.

29. Serio SJ, Schafer P, Merchant AM. Incarcerated inguinal hernia and small bowel obstruction as a rare complication of a penile prosthesis. Hernia 2013;17(6):809–12.

30. Leroy J, Saussine C, Marescaux J. TAPP laparoscopic repair of right inguinal hernia after artificial sphincter placement for post-prostatectomy urinary incontinence. 2013. Available at: http://www.websurg.com/doi-vd01en3879.htm. Accessed July 30, 2015.

31. Johnson MH, Johnson FE. Small bowel obstruction from a displaced penile prosthesis reservoir: case report and review of the literature. Br J Med Med Res 2014;4(22):4025.

32. Luks FI, Huntley HN, Tula JC, et al. Small-bowel obstruction by an inflatable penile prosthesis reservoir. Surgery 1989;106(1):101–4.

33. da Justa DG, Bianco FJ Jr, Ogle A, et al. Deep venous thrombosis due to compression of external iliac vein by the penile prosthesis reservoir. Urology 2003;61(2):462.

34. Brison D, Ilbeigi P, Sadeghi-Nejad H. Reservoir repositioning and successful thrombectomy for deep venous thrombosis secondary to compression of pelvic veins by an inflatable penile prosthesis reservoir. J Sex Med 2007;4(4ii):1185–7.

35. Deho' F, Henry GD, Marone EM, et al. Severe vascular complication after implantation of a three-piece inflatable penile prosthesis. J Sex Med 2008;5(12):2956–9.

36. Cefalu CA, Deng X, Zhao LC, et al. Safety of the "drain and retain" option for defunctionalized urologic prosthetic balloons and reservoirs during artificial urinary sphincter and inflatable penile prosthesis revision surgery: 5-year experience. Urology 2013;82(6):1436–9.

37. Boateng AA, Mohamed MA, Mahdy AE. Novel management approach to connecting tube erosion of artificial urinary sphincter. Can J Urol 2014;21(2):7246–7.
38. Singla N, Singla AK. Review of single-surgeon 10-year experience with artificial urinary sphincter with report of sterile cuff erosion managed nonsurgically. Urology 2015;85(1):252–7.

Pediatric Urology for the General Surgeon

David J. Chalmers, MD[a],*, Vijaya M. Vemulakonda, MD, JD[b]

KEYWORDS

- Pediatric urology • Inguinal hernia • Hydrocele • Cryptorchidism • Circumcision
- Genitourinary trauma

KEY POINTS

- The decision to perform pediatric inguinal herniorrhaphy depends on accurately distinguishing between a true inguinal hernia, communicating hydrocele, and simple hydrocele.
- Timely orchiopexy for the undescended testis best preserves fertility and endocrine function, while protecting against trauma and minimizing malignancy potential.
- The benefits of neonatal circumcision modestly outweigh the risks of the procedure, thus justifying access to fully informed families.
- Trauma to the genitourinary tract can typically be managed conservatively, recognizing key indications for surgical intervention.

INTRODUCTION

There are several common pediatric urologic conditions that could potentially impact the general surgeon. Particularly in rural areas, access to pediatric urology expertise may be limited. A working knowledge of a few common problems may obviate patient referrals or help the surgeon determine what care can be safely delivered without urology subspecialty. This article reviews the pathophysiology of several problems commonly encountered by pediatric urologists and describes a practical approach for the general surgeon, including the pediatric inguinal hernia or hydrocele, the cryptorchid testis, and circumcision. Additional focus is devoted to genitourinary trauma to help guide management in acute, emergent situations that lack on-site subspecialty expertise.

HERNIA/HYDROCELE
Background

The pediatric inguinal hernia may be most familiar to the general surgeon because of the similar anatomy encountered during indirect inguinal hernias in adults. In utero, the

Disclosure Statement: The authors have nothing to disclose.
[a] Division of Urology, Maine Medical Center, Tufts University School of Medicine, 22 Bramhall Street, Portland, ME 04102, USA; [b] Department of Pediatric Urology, Children's Hospital Colorado, 12123 East 16th Avenue, Aurora, CO 80045, USA
* Corresponding author. 100 Brickhill Avenue, South Portland, ME 04106.
E-mail address: dchalmers@mmc.org

processus vaginalis allows the testes to pass through the inguinal canal between 20 to 28 weeks gestation[1] and typically obliterates after testis passage. Persistent patency of the processus may result in a symptomatic hernia or hydrocele. The term "hernia" suggests the passage of abdominal contents, such as bowel or omentum, through the inguinal canal. The term "communicating hydrocele" suggests a smaller opening that allows passage of fluid alone. The incidence of patent processus vaginalis in the pediatric population is between 1% and 5% and occurs more commonly in males.[2,3] Significant risk factors for inguinal hernia include cryptorchidism, prematurity, and low birth weight.[2–4] There is also an increased familial risk and in a variety of syndromes.[2,5] These conditions are distinct from the simple hydrocele, meaning that fluid is present within the scrotum, but does not communicate.

Diagnosis

The typical presentation of pediatric inguinal hernia or hydrocele is scrotal or inguino-scrotal swelling. Pain or nausea symptoms are rare, even with tense distention of the scrotum, and testis viability is not compromised. Diurnal size variation of the scrotum is a key diagnostic feature of a communicating hydrocele, classically enlarging after physical activity or toward the end of the day and diminishing by the morning. Swelling that extends into the inguinal canal is more likely to indicate a hernia. Occasionally, abdominal contents can be palpated and manually reduced. Other notable physical examination findings include the "silk glove" sign, which entails palpating the layers of the patent processus vaginalis slipping over each other, and transillumination of the scrotum with a penlight (**Fig. 1**). If the physical examination is normal and the family cannot give a clear history of diurnal size fluctuation, it is reasonable to repeat the examination in follow-up and ask the family to further observe the scrotal size in the mornings and evenings.

It may be challenging to differentiate between a communicating hydrocele and a true inguinal hernia; however, the difference is important. The primary concern with hernia is the risk of bowel incarceration. The signs and symptoms of an incarcerated hernia include erythema, a firm bulge, and pain over the inguinal canal. This condition is an emergency because of the risk of strangulation and peritonitis. This risk should be absent with communicating hydroceles because the patent processus vaginalis is so narrow.

If the ipsilateral testis is not palpable because of a tense, distended scrotum, ultrasonography can confirm the presence of the testis and rule out secondary hydrocele

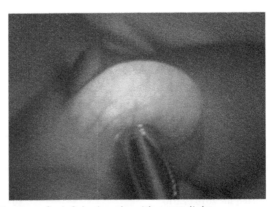

Fig. 1. Transillumination of a left hydrocele with a pen light.

from a testis tumor. If the testis is palpably normal, imaging is not necessary. Simple hydroceles (noncommunicating) that are not associated with hernia should be considered differently. Simple hydrocele is common in male neonates, presumably from delayed closure of the processus that traps fluid within the scrotum.[6] The natural history of the simple hydrocele in the perinatal period is for the fluid to slowly resorb over time. Similarly, simple hydroceles presenting in the postpubertal period can be observed in hopes of spontaneous resolution.

Management

Surgical repair has been the historic mainstay of treatment of pediatric inguinal hernias and communicating hydroceles, although there may be a role for observation in the latter. Hernia repair is normally performed promptly following the diagnosis and can be performed as an outpatient procedure as long as the adjusted gestational age is great enough (typically >50 weeks). The timing of hernia repair is controversial when the diagnosis is made in the neonatal period, and entails balancing the risks of anesthesia in the neonatal period versus the risk of bowel incarceration. Hernias may be present in approximately 15% of premature infants and the risk of incarceration rises the longer it remains untreated.[7,8] For this reason, hernias in premature and low-birth-weight infants are commonly fixed before hospital discharge, although the decision to defer surgery is reasonable if the caretakers can be educated and have the capacity to seek urgent medical attention in case of incarceration.[9] This is an ongoing controversy that is the impetus for an ongoing prospective trial.[10]

Communicating hydroceles have historically been treated similarly to true hernias. However, recent data suggest they can be safely managed conservatively. A variety of small studies have suggested that most communicating hydroceles spontaneously resolve if given enough time.[11,12] Current practice patterns from the American Academy of Pediatrics Section on Surgery vary widely, including prompt treatment similar to hernia versus waiting up to 2 years of age.[13]

Surgery

An inguinal approach to hernia/hydrocele repair is traditional because of a low complication rate, low morbidity, good cosmesis, and the ability to successfully achieve a high ligation of the hernia sac at the level of the internal inguinal ring to minimize the risk of recurrence.[14] Key components of the surgery include exposing the external oblique fascia, sharp incision of the fascia to preserve the ilioinguinal nerve, and careful dissection of the sac away from the spermatic cord structures. With this approach, postoperative complications are rare, including bleeding, wound infection, reactive hydrocele, and injury to the genital tract (testis atrophy, secondary cryptorchidism, vas deferens injury). Hernia recurrence is about 1%.[14,15]

Laparoscopic and scrotal approaches to pediatric inguinal hernia repair have also been described. The potential concern regarding the scrotal approach is the ability to achieve a high sac ligation. However, numerous series have demonstrated successful outcomes with similar recurrence risk, decreased operative time, and improved cosmesis.[16,17] Meanwhile, laparoscopic hernia repair has also been successful via a peritoneal closure[18] and extraperitoneal approach.[19,20] A potential advantage is the ability to easily assess and address the contralateral inguinal ring, which may be patent in about 40% of children with clinical unilateral hernias, and presents clinically in about 10% of patients.[21,22] Exploration of the contralateral ring via open approaches is no longer common because of the unlikely clinical significance.

CRYPTORCHIDISM
Background

Cryptorchidism, or undescended testis, is commonly treated by pediatric urologists or pediatric surgeons. The incidence is approximately 3% to 5% of newborn males and increases to 30% in premature infants.[23–25] The primary reasons for treating the condition are the risk of fertility decline in the affected testis, decline in hormonal function of the affected testis, an increased risk for testicular torsion or trauma, and the increased risk of testicular malignancy. Spontaneous descent postnatally occurs, but further descent is unlikely beyond 6 months of age[26] and observation should not delay prompt treatment. Timely orchiopexy in infancy has been shown to preserve testicular function and likely diminish the risk of malignancy.[27,28] Although men with bilateral cryptorchidism have significantly reduced fertility rates of approximately 62%,[29] unilateral cryptorchidism leads to a fertility rate of approximately 90%, which is not significantly different from the general population.[30]

Diagnosis

The most important aspects of the history are determining if the family ever notices the testis in an intrascrotal position, particularly in relaxed, warm environments, such as the bathtub, where the testis location would likely be maximally descended. Additional history should note premature delivery, which increases the risk for cryptorchidism, and previous inguinal surgery, a risk factor for secondary ascent.

A thorough physical examination typically starts with the child in a supine position, although sitting cross-legged can also be tried. Examination is most commonly started with a sweeping motion of the nondominant hand from the anterior superior iliac spine inferomedially toward the groin. If the testis is palpable, the dominant hand can attempt to grasp the testis. With a combination of sweeping and pulling, the testis can often be drawn into the scrotum. Palpable undescended testes can be classified by their location in the upper scrotum, the superficial pouch, or the inguinal canal. A nonpalpable testis should be considered intra-abdominal until proven otherwise.

It is challenging to distinguish testicular retraction from a truly undescended testis. The cremasteric reflex frequently draws testes into seemingly inguinal locations, particularly in toddler-aged boys. If there is a question of retractile versus undescended testis, the testis should be held in a dependent intrascrotal position for 30 seconds to fatigue the cremaster muscle. If the testis remains in a dependent position after release, then it is safely considered retractile. If it immediately ascends out of the scrotum, it should be considered undescended. This assessment is critical because it determines the need for surgery. The natural history of the retractile testis is to gradually descend into a more obvious scrotal position with age and testis size increase.

Imaging and laboratory tests are typically unnecessary in boys with cryptorchidism. The diagnostic accuracy of ultrasound or computed tomography (CT) imaging declines significantly in cases of intra-abdominal testes when imaging may be theoretically most helpful.[31] More importantly, results of imaging studies do not influence management decisions. Diagnostic laparoscopy or open surgery is necessary regardless of whether or not the study identifies a testis. Indications for laboratory evaluation are also uncommon. The most important exception is concurrent hypospadias and cryptorchidism, which is concerning for possible disorder of sex differentiation. Karyotype and referral for endocrine evaluation is appropriate.

Treatment

The mainstay of treatment of the undescended testis is surgery. Hormonal therapy with human chorionic gonadotropin or gonadotropin-releasing hormone has been used historically with the aim of stimulating descent through androgen production. However, multiple series have demonstrated suboptimal outcomes and this approach is no longer recommended in the United States.[32] Surgery is optimally performed between 6 and 18 months of age when the risks of anesthesia have reached a nadir, but the timing is early enough to avoid histologic degradation.[33]

The surgical approach depends on the location of the testis and the first step to any orchiopexy procedure is to re-examine the patient under anesthesia. A previously nonpalpable testis may become palpable in about 20% of cases, obviating abdominal exploration. For the palpable undescended testis, an incision over the inguinal canal is most common. Key principles of the procedure include protecting the cord structures, including the vessels and vas deferens; transecting the cremaster muscle fibers; and dividing the spermatic fascial attachments to the testis and cord. Undescended testes are frequently associated with an inguinal hernia. The most important maneuver to achieve mobility of the testis is to isolate the patent or obliterated processus vaginalis off of the anteriomedial surface of the cord and ligate it proximally. The testis is then fixated into the ipsilateral hemiscrotum as dependently as possible with a fixation suture or with a sutureless subdartos pouch. Fixation sutures may position the testis more securely but risk parenchymal damage.[34] With this approach, success rates may exceed 95% with rare testicular atrophy or secondary ascent. More recently, a primary scrotal approach has also proved to be successful,[35,36] although many surgeons reserve this approach for testes that are close to or can be drawn into the scrotum.

In cases of nonpalpable testes, abdominal exploration is indicated. Diagnostic laparoscopy has replaced open exploration and most commonly reveals the following situations:

1. Blind-ending gonadal vessels above the internal inguinal ring indicate a "vanishing testis" that likely suffered an early prenatal vascular event. There is no need to proceed at this point (**Fig. 2**).
2. A viable intra-abdominal testis is discovered. Depending on the location and comfort level of the surgeon, options include primary laparoscopic orchiopexy, a one-stage Fowler-Stephens orchiopexy where the spermatic artery is divided and the testis survives on the vas deferens and cremasteric arteries,[37] or a two-stage Fowler-Stephens procedure where the artery is divided in the first stage and the testis is repositioned 6 months later using additional collateral vessels (**Fig. 3**).
3. Cord structures are seen entering the internal ring, indicating either a testis that was missed on examination or a testicular nubbin within the canal or scrotum. Nubbins or dysplastic-appearing testes are usually excised because of concern of future malignancy (**Fig. 4**).

Laparoscopic orchiopexy is a challenging procedure, particularly if the testis is located superiorly in the abdomen. Success rates may diminish to 80% or lower.[38]

CIRCUMCISION

Background

Circumcision is one of the oldest surgical procedures, dating back to antiquity.[39] It is routinely performed for social, religious, and cultural reasons and the prevalence

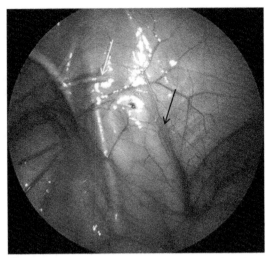

Fig. 2. Right internal ring with blind ending vas (*yellow arrow*) and vessels (*black arrow*).

highly depends on the geographic region.[39] Providers who counsel families about the decision to circumcise should provide objective information regarding the potential benefits of being circumcised and the risks of the surgical procedure. In the United States, approximately 60% of male newborns undergo neonatal circumcision,[40] but it may be deferred because of low birth weight, unfavorable anatomy (buried penis, incomplete foreskin), or comorbid conditions. Indications for circumcision later in life include urinary tract infections (UTIs) or sequela related to phimosis.

Circumcision Benefits

Circumcision reduces the bacteria that accumulates under the prepuce and reduces the risk of UTI in the infant period.[41] Given the low risk of UTI in infant males (~1%), the number of circumcisions needed to prevent a UTI is approximately 100; however, there may be a more substantial benefit in children at increased risk for UTI. There

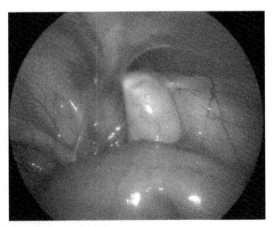

Fig. 3. "Peeping" intra-abdominal testis.

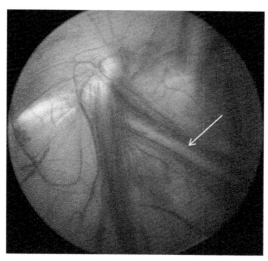

Fig. 4. Closed internal inguinal ring with vas deferens (*arrow*) and vessels.

are a variety of proposed reasons why circumcision may influence the risk of infection. The prepuce is thin and may be more susceptible to microabrasions, there may be entrapment of pathogens within the uncircumcised prepuce, and the prepuce has a particularly high concentration of CD4 T cells.[42–44]

Other infectious benefits include reducing the risk of human immunodeficiency virus transmission[45] and a lower prevalence of human papillomavirus infection[46] and herpes simplex virus type 2 transmission.[47] Other sexually transmitted infections do not seem to be significantly affected by circumcision status.[48] Additional benefits of male circumcision include decreasing the risk of invasive penile cancer.[49] Because the incidence of penile cancer is already low, it would likely require thousands of circumcisions to prevent one case. Improved hygiene of the uncircumcised penis is likely a better preventive strategy because it avoids procedure complications. Finally, there seems to be a modest protective effect of male circumcision against cervical cancer in the respective female partners[50] likely related to the difference in human papillomavirus infection transmission.

Neonatal Circumcision

There are three common techniques for performing circumcision in the neonatal period: (1) the Gomco clamp, (2) the Plastibell, and (3) the Mogen clamp. Key components to all three techniques include adequate local anesthesia (dorsal penile nerve block or penile ring block typically), estimating an appropriate amount of prepuce to be removed, reducing penile adhesions to visualize the glans, correctly placing the device, leaving the device in place long enough to provide hemostasis, and removal of the redundant prepuce. Each technique is performed safely with low complication rates of 0.2% to 3% depending on the definition.[51,52] Contraindications include some anatomic congenital anomalies, including hypospadias (**Fig. 5**), buried penis syndrome (**Fig. 6**), or ambiguous genitalia. Bleeding diatheses or failure to administer Vitamin K in the neonatal period are relative contraindications. Bleeding is the most common complication that can typically be controlled by a compression dressing. Major complications, such as glans amputation or urethral injury, are very rare. Late complications, including excessive residual skin (incomplete circumcision), penile

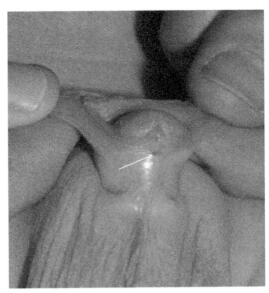

Fig. 5. Hypospadias (true meatus marked with arrow) with dorsal hooded foreskin.

adhesions, skin bridges, meatal stenosis, cicatrix scar formation, and epithelial inclusion cysts, are more common and can be treated electively.

Postnewborn Circumcision

The incidence of circumcision complications is significantly higher outside of the neonatal period.[53] The risk of significant bleeding, infection, and cosmetic defects is

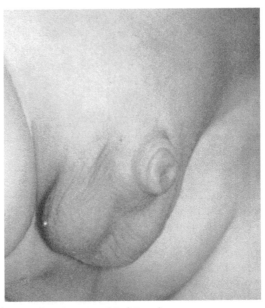

Fig. 6. Buried penis, prominent suprapubic fat pad.

substantially greater compared with neonatal circumcision. Furthermore, general anesthesia is required because the procedure takes longer and involves ensuring hemostasis and suturing skin edges. General anesthesia carries a low risk of significant morbidity or mortality (1 death per 400,000)[54] and is minimized by ensuring patients are in an optimal state of health. Specifically, general anesthesia should be performed in a facility familiar with pediatric anesthesia and should not be performed with active airway disease or recent upper respiratory infection.[55]

Risk-Benefit Assessment

It is currently not possible to fully weigh the medical benefits of circumcision against the risks associated with the procedure. The Centers for Disease Control and Prevention study found that male circumcision before the first sexual encounter was cost-effective for the prevention of human immunodeficiency virus in the United States.[56] This study did not take into account the other potential infectious benefits of circumcision and did not attempt to assess the significance of the surgical complications. The optimal time to perform circumcision seems to be in the neonatal period when the risk profile is lowest and an operative procedure under general anesthesia can be avoided. Ideally, parents should receive factually correct, nonbiased information about circumcision before delivery so a fully informed decision is made in the neonatal period. For these reasons, the American Academy of Pediatrics takes the position that the preventive and public health benefits associated with newborn male circumcision outweigh the risks, and this should justify access to this procedure for those families who choose it.[57]

GENITOURINARY TRAUMA
Introduction

Trauma is the leading cause of mortality in the pediatric population, largely from motor vehicle accidents.[58–60] Fortunately, injuries to the genitourinary tract are rare, but can be responsible for significant morbidity.[61] Similar to any evaluation of the trauma patient, a comprehensive history and physical examination should be performed as quickly as possible. In a child with blunt or penetrating abdominal trauma, key details for the urology perspective include the mechanism of injury; associated multiorgan injury; and the presence of hematuria, abdominal or flank tenderness, rib fractures, and abdominal contusions or abrasions. Penetrating injury to the flank or abdomen is particularly worrisome for genitourinary injury and a likely indication for further imaging. The presence of multisystem trauma, gross hematuria, and substantial microscopic hematuria are additional details that also warrant further investigation.[62–64]

Unlike in the adult trauma setting, blood pressure and heart rate are not sensitive indicators of shock in children. Tachycardia may be a result of anxiety or pain from the trauma and children are capable of compensating for significant blood loss through vasoconstriction and increased cardiac output. If an injured child's blood pressure does decrease because of hypovolemia, it is a late sign of instability. For this reason, adults with blunt trauma and microhematuria without hypotension are often observed. However, because hypotension is an unreliable predictor of pediatric renal injury, all children with a history of significant blunt abdominal trauma and any degree of hematuria should undergo imaging of the urinary tract regardless of vital signs.

The physical examination should focus on abdominal and genital signs of injury. A mass or ecchymosis of the flank may represent a perinephric hematoma or urinoma. Eccymosis of the perineum in a butterfly configuration indicates blood tracking within Colles fasica. Scrotal or labial hematoma or edema can result from genital trauma or pelvic injury. Blood at the urethral meatus or urinary retention must raise suspicion for urethral injury. The presence of these findings warrants further evaluation in the stable patient.

Renal Trauma

The kidney is the most common site of genitourinary injury, resulting in approximately half of all genitourinary injuries in children. Most (>80%) injuries to the kidney are from blunt trauma, whereas the remaining injuries are penetrating in nature.[61] Notably, renal injury seldom occurs in isolation. Approximately 80% of all grades of renal injury have other associated organ injuries.[58,65] Current management of renal injuries has shifted toward a nonoperative approach with up to 85% of blunt renal injuries managed non-operatively.[61] Goals of either a conservative or surgical approach should focus on preservation of renal tissue and kidney function while minimizing the morbidity and mortality of the injury to the child.

Hematuria is an important indicator of injury to the kidney; however, more than 50% of children sustaining renal trauma may fail to demonstrate hematuria on presentation and the degree of hematuria does not correlate with injury severity.[66–68] Children's higher sympathetic tone and the less reliable correlation between hematuria and injury dictate a greater reliance on the clinical history and the presence of associated injuries compared with adults.

Indications for radiographic work-up in the pediatric trauma patient include penetrating injury to the abdomen or flank; blunt trauma resulting from significant deceleration, such as a high-velocity motor vehicle collision or fall; blunt trauma leading to other significant multiorgan injuries; and gross hematuria or microscopic hematuria greater than 50 red blood cells per high-power field.

Contrast-enhanced CT is the primary imaging modality used to assess injury to the urinary tract and is necessary to properly stage renal injury. Most emergency departments have an established renal protocol including noncontrast, contrast, and delayed phases to evaluate the renal blood vessels, parenchyma, and the entire collecting system, respectively. Conversely, ultrasonography is not reliable in renal trauma situations. Ultrasonography misses an unacceptable proportion of renal lacerations and low-grade renal injuries.[69] Ultrasound is accurate in monitoring perinephric fluid, such as urinoma or hematoma, however. For this reason, it may be more appropriate to monitor defined injuries periodically with ultrasound rather than reimaging with CT scan as is common following adult trauma.[70,71] The modality and timing of reimaging following renal trauma is physician dependent, but generally not necessary for low-grade trauma.

The degree of renal injury is assessed by a grading scale (**Table 1**)[72] and is a critical tool in determining appropriate management. Renal contusions or hematomas are considered grade 1 injuries and are the most common injuries to the kidney constituting 80% of renal trauma.[73,74] Grade II and III renal injuries occur when the renal parenchyma tears. Tears less than 1 cm are considered grade II and greater than 1 cm are grade III. These lacerations are considered minor if they are limited to the parenchyma of the kidney and do not extend into the collecting system. These injuries likely produce more pain and nausea than contusion and may lead to extensive perinephric hematomas, but there should not be urinary extravasation. Conservative management is appropriate for lower grades of renal injury (I–III) and commonly involves bed rest until hematocrit measurements have stabilized and hematuria has resolved. Re-evaluation with ultrasound can reliably detect an expanding urinoma or hematoma. Following discharge, limited activity should be recommended for 2 to 6 weeks according to the clinician's impression. This approach has proved to be highly successful in

Table 1
Renal injury grading scale

Grade	Injury	CT Appearance
I	Contusion	Microscopic or gross hematuria
	Hematoma	Subcapsular, nonexpanding without parenchymal tear
II	Hematoma	Nonexpanding perirenal hematoma
	Laceration	<1.0-cm parenchymal depth of renal cortex without collecting system rupture or urinary extravagation
III	Laceration	>1.0-cm parenchymal depth of renal cortex without collecting system rupture or urinary extravagation
IV	Laceration	Parenchymal laceration extending through renal cortex, medulla, and collecting system
	Vascular	Main renal artery or vein injury with contained hemorrhage
V	Laceration	Completely shattered kidney
	Vascular	Avulsion of renal hilum, with devascularized kidney

avoiding long-term complications, such as hypertension, loss of renal function, and hydronephrosis.[75] Patients that decline clinically or are unstable may require additional CT imaging and possible intervention, such as exploration with an attempt at renal repair, placement of a ureteral stent, or angiographic embolization.

Severe lacerations that extend into the kidney and disrupt the collecting system are considered grade IV injuries. Bleeding can be extensive and may fill the Gerota fascia space completely. Although the amount of blood may be impressive, this is not necessarily an indication to intervene surgically. As the space within Gerota fascia fills with blood, blood loss may be contained and tamponaded by the hematoma itself. The diagnosis of urinary extravasation also indicates a grade IV injury and requires delayed imaging by CT scan for accurate diagnosis. Grade IV injury may also result from injury to the hilar vessels with contained hemorrhage.

Wide separation of multiple renal fragments indicates a "shattered kidney" and is the most common appearance of a grade V injury. It can be difficult to determine what segments are poorly perfused because of severe contusion and what tissue may be truly devitalized. Massive bleeding and extravasation within Gerota fascia is common. Major hilar injury leading to devascularization also defines grade V renal injuries. The warm ischemia time inherent to this type of injury makes salvage unlikely and surgery is generally reserved for nephrectomy to stabilize active hemorrhage. Even under ideal circumstances, salvage rates for kidneys with renal pedicle injuries are less than 30%.[76,77]

The management of severe renal injury (grades IV–V) is more controversial and requires an individualized approach. A significant consideration is that surgical intervention may lead to nephrectomy rates higher than 85%.[78] Patients who are hemodynamically stable with isolated high-grade renal injuries are candidates for nonoperative management. Nonetheless, surgery is indicated for patients with a vascular pedicle injury or shattered kidney that place the patient at risk for life-threatening hemorrhage. Absolute indications for operative intervention also include an expanding or pulsatile retroperitoneal hematoma and the inability to stop hemorrhage by selective angioembolization. Relative indications for exploration are significant urinary extravasation, nonviable renal tissue, arterial injury, and expanding hematoma or if accurate staging is not possible. Surgical management should first focus on control of the renal pedicle and aorta. When hemostasis is achieved, inspection of the kidney and collecting system can be performed. Devitalized tissue should be debrided and any defects in the parenchyma closed and covered if possible. Urinary extravasation can be managed with a ureteral stent or nephrostomy tube. A successful outcome for emergency repair of a severe pedicle injury or thrombosis is unlikely given the amount of warm ischemia the injured kidney undergoes during the evaluation and resuscitation of the patient. Attempts at salvage in these situations should be limited to extreme circumstances, such as a solitary kidney or bilateral renal injuries.

There is a variety of important complications associated with renal injury. The most significant early complications include bleeding, infection, and urinary extravasation or urinoma. The risk of bleeding is highest immediately following the trauma and admission for close observation is necessary. Strict bed rest and serial hematocrits are the mainstay of treatment for conservative management of low-grade renal injuries. Signs of hemodynamic instability, including hypovolemia and severe hypotension that does not respond to blood transfusion, should prompt consideration of surgical exploration or angiography with potential embolization. Primary angioembolization may reduce the morbidity associated with surgical exploration, and is useful for segmental artery bleeding or delayed hemorrhage. The risk of delayed hemorrhage may be 25% of patients with grade III to IV renal trauma who are managed conservatively.[79–81]

Ureteral Trauma

The incidence of ureteral injury is uncommon, constituting less than 3% of genitourinary trauma.[82] The ureter is largely protected by its anatomic location and is also a small target with inherent mobility. Severe blunt injury, classically from significant deceleration, may cause disruption of the ureteropelvic junction. Penetrating injury, such as gunshot wounds or stab wounds, is more common and is associated with other organ injury in 97% of cases.[83] Gunshot wounds, in particular, are capable of injuring the ureter even if it is outside the path via a blast effect. Finally, iatrogenic injury is possible in laparoscopic, pelvic, or endoscopic procedures. Recognition at the time of injury is critical to minimize sequelae.

A high index of suspicion for ureteral injury must be maintained to avoid missing the diagnosis. Hematuria may be present in only 23% to 45% of cases and CT scans may miss up to 75% of cases, particularly without delayed imaging to visualize contrast throughout the collecting system.[84,85]

The timing and specific intervention for ureteral injury depend on such factors as the timing of diagnosis, the severity of injury, and the patient's overall condition. Early recognition of an injury, such as an intraoperative iatrogenic injury, should prompt immediate repair. Key features of an appropriate ureteral repair consist of a tension-free, spatulated anastomosis over a ureteral stent. Devitalized segments should be excised to reapproximate healthy edges. In cases where direct reanastamosis is not possible, options include further mobilization of the kidney and ureter, psoas hitch or Boari flap with or without ureteral reimplantation, and transureteroureterostomy. These considerations may be dictated by the location and extent of the injury. Nephrectomy is avoided even for the longest ureteral insults by ileal transposition.

Delayed recognition of ureteral injuries is common and presents a more complex management problem. If the injury is recognized within 5 to 7 days, surgical intervention remains an option. If outside of this window, reconstruction should be delayed several months. Temporary diversion with a nephrostomy tube or internal stenting can bridge this gap or be used in an unstable patient unfit for surgery.

If a significant ureteral injury is not addressed properly, the primary complication is urinary extravasation into the retroperitoneum resulting in urinoma or abscess formation. Initial management in this situation includes drainage with a nephrostomy tube or prolonged ureteral stent with percutaneous drainage of the urinoma or abscess. Ureteral strictures are a particularly troublesome long-term complication. Their presentation may be insidious and serial ultrasound imaging following ureteral injury is imperative to rule out progressive hydronephrosis and signs of obstruction.

Bladder and Urethral Injury

Pediatric bladder and urethral trauma are usually associated with other severe injuries that include pelvic fracture. Consequently, mortality rates are higher. Motor vehicle collisions are a leading cause of pelvic blunt trauma and inappropriately fastened lap belts may increase the risk of bladder injury. Compared with the adult setting, the bladder in a child is located in a more abdominal position, particularly when full. This anatomic difference makes the pediatric bladder more susceptible to external injury. The less developed rectus abdominal muscles also offer less protection. Bladder and urethral injuries are capable of producing a considerable amount of blood loss into the pelvis and perineum. Large pelvic hematomas may cause a mass effect significant enough to cause urinary retention.

The hallmark signs of bladder and urethral injury are suprapubic pain, tenderness, inability to urinate, gross hematuria, and blood at the urethral meatus. Indications for imaging the bladder include the presence of gross hematuria and/or urinary retention in conjunction with a pelvic fracture. All penetrating injury concerning for bladder injury should prompt imaging to rule out bladder injury.

Most urethral injuries from a straddle mechanism do not cause significant extravasation of urine because the urethra is crushed as opposed to lacerated. However, bleeding into the perineum can be substantial and leads to the pathognomonic "butterfly pattern" by spreading within the limits of Colles fascia. Although digital rectal examination has historically been performed to assess for the presence of the concurrent rectal or prostatic injury, recent studies have shown that digital rectal examination is less than 15% accurate in diagnosing either a displaced prostate injury or rectal injury.[86,87]

The initial trauma CT scan may not be adequate to completely characterize lower urinary tract injury. The urethra will not have contrast material within it and delayed-phase imaging must demonstrate an adequately full bladder. Other modalities to assess bladder injury include cystography or intravenous pyelography. Oblique and postdrainage films should be included. CT cystography is perhaps the most sensitive and specific test but involves significant radiation exposure and should be used judiciously. No matter which modality is chosen, the bladder should be filled to at least 50% capacity and should stop at the maximum of estimated bladder capacity. Common equations for estimating the pediatric bladder capacity are (Age + 2) × 30 mL and Kilograms × 7 mL in infants less than 1 year old. The classic appearance of an intraperitoneal bladder injury on cystogram is a starburst pattern of contrast outlining loops of bowel.

The retrograde urethrogram is the best imaging study for investigating the urethra. Oblique views are necessary to rule out posterior extravasation and complete continuity of the urethra. A Foley catheter may be placed into the bladder under radiographic guidance in cases of an intact urethra with a small tear. If a catheter has been placed previously, it should not be removed. A feeding tube can be placed in the meatus alongside the catheter to perform the study and assess injury. Alternatively, if the patient has already voided and examination does not suggest urethral injury, a urethral catheter can be placed immediately without a retrograde study.

The primary clinical distinction in bladder injury is determining an intraperitoneal versus extraperitoneal injury site. Intraperitoneal rupture accounts for approximately one-third of cases.[88] Children with intraperitoneal rupture may develop hyponatremia, hypokalemia, and elevated serum urea and creatinine. Intraperitoneal rupture is less common and typically occurs at the dome of the bladder. Although intraperitoneal rupture is generally an indication for operative intervention, this decision is somewhat controversial in children. Successful nonoperative management may be reasonable for small, isolated injuries.[89,90] This decision may be an option for stable patients with small injuries who can be observed carefully. Laparotomy for other associated injuries is an opportunity to inspect the bladder and repair any injuries.

Extraperitoneal rupture is more commonly associated with pelvic fracture.[91] This incidence is significantly lower in children, which is attributed to more elastic pelvic attachments. Most extraperitoneal injuries are managed by catheter drainage alone. If gross hematuria persists or worsens during this period, open repair can be considered. Furthermore, the presence of a bony spicule necessitates operative intervention.

Conservative management should be similar regardless of the injury site. Continuous bladder drainage is typically continued for 10 to 14 days in cases of conservative management or following operative repair. Confirmation of adequate healing can be confirmed by a negative cystogram before catheter removal.

The most important acute goals for urethral injury are minimizing infectious complications with broad-spectrum antibiotics and establishing urinary drainage. If possible, placement of a urethral catheter helps alignment and provides bladder drainage. In cases of complete disruption and urethral disassociation, urethral catheter placement may not be possible. Appropriate management in this scenario remains controversial, with accepted options including immediate primary realignment of the urethra or suprapubic drainage and delayed reconstruction.

Penile Trauma

Patterns of penile injury are largely determined by patient age and are rarely subtle. Penile injuries in the neonate are most commonly iatrogenic from neonatal circumcision injury. Zipper injuries may result in contusion or pressure necrosis of the prepuce.[92] The "hair tourniquet" may lead to preputial edema and inflammation. As children reach toddler age and begin toilet training, toilet seat injuries become common.[93] Penile lacerations and amputations have been reported from dog or other animal bites.[94] Animal attacks may be the most significant injuries seen in childhood. Verification of the animal's tetanus and rabies vaccination status is necessary.

Superficial contusions and lacerations can typically be managed with topical antibiotic ointments, but may require minor debridement and skin approximation depending on the mechanism, patient anxiety level, and severity of injury. Empiric antibiotics may be prescribed to decrease the risk of cellulitis. Most circumcision injury can be managed by healing through secondary and antibiotic ointment.[95] Zipper injuries to the penis more commonly occur in uncircumcised boys and may be treated with mineral oil to slip the trapped skin from the zipper or by cutting of the median bar of the zipper with bone cutters.[96]

Amputation injuries may be managed with primary reanastamosis up to 8 hours after injury.[97] Partial amputation injuries may be treated nonoperatively with intermittent application of epinephrine-soaked sponges to control hemorrhage in the absence of associated urethral injury. As with any other body part, the amputated penis should be cooled as quickly as possible to reduce ischemic injury.

Genital injury caused by animal bite should be assessed under anesthesia to fully assess the extent of trauma. Broad-spectrum antibiotics and tetanus prophylaxis should be administered before treatment. Debridement of devitalized tissue and aggressive irrigation of the wound have been shown to reduce the risk of wound infection from 59% to 12%.[98] Split-thickness skin grafts should be applied to denuded areas to minimize wound contraction. Investigation for potential abuse or neglect should be initiated in these cases to reduce the risk of future injury.

Scrotal/Testicular Trauma

Injury to the testis is commonly associated with straddle injury, where the testis is forced against the pubic ramus, causing tearing of the tunica albuginea. Injuries may also result from hits or kicks to the scrotum during sporting events or rough-housing. Trauma to the scrotum without underlying testicular injury tends to resolve within a short time. In patients with pain that initially resolves after a short period but recurs after several days, traumatic epididymitis should be considered. However, pain persisting greater than 2 hours after trauma is suspicious for more significant testicular injuries, including testicular torsion or rupture. Testicular torsion associated with scrotal injury, although uncommon, has been reported.[99,100] A history of trauma is the presenting symptom in 4% to 8% of all cases of testicular torsion.[101] Acute scrotal swelling may also be associated with intraperitoneal pathology, such as appendicitis, peritonitis, liver laceration, or splenic rupture.[102–104]

If physical examination and imaging, such as ultrasound, are indeterminate or suggest significant testicular injury, early scrotal exploration is recommended. Rates of salvage in cases of testicular rupture have been reported at 90% if performed within 72 hours[105] and may also decrease convalescence. In cases of penetrating scrotal injury, a careful physical examination should be performed to determine the depth of penetration and to ensure adequate cleansing and debridement.

Cases of isolated hematocele may be followed nonoperatively in the absence of impaired testicular flow. Isolated epididymitis may also be treated with supportive care including scrotal elevation and nonsteroidal analgesics. In the absence of ischemic changes, testicular fracture without disruption of the tunica albuginea may be observed. If nonoperative management is selected, follow-up with physical examination and ultrasonography should be used to monitor resolution of injury.

Vaginal Trauma

Vaginal injuries are relatively rare in the pediatric population and are typically caused by straddle injuries.[106,107] Pelvic fractures may result in penetrating injury caused by bone spicules and traction injury caused by shear forces.[108] Because of the proximity of the urethra and vagina and the susceptibility of the urethrovaginal septum to injury, traumatic urethral injuries in girls should prompt an evaluation for associated vaginal injuries.[109]

Prompt diagnosis is essential to avoid fistulae, stenosis, or other long-term complications of unrecognized vaginal injuries.[110,111] Physical examination may show evidence of labial bruising, bleeding at the introitus, vulvar edema, or hematuria. Examination in the emergency room can underestimate the extent of injuries. Lighting may be inadequate and patients are often unable to fully cooperate with a sensitive or uncomfortable examination, leading to an incomplete examination.[112] Based on these findings, examination under anesthesia should be performed when any doubt exists as to the extent of the injury.

Operative management is seldom required for genital trauma in young girls. However, sexual abuse or assault may be identified in 25% of girls with genital injury.[113] Cystoscopy, vaginoscopy, and rectal examination should be performed to fully evaluate associated injuries. For more extensive vaginal lacerations, primary repair should be performed to reduce the rate of vaginal stenosis and urethrovaginal fistulae. Vaginal lacerations may be repaired in layers with absorbable sutures. Perioperative use of antibiotics may help reduce the risk of secondary infection and wound dehiscence. Postoperative care includes the avoidance of extreme lower extremity abduction, sitz bathing, and the use of topical antibiotic ointments. For injuries that extend into the introitus, the use of permanent monofilament sutures in an interrupted fashion is recommended to reduce postrepair dehiscence risk.

REFERENCES

1. Barteczko KJ, Jacob MI. The testicular descent in human. Origin, development and fate of the gubernaculum Hunteri, processus vaginalis peritonei, and gonadal ligaments. Adv Anat Embryol Cell Biol 2000;156:III–X, 1–98.
2. Jones ME, Swerdlow AJ, Griffith M, et al. Risk of congenital inguinal hernia in siblings: a record linkage study. Paediatr Perinat Epidemiol 1998;12(3):288–96.
3. Brandt ML. Pediatric hernias. Surg Clin North Am 2008;88(1):27–43, vii–viii.
4. Kapur P, Caty MG, Glick PL. Pediatric hernias and hydroceles. Pediatr Clin North Am 1998;45(4):773–89.
5. Gong Y, Shao C, Sun Q, et al. Genetic study of indirect inguinal hernia. Med Genet 1994;31(3):187–92.
6. Osifo OD, Osaigbovo EO. Congenital hydrocele: prevalence and outcome among male children who underwent neonatal circumcision in Benin City, Nigeria. J Pediatr Urol 2008;4(3):178–82.
7. Phelps S, Agrawal M. Morbidity after neonatal inguinal herniotomy. J Pediatr Surg 1997;32(3):445–7.
8. Rajput A, Gauderer MW, Hack M. Inguinal hernias in very low birth weight infants: incidence and timing of repair. J Pediatr Surg 1992;27(10):1322–4.
9. Lautz TB, Raval MV, Reynolds M. Does timing matter? A national perspective on the risk of incarceration in premature neonates with inguinal hernia. J Pediatr 2011;158(4):573–7.
10. Blakely ML, Tyson JE. ClinicalTrials.gov [Internet]. Timing of inguinal hernia repair in premature infants. Bethesda (MD): National Library of Medicine (US); 2000. Available at: http://clinicaltrials.gov/show/NCT01678638 NLM Identifier: NCT01678638. Accessed January 17, 2015.
11. Koski ME, Makari JH, Adams MC, et al. Infant Communicating Hydroceles- do they need immediate repair or might some clinically resolve? J Pediatr Surg 2010;45(3):590–3.
12. Hall NJ, Ron O, Eaton S, et al. Surgery for hydrocele in children-an avoidable excess? J Pediatr Surg 2011;46(12):2401–5.
13. Antonoff MB, Kreykes NS, Saltzman DA, et al. American Academy of Pediatrics Section on Surgery hernia survey revisited. J Pediatr Surg 2005;40(6):1009–14.
14. Grosfeld JL, Minnick K, Shedd F, et al. Inguinal hernia in children: factors affecting recurrence in 62 cases. J Pediatr Surg 1991;26(3):283–7.
15. Vogels HD, Bruijnen CJ, Beasley SW. Predictors of recurrence after inguinal herniotomy in boys. Pediatr Surg Int 2009;25(3):235–8.
16. Fearne CH, Abela M, Aquilina D. Scrotal approach for inguinal hernia and hydrocele repair in boys. Eur J Pediatr Surg 2002;12(2):116–7.
17. Gökçora IH, Yagmurlu A. A longitudinal follow-up using the high trans-scrotal approach for inguinal and scrotal abnormalities in boys. Hernia 2003;7(4):181–4.

18. Schier F. Laparoscopic inguinal hernia repair-a prospective personal series of 542 children. J Pediatr Surg 2006;41(6):1081–4.
19. Takehara H, Yakabe S, Kameoka K. Laparoscopic percutaneous extraperitoneal closure for inguinal hernia in children: clinical outcome of 972 repairs done in 3 pediatric surgical institutions. J Pediatr Surg 2006;41(12):1999–2003.
20. Endo M, Watanabe T, Nakano M, et al. Laparoscopic completely extraperitoneal repair of inguinal hernia in children: a single-institute experience with 1,257 repairs compared with cut-down herniorrhaphy. Surg Endosc 2009;23(8): 1706–12.
21. Miltenburg DM, Nuchtern JG, Jaksic T, et al. Laparoscopic evaluation of the pediatric inguinal hernia-a meta-analysis. J Pediatr Surg 1998;33(6):874–9.
22. Ron O, Eaton S, Pierro A. Systematic review of the risk of developing a metachronous contralateral inguinal hernia in children. Br J Surg 2007;94(7):804–11.
23. Scorer CG. The descent of the testis. Arch Dis Child 1964;39:605–9.
24. Berkowitz GS, Lapinski RH, Dolgin SE, et al. Prevalence and natural history of cryptorchidism. Pediatrics 1993;92(1):44–9.
25. Scorer CG, Farrington HG. Congenital deformities of the testis and epididymis. London: Butterworths; 1971.
26. Wenzler DL, Bloom DA, Park JM. What is the rate of spontaneous testicular descent in infants with cryptorchidism? J Urol 2004;171(2 Pt 1):849–51.
27. Chilvers C, Dudley NE, Gough MH, et al. Undescended testis: the effect of treatment on subsequent risk of subfertility and malignancy. J Pediatr Surg 1986; 21(8):691–6.
28. Kollin C, Granholm T, Nordenskjöld A, et al. Growth of spontaneously descended and surgically treated testes during early childhood. Pediatrics 2013;131(4):e1174–80.
29. Lee PA, O'Leary LA, Songer NJ, et al. Paternity after unilateral cryptorchidism: a controlled study. Pediatrics 1996;98(4 Pt 1):676–9.
30. Lee PA, Coughlin MT, Bellinger MF. Paternity and hormone levels after unilateral cryptorchidism: association with pretreatment testicular location. J Urol 2000; 164(5):1697–701.
31. Hrebinko RL, Bellinger MF. The limited role of imaging techniques in managing children with undescended testes. J Urol 1993;150(2 Pt 1):458–60.
32. Kolon TF, Herndon CD, Baker LA, et al. Evaluation and treatment of cryptorchidism: AUA guideline. J Urol 2014;192(2):337–45.
33. Tasian GE, Hittelman AB, Kim GE, et al. Age at orchiopexy and testis palpability predict germ cell loss: clinical predictors of adverse histological features of cryptorchidism. J Urol 2009;182:704–9.
34. Bellinger MF, Abromowitz H, Brantley S, et al. Orchiopexy: an experimental study of the effect of surgical technique on testicular histology. J Urol 1989; 142(2 Pt 2):553–5 [discussion: 572].
35. Gordon M, Cervellione RM, Morabito A, et al. 20 years of transcrotal orchidopexy for undescended testis: results and outcomes. J Pediatr Urol 2010;6(5): 506–12.
36. Dayanc M, Kibar Y, Irkilata HC, et al. Long-term outcome of scrotal incision orchiopexy for undescended testis. Urology 2007;70(4):786–8 [discussion: 788–9].
37. Fowler R, Sephens FD. The role of testicular vascular anatomy in the salvage of high undescended testes. Aust N Z J Surg 1959;29:92–106.
38. Docimo S, Moore RG, Kavoussi LR. Laparoscopic orchiopexy. Urology 1995; 46(5):715.

39. Niku SD, Stock JA, Kaplan GW. Neonatal circumcision. Urol Clin North Am 1995; 22(1):57–65.
40. Centers for Disease Control and Prevention (CDC). Trends in in-hospital newborn male circumcision—United States, 1999-2010. MMWR Morb Mortal Wkly Rep 2011;60(34):1167–8.
41. Shaikh N, Morone NE, Bost JE, et al. Prevalence of urinary tract infection in childhood: a meta-analysis. Pediatr Infect Dis J 2008;27(4):302–8.
42. Günşar C, Kurutepe S, Alparslan O, et al. The effect of circumcision status on periurethral and glanular bacterial flora. Urol Int 2004;72(3):212–5.
43. Aridogan IA, Ilkit M, Izol V, et al. Glans penis and prepuce colonisation of yeast fungi in a paediatric population: pre and postcircumcision results. Mycoses 2009;52(1):49–52.
44. Serour F, Samra Z, Kushel Z, et al. Comparative periurethral bacteriology of uncircumcised and circumcised males. Genitourin Med 1997;73(4):288–90.
45. Gray RH, Kigozi G, Serwadda D, et al. Male circumcision for HIV prevention in men in Rakai, Uganda: a randomised trial. Lancet 2007;369(9562):657–66.
46. Tobian AA, Serwadda D, Quinn TC, et al. Male circumcision for the prevention of HSV-2 and HPV infections and syphilis. N Engl J Med 2009;360(13):1298–309.
47. 2010 sexually transmitted diseases surveillance: other sexually transmitted disease—herpes simplex virus. Atlanta, GA. Centers for Disease Control and Prevention. Available at: www.cdc.gov/std/stats10/other.htm. Accessed November 17, 2011.
48. Sobngwi-Tambekou J, Taljaard D, Nieuwoudt M, et al. Male circumcision and *Neisseria gonorrhoeae, Chlamydia trachomatis* and *Trichomonas vaginalis*: observations after a randomized controlled trial for HIV prevention. Sex Transm Infect 2009;85(2):116–20.
49. Daling JR, Madeleine MM, Johnson LG, et al. Penile cancer: importance of circumcision, human papillomavirus and smoking in in situ and invasive disease. Int J Cancer 2005;116(4):606–16.
50. Castellsagué X, Bosch FX, Muñoz N, et al, International Agency for Research on Cancer Multicenter Cervical Cancer Study Group. Male circumcision, penile human papillomavirus infection, and cervical cancer in female partners. N Engl J Med 2002;346(15):1105–12.
51. Wiswell TE, Geschke DW. Risks from circumcision during the first month of life compared with those for uncircumcised boys. Pediatrics 1989;83(6):1011–5.
52. O'Brien TR, Calle EE, Poole WK. Incidence of neonatal circumcision in Atlanta, 1985-1986. South Med J 1995;88(4):411–5.
53. Wiswell TE, Tencer HL, Welch CA, et al. Circumcision in children beyond the neonatal period. Pediatrics 1993;92(6):791–3.
54. Kakavouli A, Li G, Carson MP, et al. Intraoperative reported adverse events in children. Paediatr Anaesth 2009;19(8):732–9.
55. Hackel A, Badqwell JM, Binding RR, et al. Guidelines for the pediatric perioperative anesthesia environment. American Academy of Pediatrics. Section on Anesthesiology. Pediatrics 1999;103(2):512–5.
56. Sansom SL, Prabhu VS, Hutchinson AB, et al. Cost-effectiveness of newborn circumcision in reducing lifetime HIV risk among U.S. males. PLoS One 2010; 5(1):e8723.
57. American Academy of Pediatrics Task Force on Circumcision. Circumcision policy statement. Pediatrics 2012;130(3):585–6.
58. McAleer IM, Kaplan GW, Scherz HC, et al. Genitourinary trauma in the pediatric patient. Urology 1993;42:563–7 [discussion: 567–8].

59. Levine PM, Gonzales ET Jr. Genitourinary trauma in children. Urol Clin North Am 1895;12:53–65.
60. Buckley JC, McAninch JW. The diagnosis, management and outcomes of pediatric renal injuries. Urol Clin North Am 2006;33:33–40.
61. Buckley JC, McAninch JW. Pediatric renal injuries: management guidelines from a 25-year experience. J Urol 2004;172:687–90 [discussion: 690].
62. Cass AS. Blunt renal trauma in children. J Trauma 1983;23:123–7.
63. Carpio F, Morey AF. Radiographic staging of renal injuries. World J Urol 1999;17: 66–70.
64. Morey AF, Bruce JE, McAninch JW. Efficacy of radiographic imaging in pediatric blunt renal trauma. J Urol 1996;156:2014–8.
65. Stein JP, Kaji DM, Eastham J, et al. Blunt renal trauma in the pediatric population: indications for radiographic evaluation. Urology 1994;44:406.
66. Mee SL, McAninch JW, Robinson AL, et al. Radiographic assessment of renal trauma: a 10-year prospective study of patient selection. J Urol 1989;141: 1095–8.
67. Heyns C. Renal trauma: indications for imaging and surgical exploration. BJU Int 2004;93:1165–70.
68. Santucci R, Langenburg S, Zachareas M. Traumatic hematuria in children can be evaluated as in adults. J Urol 2004;171:822–5.
69. McGahan JP, Richards JR, Jones CD, et al. Use of ultrasonography in the patient with acute renal trauma. J Ultrasound Med 1999;18:207.
70. Al-Qudah H, Santucci R. Complications of renal trauma. Urol Clin North Am 2006;33:41–53.
71. Malcom J, Derweesh I, Mehrazin R, et al. Nonoperative management of renal trauma: is routine early follow-up imaging necessary? BMC Urol 2008;8:11–7.
72. Moore EE, Cogbill TH, Malangoni MA, et al. Organ injury scaling. Surg Clin North Am 1995;75:293–303.
73. Abou-Jaoude WA, Sugarman JM, Fallat ME, et al. Indicators of genitourinary tract injury or anomaly in cases of pediatric blunt trauma. J Pediatr Surg 1996;31:86–9 [discussion: 90].
74. Taylor GA, Eichelberger MR, Potter BM. Hematuria: a marker of abdominal injury in children after blunt trauma. Ann Surg 1988;208:688.
75. Broghammer JA, Langenburg SE, Smith SJ, et al. Pediatric blunt renal trauma: its conservative management and patterns of associated injuries. Urology 2006; 67:823–7.
76. Cass AS, Luxenberg M. Management of renal artery injuries from external trauma. J Urol 1987;138:266.
77. Abdalati H, Bulas DI, Sivit CJ, et al. Blunt renal trauma in children: healing of renal injuries and recommendations for imaging follow-up. Pediatr Radiol 1994;24:573.
78. Wright JL, Nathens AB, Rivara FP, et al. Renal and extrarenal predictors of nephrectomy from the national trauma data bank. J Urol 2006;175:970–5 [discussion: 975].
79. Wessells H, Deirmenjian J, McAninch J. Preservation of renal function after reconstruction for trauma: quantitative assessment with radionuclide scintigraphy. J Urol 1997;157:1583–6.
80. Dinkel H, Danuser H, Triller J. Blunt renal trauma: minimally invasive management with microcatheter embolization experience in nine patients. Radiology 2002;223:723–30.

81. Kansas B, Eddy M, Mydlo J, et al. Incidence and management of penetrating renal trauma in patients with multiorgan injury: extended experience at an inner city trauma center. J Urol 2004;172:1355–60.

82. Corriere JN Jr. Ureteral injuries. In: Gillenwater JY, Grayhack JT, Howards SS, et al, editors. Adult and pediatric urology. 3rd edition. St Louis (MO): Mosby; 1996. p. 554–62.

83. Bright TC, Peters PC. Ureteral injuries due to external violence: 10 years experience with 59 cases. J Trauma 1977;17:616.

84. Perez-Brayfield MR, Keane TE, Krishnan A, et al. Gunshot wounds to the ureter: a 40-year experience at Grady Memorial Hospital. J Urol 2001;166:119.

85. Elliott SP, McAninch JW. Ureteral injuries from external violence: the 25-year experience at San Francisco General Hospital. J Urol 2003;170:1213.

86. Shlamovitz G, Mower W, Bergman J, et al. Lack of evidence to support routine digital rectal examination in pediatric trauma patients. Pediatr Emerg Care 2007; 23:537–43.

87. Shlamovitz G, Mower W, Bergman J, et al. Poor test characteristics for the digital rectal examination in trauma patients. Ann Emerg Med 2007;50:25–33.

88. Corriere JN, Sandler CM. Bladder rupture from external trauma: diagnosis and management. World J Urol 1999;17:84–9.

89. Osman Y, El-Tabey N, Mohsen T, et al. Nonoperative treatment of isolated post-traumatic intraperitoneal bladder rupture in children: is it justified? J Urol 2005; 173:955–7.

90. Richardson JR, Leadbetter GW. Non-operative treatment of the ruptured bladder. J Urol 1975;114:213.

91. Tarman GJ, Kaplan GW, Lerman SL, et al. Lower genitourinary injury and pelvic fractures in pediatric patients. Urology 2002;59:123–6 [discussion: 126].

92. Kanegaye JT, Schonfeld N. Penile zipper entrapment: a simple and less threatening approach using mineral oil. Pediatr Emerg Care 1993;9:90–1.

93. Adams JA. Guidelines for medical care of children evaluated for suspected sexual abuse: an update for 2008. Curr Opin Obstet Gynecol 2008;20:435–41.

94. Donovan JF, Kaplan WE. The therapy of genital trauma by dog bite. J Urol 1989; 141:1163–5.

95. Sotolongo JR Jr, Hoffman S, Gribetz ME. Penile denudation injuries after circumcision. J Urol 1985;133:102–3.

96. Nakagawa T, Toguri AG. Penile zipper injury. Med Princ Pract 2006;15:303–4.

97. Sherman J, Borer JG, Horowitz M, et al. Circumcision: successful glanular reconstruction and survival following traumatic amputation. J Urol 1996;156: 842–4.

98. Callaham ML. Treatment of common dog bites: infection risk factors. JACEP 1978;7:83–7.

99. King LM, Sekaran SK, Sauer D, et al. Untwisting in delayed treatment of tosion of the spermatic cord. J Urol 1974;112:217–21.

100. Jackson RH, Craft AW. Bicycle saddles and torsion of the testis. Lancet 1978;1: 983–4.

101. Seng YJ, Moissinac K. Trauma induced testicular torsion: a reminder for the unwary. J Accid Emerg Med 2000;17:381–2.

102. Nagel P. Scrotal swelling as the presenting symptom of acute perforated appendicitis in an infant. J Pediatr Surg 1984;19:177–8.

103. Udall DA, Drake DJ Jr, Rosenberg RS. Acute scrotal swelling: a physical sign of primary peritonitis. J Urol 1981;125:750–1.

104. Sujka SK, Jewett TC Jr, Karp MP. Acute scrotal swelling as the first evidence of intraabdominal trauma in a battered child. J Pediatr Surg 1988;23:380.
105. Munden MM, Trautwein LM. Scrotal pathology in pediatrics with sonographic imaging. Curr Probl Diagn Radiol 2000;29:185–205.
106. Okur H, Kucikaydin M, Kazez A, et al. Genitourinary tract injuries in girls. Br J Urol 1996;78:446–9.
107. Iqbal CW, Jrebi NY, Zielinski MD, et al. Patterns of accidental genital trauma in young girls and indications for operative management. J Pediatr Surg 2010;45: 930–3.
108. Boos SC, Rosas AJ, Boyle C, et al. Anogenital injuries in child pedestrians run over by low-speed motor vehicles: four cases with findings that mimic child sexual abuse. Pediatrics 2003;112:e77–84.
109. Merchant WC 3rd, Gibbons MD, Gonzales ET Jr. Trauma to the bladder neck, trigone and vagina in children. J Urol 1984;131:747–50.
110. Pode D, Shapiro A. Traumatic avulsion of the female urethra: case report. J Trauma 1990;30:235–7.
111. Patil U, Nesbitt R, Meyer R. Genitourinary tract injuries due to fracture of the pelvis in females: sequelae and their management. Br J Urol 1982;54:32–8.
112. Lynch JM, Gardner MJ, Albanese CT. Blunt urogenital trauma in prepubescent female patients: more than meets the eye! Pediatr Emerg Care 1995;11:372–5.
113. Jones JG, Worthington T. Genital and anal injuries requiring surgical repair in females less than 21 years of age. J Pediatr Adolesc Gynecol 2008;21:207–11.

The Use of Bowel in Urologic Reconstructive Surgery

Moritz H. Hansen, MD*, Matthew Hayn, MD, Patrick Murray, MD

KEYWORDS

- Urinary diversion • Bladder substitution • Neobladder • Ileal ureter
- Bladder augmentation • Appendicovesicostomy • Metabolic changes

KEY POINTS

- Urologists routinely use intestinal segments for reconstructive procedures and surgeons often encounter such reconstructions of the urinary tract.
- Surgeons should have a clear understanding of the most common urinary reconstructions using intestinal segments.
- Urinary tract reconstructions using intestinal segments can result in a variety of metabolic and electrolyte abnormalities.

Intestinal surgery involves an operative space shared by both general surgeons and urologists and is a border region where these 2 surgical disciplines often intersect. Urologists routinely use both small and large bowel for reconstructive procedures and surgeons often encounter such reconstructions of the urinary tract. It is therefore essential for surgeons to have a clear understanding of the urologic indications for using intestinal segments for reconstructive procedures, the variety of such reconstructions, the anatomic landmarks and potential pitfalls that should be considered when intraoperatively encountering such reconstructions, and the potential metabolic consequences associated with the incorporation of bowel segments into the urinary collecting system.

URINARY DIVERSION

Urinary diversion involves the separation of the ureters from the bladder and the development of an alternate route of urinary evacuation. The goal of urinary diversion is to provide a convenient and reliable drainage system when the native bladder is

Disclosure: None.
Division of Urology, Maine Medical Center, Tufts University School of Medicine, 100 Brickhill Avenue, South Portland, ME 04106, USA
* Corresponding author.
E-mail address: hansemo@mmc.org

Surg Clin N Am 96 (2016) 567–582
http://dx.doi.org/10.1016/j.suc.2016.02.011
0039-6109/16/$ – see front matter © 2016 Elsevier Inc. All rights reserved.
surgical.theclinics.com

no longer able to serve this function. Common indications for urinary diversion include:

- Bladder or other pelvic malignancies requiring removal of the bladder
- Congenital anomalies of bladder development
- Intractable urinary incontinence
- Intractable bladder hemorrhage

Although a full description of all variants of urinary reconstruction involving intestinal segments is beyond the scope of this article, it is informative to understand the historical evolution of these procedures, the anatomic principles fundamental to each procedure, and the most common variations that surgeons can expect to encounter.

URETEROSIGMOIDOSTOMY

In 1852, Simon[1] described the first urinary diversion after performing a ureterosigmoi-dostomy on a patient with congenital bladder exstrophy. Ureterosigmoidostomy involves the implantation of the ureters into the tenia of the sigmoid colon, resulting in a combined evacuation of urine and feces per rectum. This procedure remained the most common form of urinary diversion for nearly a century. However, with longer-term follow-up it became clear that ureterosigmoidostomy often led to significant complications, to include:

- Chronic diarrhea and consequent electrolyte abnormalities
- Upper urinary tract obstruction
- Chronic pyelonephritis, renal scarring, and renal insufficiency
- Secondary malignant neoplasms occurring at the ureterocolonic implantation site[2]

This realization led to further investigations in which the ureters were implanted into a variety of other bowel segments that were separated from the fecal stream.

CONDUIT URINARY DIVERSIONS

In 1950, Bricker[3] ushered in a new era in urinary diversion with his description of the intestinal conduit urinary diversion with cutaneous drainage. Although conduit urinary diversion had conceptually been described earlier by Zaayer[4] in 1911, it was Bricker's[3] simple and straightforward description of the ileal conduit diversion that popularized this procedure.

ILEAL CONDUIT

The ileal conduit remains the most common form of urinary diversion in the world and it is therefore often encountered by surgeons. It is generally constructed from a ~20-cm segment of ileum with its distal end ~20 cm proximal to the ileocecal junction (**Fig. 1**). In general, when urologists harvest a segment of small bowel for reconstructive purposes the remaining bowel is brought cephalad to it and continuity is reestablished. Ileal conduits are most often placed in the right lower quadrant of the abdomen rather than the left because of limitations of the length of the distal ileal mesentery. The ureteroileal anastomosis may be performed in the following 2 ways:

- The Bricker[3] technique, in which the ureters are reimplanted individually in an end-to-side fashion to the proximal end of the ileal conduit (**Fig. 2**).

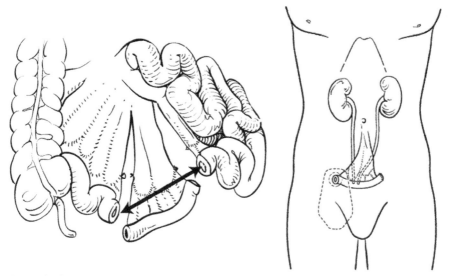

Fig. 1. Ileal conduit urinary diversion. (*From* Parekh DJ, Donat SM. Urinary diversion: options, patient selection, and outcomes. Semin Oncol 2007;34(2):98–109; with permission.)

- The Wallace[5] technique, in which the ureters are spatulated and then joined together in an end-to-end fashion (**Fig. 3**).

The proximal end of the ileal conduit is usually fixed to the posterior peritoneum to prevent volvulus of the conduit. The lateral aspect of the ureter may also be fixed to the lateral edge of the peritoneum to prevent intestinal herniation of bowel lateral to the

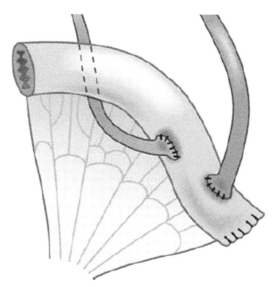

Fig. 2. Bricker technique for ureteroileal anastomosis. (*From* Manoharan M, Tunuguntla HS. Standard reconstruction techniques: techniques of ureteroneocystostomy during urinary diversion. Surg Oncol Clin N Am 2005;14(2):367–79; with permission.)

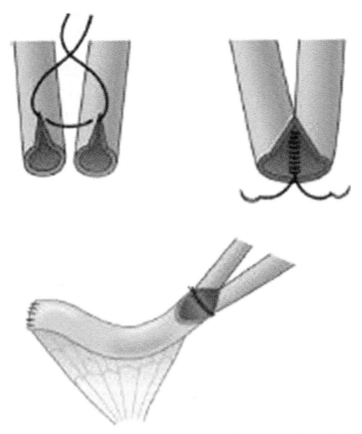

Fig. 3. Wallace technique for ureteroileal anastomosis. (*From* Manoharan M, Tunuguntla HS. Standard reconstruction techniques: techniques of ureteroneocystostomy during urinary diversion. Surg Oncol Clin N Am 2005;14(2):367–79; with permission.)

conduit. The distal end of the conduit is brought through the rectus abdominis muscle, anchored to the fascia, and everted and matured into a cutaneous stoma.

JEJUNAL CONDUIT

Conduit urinary diversions using jejunum are only used if no other bowel segment is available. Although construction of a jejunal conduit is technically identical to the construction of an ileal conduit, the use of jejunum results in significant electrolyte abnormalities, which limits its usefulness in reconstructive urologic procedures.

COLON CONDUITS

Although urologists primarily use small bowel segments for urinary reconstruction there are multiple scenarios in which small bowel is not available, or has been previously irradiated, or when large bowel is anatomically preferable. Colon conduits using either transverse or sigmoid colon are therefore an important alternative option for urinary diversion.

TRANSVERSE COLON CONDUIT

A transverse colon conduit is an excellent option for patients who have previously undergone extensive pelvic irradiation limiting the use of small bowel. In addition, when there is limited ureteral length the proximity of the transverse colon to the upper ureters allows even short ureteral segments to be implanted to form a transverse colon conduit. Transverse colon conduit stomas are generally placed high on either side of the patient's abdomen.

Note that, unlike other small and large bowel conduits, after harvesting a segment of transverse colon for reconstructive purposes the remaining bowel is usually brought caudad to it and continuity reestablished.

SIGMOID COLON CONDUIT

The sigmoid colon is generally the intestinal segment used for a urinary conduit if the ileum is not available. It is also a good choice in patients undergoing pelvic exenteration with colostomy placement, because no bowel anastomosis needs to be made. Although a double-barreled stoma may be performed,[6,7] the fecal and urinary stoma sites are generally separated (**Fig. 4**). The sigmoid colon conduit is placed in the left lower quadrant of the abdomen lateral to the reapproximated sigmoid colon. The ureters are separately reimplanted end to side into the tenia of the colon, and the proximal end of the colon conduit fixed to the posterior peritoneum.

For sigmoid conduits, note that surgeons can generally follow the course of the tenia to identify the location of the ureteroileal anastomoses.

CONTINENT URINARY DIVERSION

In 1982, Koch and colleagues[8] first reported on an ileal reservoir urinary diversion with a cutaneous catheterizable stoma. This report generated great interest and encouraged the development of a variety of continent urinary diversions based on both small

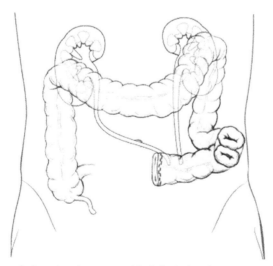

Fig. 4. Double-barreled wet colostomy with inferiorly placed sigmoid colon conduit. (*From* Chokshi RJ, Kuhrt MP, Schmidt C, et al. Single institution experience comparing double-barreled wet colostomy to ileal conduit for urinary and fecal diversion. Urology 2011;78(4):856–62; with permission.)

and large bowel urinary reservoirs. Although there is no single ideal continent urinary diversion, they all share in common the following 2 elements:

- A reservoir pouch constructed of a detubularized bowel segment. Detubularization is intended to reduce peristaltic high-pressure contractions, which in turn can lead to chronically increased intrarenal pressures, renal insufficiency, as well as stomal incontinence.
- An efferent continent limb that is brought to the skin surface and through which clean intermittent catheterization can be performed.

Although a large variety of continent urinary diversions have been described, the most common continent urinary diversions are based on the right-sided ascending colon and terminal ileum, and are commonly referred to as an Indiana pouch.[9] The cecum and ascending colon are detubularized and then folded over in a clam-shell fashion to create a spherical reservoir (**Fig. 5**). The ureters are separately reimplanted end to side into the tenia of the colon. The right-colon pouch is secured to the right anterior abdominal wall and the distal ileum is tapered and brought to the skin in the right lower quadrant of the abdomen as a cutaneous catheterizable stoma. Urinary continence is based on the ileocecal valve, although it may also be reinforced by imbricating sutures placed at the ileocecal junction.

Surgical considerations when operating on patients with conduits or urinary diversions:

- In patients with a conduit or continent diversion stoma the contralateral ureter is brought under the sigmoid colon mesentery in the avascular plane above the sacrum.
- The proximal end of an intestinal conduit, which is generally the location of the ureteroileal anastomosis, is often fixed to the posterior peritoneum and adherent to the region of the common iliac vessels. This point can serve as a landmark, but can also make dissection in this region more difficult.
- For inadvertent injuries to a conduit or continent urinary diversion, urologic consultation is recommended. If a urologist is not available, the injury should be repaired in a running fashion with absorbable suture (eg, 2-0 polyglactin) in 2 layers. The repair should be tested by gentle normal saline irrigation via the stoma. A catheter should be placed via the stoma (eg, 16 Fr) and left in place to provide maximal low-pressure drainage. A closed suction pelvic drain should also be placed. The drain may be removed once output is minimal, and if the drain fluid creatinine level is equivalent to the serum creatinine level (ie, consistent with serous fluid rather than urine).

Although continent urinary diversion with a catheterizable stoma is an excellent option for a patient who does not wish to have a conduit diversion, the popularity of the procedure has dramatically decreased over the past several decades with the emergence of orthotopic bladder substitution.

BLADDER SUBSTITUTION (COMMONLY REFERRED TO AS A NEOBLADDER)

In 1979, Camey and LeDuc[10] first described the technique of bladder substitution in which the ureters were anastomosed to one end of a segment of ileum, and the other end was directly anastomosed to the urethra.[10,11] Further modifications have included folding detubularized segments of ileum into J-shaped or W-shaped reservoirs.[12,13] In general, 40 to 60 cm of distal ileum are harvested for the bladder

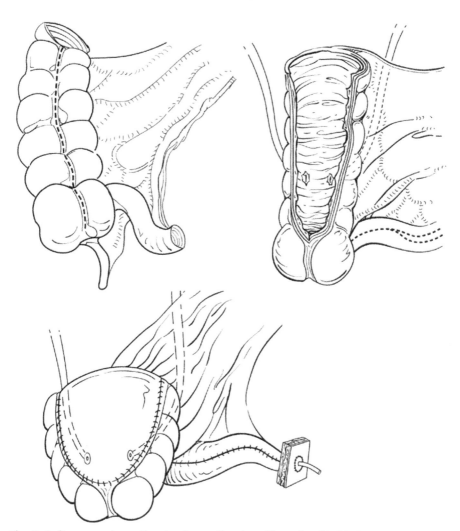

Fig. 5. Indiana pouch continent urinary diversion. (*From* Parekh DJ, Donat SM. Urinary diversion: options, patient selection, and outcomes. Semin Oncol 2007;34(2):98–109; with permission.)

substitution, with ~20 cm of terminal ileum left in place. For a J-pouch the ileal segment is detubularized except for a proximal 5-cm to 10-cm chimney segment to which the ureters are anastomosed (**Fig. 6**). For a W-pouch the ileal segment is either completely detubularized and the ureters are reimplanted into the posterior wall of the reservoir, or the proximal segment of ileum is not detubularized and the ureters are anastomosed to a chimney segment as in a J-pouch (**Fig. 7**). In either case the ileal bladder substitution is directly anastomosed to the urethra. Bladder substitutions lie predominantly in the midline, and most often extend toward the right side, but sometimes lie toward the left depending on the orientation of the small bowel mesentery. Continence is provided by the patients' native continence mechanism, thereby allowing patients to either void per urethra, or to perform clean intermittent catheterization per urethra.

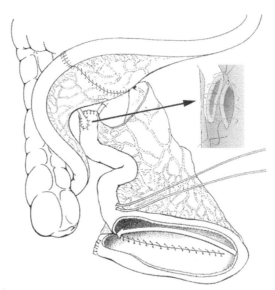

Fig. 6. J-pouch ileal bladder substitution. End-to-side ureteroileal anastomoses to proximal chimney. Detubularized portion of ileum has been folded into a J configuration. The posterior wall has been sutured together, whereas the anterior wall closure and urethral anastomosis remain to be completed. (*From* Thoeny HC, Sonnenschein MJ, Madersbacher S, et al. Is ileal orthotopic bladder substitution with an afferent tubular segment detrimental to the upper urinary tract in the long term? J Urol 2002;168(5):2030–4. [discussion: 2034]; with permission.)

Surgical considerations when operating on patients with bladder substitutions:

- Before making an abdominal incision a urethral catheter should be placed in a sterile fashion in order to decompress the bladder substitution. This technique also allows for intraoperative filling of the bladder substitution to facilitate anatomic dissection as well as identification of inadvertent injuries to it.
- Intestinal bladder substitutions may produce significant mucus, which can cause mucous plugging of catheters, poor drainage, and over distention. For this reason, large-caliber catheters (eg, 20–22 Fr) should ideally be placed. Note that anastomotic scarring at the ileal-urethral junction may only allow placement of a smaller-caliber catheter. If the catheter is to remain in place postoperatively, it should be gently irrigated with ~ 30 mL of sterile water or saline 4 times daily, and as needed, to prevent mucous plugging. Note that perforation of a bladder substitution is an intraperitoneal perforation, and is a potentially fatal complication.
- Intestinal bladder substitutions generally lie low in the midline abdomen and pelvis, and are often encountered when performing a low midline abdominal incision.
- Although ileal bladder substitutions predominantly lie in the midline, if a proximal chimney has been preserved the ureteroileal anastomosis most often extends toward the right side and is often adherent to the region of the common iliac vessels.
- For pelvic trauma that has disrupted the urethra, a large-caliber suprapubic tube (eg, 20–22 Fr) may be directly placed into the anterior bladder substitution. This catheter should also be routinely irrigated to prevent mucous plugging.

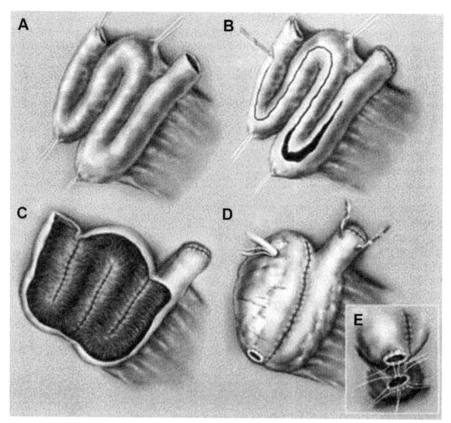

Fig. 7. W-pouch ileal bladder substitution. End-to-side ureteroileal anastomosis through posterior wall of W-pouch. (*A*) Ileal neobladder is constructed by Removed 68 cm. long ileal segment and orientating it into W shape with 4, 15 cm limbs. (*B*) Most proimal 8 to 12cm of ileal segment are not detubularized and remaining 60 cm of bowel are opened along anti-mesenteric border. (*C*) Posterior plate of W is sewn together. (*D*) Pouch is closed. (*E*) Ileal ure-thral anastomosis. (*From* Hollowell CM, Christiano AP, Steinberg GD. Technique of Hautmann ileal neobladder with chimney modification: interim results in 50 patients. J Urol 2000;163(1):47–50. [discussion: 50–1]; with permission.)

- For inadvertent injuries to a bladder substitution, urologic consultation is recommended. If a urologist is not available, the injury to the bladder substitution should be repaired in a running fashion with absorbable suture (eg, 2-0 polyglactin) in 2 layers. The repair should be tested by irrigating the previously placed catheter. The catheter should be left in place to provide maximal low-pressure drainage. A closed suction pelvic drain should also be placed. The drain may be removed once output is minimal, and if the drain fluid creatinine level is equivalent to the serum creatinine level (ie, consistent with serous fluid rather than urine.)

BLADDER AUGMENTATION/CYSTOPLASTY

Bladder augmentation (addition), or cystoplasty, is performed in patients with small-capacity, high-pressure bladders. This procedure is most often done in children, especially those with spina bifida or other spinal dysraphism. The terminal ileum was the first bowel segment described for cystoplasty, and is the most commonly used bowel segment[14] (**Fig. 8**). The cecum, sigmoid colon, and stomach (gastrocystoplasty) can also be used (**Fig. 9**). In essence, a segment of detubularized bowel is used to increase the capacity of the bladder. The bladder is opened, and the segment of intestine is sutured to the bladder.

Short-term complications of bladder augmentation include anastomotic leak, most of which heals with conservative management. Occasionally, prolonged catheter drainage and bilateral nephrostomy tubes are necessary to allow the leak to heal. Long-term complications include:

- Recurrent urinary tract infections
- Bladder stones (10%–50%)
- Bladder perforation, carcinoma
- Metabolic disorders

The bowel segments used in cystoplasty continue to make mucus, which may require occasional bladder irrigation. As with a perforated bladder substitution, perforation of an augmented bladder is a potentially fatal complication. Acute abdominal pain is the most common presenting symptom; other symptoms include nausea, vomiting, oliguria, and fever. In addition, patients with neurogenic bladders often have impaired sensation, which may delay the diagnosis. A high index of suspicion should be maintained in these patients. For patients who present with a suspected perforation of an augmented bladder, computed tomography cystogram is the study of choice. Treatment of bladder perforation includes immediate catheter drainage and operative repair of the perforation. Urologic consultation should be obtained. If a urologist is not available, the bladder should be repaired in 2 layers with absorbable suture. The bladder repair should be tested to make sure it is watertight.[15]

APPENDICOVESICOSTOMY

Patients with neurogenic bladder dysfunction often have physical limitations that prevent easy access to the urethra, particularly if they are wheelchair bound. In addition,

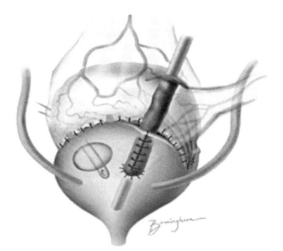

Fig. 8. Ileal cystoplasty. (*From* Gundeti MS, Acharya SS, Zagaja GP, et al. Pediatric robotic-assisted laparoscopic augmentation ileocystoplasty and Mitrofanoff appendicovesicostomy (RALIMA): feasibility of and initial experience with the University of Chicago technique. BJU Int 2011;107:966; with permission.)

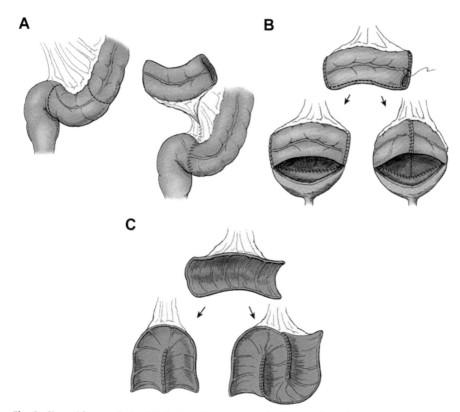

Fig. 9. Sigmoid cystoplasty. (*A*) A sigmoid segment of adequate length is removed from the gastrointestinal tract, and a colocolostomy is performed. (*B*) In the Mitchell technique the two opened ends are closed. The antimesentric border is incised, and the segment is anastomosed to the bivalved bladder. It may be rotated 180 degrees to allow an easy fit. (*C*) The opened sigmoid segment can be reconfigured into a U or S configuration, which may lower pressure. (*From* Adams MC, Joseph DB, Thomas JC. Urinary tract reconstruction in children. In: Wein AJ, editor. Campbell-Walsh urology. 11th edition. Elsevier: Philadelphia; 2016. p. 145, 3330–67.e10; with permission.)

for patients (and especially children) with normal urethral sensation, compliance with a routine catheterization schedule may be difficult to maintain. For this reason, continent catheterizable stomas are often used.

The most common type of catheterizable stoma in children is an appendicovesicostomy. The appendix is ideal for this purpose, because it is a natural tubular structure that can safely be removed from the gastrointestinal tract without significant morbidity. Typically, the distal end of the appendix is tunneled into a posterolateral position within the bladder, and the base of the appendix is brought up to the abdominal wall (**Fig. 10**).

Note that, most commonly, the base of the appendix is hidden within the umbilicus. The appendix and bladder wall are often secured to the peritoneum beneath the fascia to reduce the problem of conduit kinking with bladder filling.

Stomal stenosis is a common complication, generally occurring in 10% to 20% of patients with appendicovesicostomy.[16] Appendiceal perforation can also occur, but should heal with catheter placement (eg, 12–16 Fr) into the appendicovesicostomy.

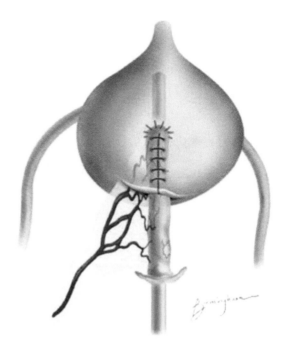

Fig. 10. Appendicovesicostomy. (*From* Wille MA, Zagaja GP, Shalhav AL, et al. Continence outcomes in patients undergoing robotic assisted laparoscopic Mitrofanoff appendicovesi-costomy. J Urol 2011;185(4):1438–43; with permission.)

ILEAL URETERAL SUBSTITUTION

In cases of pan-ureteral stricture or other cause of ureteral loss, a segment of ileum can be used to bridge the gap. The ileal ureter was first described by Shoemaker in 1909.[17] After the diseased portion of ureter is either removed or excluded, an appropriate length of ileum is used to connect either the renal pelvis or proximal ure-ter to the bladder (**Fig. 11**). In general, the mesentery for an ileal ureter has to be divided more extensively than for an ileal conduit in order to achieve maximal length and mobility.

Note that, in general, after bowel continuity has been reestablished, the ileal ureter is brought through the colonic mesentery laterally. Alternatively, on the right side, the cecum and ascending colon can be reflected superiorly to avoid the mesenteric window.

Ileal ureters are usually not performed in patients with a serum creatinine level of greater than 2 mg/dL, or if the patients have bladder dysfunction/outlet obstruction, inflammatory bowel disease, or radiation enteritis. Potential complications of an ileal ureter include:

- Urinary leak or fistula
- Mucous plugging of the ileal segment
- Bowel obstruction
- Kinking of the ileal segment[18]
- Ischemic necrosis of the ileal segment is a rare complication but should be considered in cases of an acute abdomen[19]

A   **B**   **C**

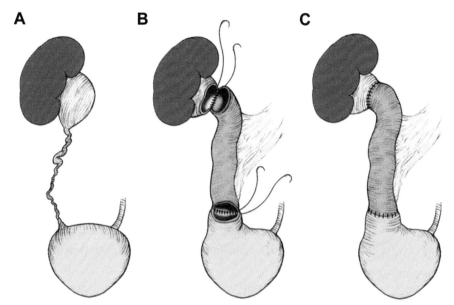

Fig. 11. Ileal ureteral substitution. (*From* Nakada SY, Best SL. Management of upper urinary tract obstruction. In: Wein AJ, editor. Campbell-Walsh urology. 11th edition. Elsevier: Philadelphia; 2016. p. 49, 1104–47.e7; with permission.)

METABOLIC COMPLICATIONS

Interposition of bowel into the urinary tract may lead to acute or chronic metabolic complications. In general, these complications can be divided into the following categories:

- Electrolyte abnormalities
- Nutritional disturbances
- Abnormal drug metabolism
- Bone disease[20]

This article focuses here on the pathophysiology, clinical presentation, and treatment of these metabolic complications.

Electrolyte Abnormalities

Stomach

A hypochloremic, hypokalemic, metabolic alkalosis may develop if the stomach is incorporated into the urinary tract because of the gastric mucosa's secretion of hydrogen, chloride, and potassium ions into the urine. This complication is rarely clinically significant in well-hydrated patients with normal renal function; however, a severe metabolic alkalosis may develop in patients who become acutely dehydrated or develop impaired renal function. Clinically, patients present with lethargy, respiratory insufficiency, and ventricular arrhythmias. Alkalosis is generally managed successfully with intravenous hydration, repletion of potassium, and H2 blockers to suppress the loss of acid into the urine. If H2 blockers fail, then a proton pump inhibitor may be used. Response rates to medical therapies are high; however, an intractable life-threatening metabolic alkalosis may require removal of the gastric segment.

Jejunum

All efforts should be made to avoid or minimize the use of the jejunum for intestinal urinary reconstruction. Interposition of this segment often leads to severe and intractable electrolyte abnormalities. The jejunum's secretion of sodium and chloride, coupled with the resorption of potassium and hydrogen, produces a hyponatremic, hyperkalemic, metabolic acidosis. Of particular concern with hyponatremia is the development of hypovolemia. In response to hypovolemia, the kidneys secrete renin. Activation of the renin-angiotensin-aldosterone system causes the kidney to resorb sodium and secrete potassium in the urine. When this low-sodium, high-potassium urine comes into contact with the jejunum, the jejunum secretes more sodium and resorbs more potassium, thereby creating a self-perpetuating cycle and worsening the metabolic derangement. When severe, these patients present with lethargy, nausea, vomiting, dehydration, weakness, and fever.[20] Treatment consists of saline administration to correct dehydration and hyponatremia, and administration of sodium bicarbonate to correct the acidosis. Note that hyperalimentation solutions should be avoided because they can exacerbate the metabolic derangement. Preventive measures consist of oral sodium chloride supplementation and adequate hydration.

Ileum and colon

A hyperchloremic metabolic acidosis may develop if ileum or colon is used for urinary tract reconstruction because of absorption of ammonium chloride and secretion of carbonic acid by the ileum or colon. Concomitant hypokalemia may also occur and is more pronounced when the colon is used because of its limited ability to absorb potassium.

If there is evidence of a hyperchloremic metabolic acidosis, even if mild, it should be treated with oral sodium bicarbonate or bicitrates. If severe, acute treatment consists of correction of the acidosis with administration of sodium bicarbonate and simultaneous potassium repletion. Concomitant potassium repletion is critical during correction of the metabolic acidosis to avoid severe hypokalemia.

Nutritional Disturbances

A variety of nutritional disturbances may occur with intestinal urinary diversion because of the loss of absorptive tissue following a bowel segment removal. When the stomach or terminal ileum is removed from the gastrointestinal tract, B_{12} deficiency may develop. This deficiency is caused by loss of the production of intrinsic factor, a cofactor necessary for B_{12} absorption within the terminal ileum. The body contains large stores of B_{12}; therefore, a clinically significant deficiency may not develop for 3 to 5 years.[21] B_{12} deficiency primarily manifests as megaloblastic anemia and sensory neuropathy. Diagnosis is based on low B_{12} levels but also increased levels of methylmalonic acid and homocysteine. Treatment consists of B_{12} injections.

If the ileum or ileocecal valve is removed, persistent diarrhea may develop because of abnormal bile salt metabolism. Bile salt is normally absorbed by the ileum and has a secretory effect on the colon that leads to chronic diarrhea. Cholestyramine, which acts to bind the bile salt, can be used to treat chronic diarrhea. Loss of the ileocecal valve also allows bacteria from the colon to reflux into the small bowel, resulting in bacteria overgrowth, fat malabsorption, and fat-soluble vitamin deficiency. Treatment consists of dietary modification with a low-fat diet and supplementation of fat-soluble vitamins if indicated.

Infection

Intestinal urinary diversion increases the risk for recurrent urinary tract infections, bacteremia, and sepsis. Although the mechanism is not fully understood, the high incidence of bacterial urinary colonization is thought to lead to bacteria dissemination into the blood stream.[20] Up to 75% of asymptomatic patients have positive urine cultures[20]; therefore, patients should not be treated without clinical signs of infection except for proteus and pseudomonas infections. These species are particularly virulent in the urinary system and mandate treatment even if the patient fails to manifest clinical symptoms. Systemically ill patients present with fever, chill, flank pain, malaise, and leukocytosis. A urine sample should be obtained via straight catheterization using sterile technique to confirm the diagnosis to minimize contamination from colonization. Urine samples obtained from a urostomy bag have an exceedingly high rate of bacterial contamination and should not be used. Treatment generally consists of intravenous fluid resuscitation, correction of electrolyte abnormalities, and antibiotic therapy based on culture sensitivity.

Abnormal Drug Metabolism

Intestinal urinary diversion increases the risk for abnormal drug metabolism leading to drug toxicity in the body. Medications normally absorbed by the gastrointestinal tract and excreted unchanged by the kidneys are most likely to become problematic.[20] Commonly problematic medications include phenytoin, lithium, β-lactam and aminoglycoside antibiotics, methotrexate, and cisplatin. Drug levels should be carefully and regularly monitored to prevent toxicity. Continuous drainage with placement of a Foley catheter should be considered if a patient requires chemotherapy treatment.

Bone Disease

Intestinal urinary diversion often leads to the development of osteomalacia and altered bone mineralization caused by chronic metabolic acidosis, vitamin D resistance, and persistent loss of calcium via the kidneys. The bones act to buffer the acidosis with the release of calcium, leading to demineralization over time. Correction of metabolic acidosis is critical to prevent bone loss and facilitate remineralization.[22] Treatment consists of correcting the metabolic acidosis and calcium supplementation. If bone density fails to improve, the active metabolite of vitamin D, 1-alpha-hydroxycholecalciferol, should be administered.

REFERENCES

1. Simon C. Ektopia vesicae: operation for diverting the orifices of the ureters into the rectum: temporary success; subsequent death; autopsy. Lancet 1857;2: 568–70.
2. Wear JB, Barquin OP. Ureterosigmoidostomy. Long term results. Urology 1973; 1(3):192–200.
3. Bricker EM. Bladder substitution after pelvic evisceration. Surg Clin North Am 1950;30:1511–21.
4. Zaayer EJ. Intra-abdominale plastieken. Ned Tijdrschr Geneeskd 1911;65:836.
5. Wallace DM. Uretero-ileostomy. Br J Urol 1970;42(5):529–34.
6. Chokshi RJ, Kuhrt MP, Schmidt C, et al. Single institution experience comparing double-barreled wet colostomy to ileal conduit for urinary and fecal diversion. Urology 2011;78:856–62.
7. Backes FJ, Tierney BJ, Eisenhauer EL, et al. Complications after double-barreled wet colostomy compared to separate urinary and fecal diversion during pelvic exenteration: time to change back? Gynecol Oncol 2013;128:60–4.

8. Kock NG, Nilson AE, Nilsson LO, et al. Urinary diversion via a continent ileal reservoir. Clinical results in 12 patients. J Urol 1982;128:469.

9. Bihrle R. The Indiana pouch continent urinary reservoir. Urol Clin North Am 1997; 24:773.

10. Camey M, LeDuc A. A procedure for avoiding reflux in uretero-ileal implantations during enterocystoplasty. Ann Urol (Fr) 1979;13:114–23.

11. Lillien OM, Camey M. 25-year experience with replacement of the human bladder (Camey procedure). J Urol 1984;132:886–91.

12. Studer U, Zingg E. Ileal orthotopic bladder substitutes. Urol Clin North Am 1997; 24:781.

13. Hautmann R, de Petriconi R, Gottfried HW, et al. The ileal neobladder: complications and functional results in 363 patients after 11 years of followup. J Urol 1999; 161:422.

14. Goodwin WE, Winter CC, Barker WF. "Cup-patch" technique of ileocystoplasty for bladder enlargement of partial substitution. Surg Gynecol Obstet 1959;108: 240–4, 13625074.

15. Taneja. Complications of urologic surgery. Chapter 49. In: Taneja, Samir, editors. Complications of bladder augmentation. Philadelphia: Saunders Elsevier; 2009. p. 571–8.

16. Harris CF, Cooper CS, Hutcheson JC, et al. Appendicovesicostomy: the Mitrofanoff procedure—a 15-year perspective. J Urol 2000;163:1922–6.

17. Shoemaker, cited by Moore EV, Weber R, Woodward ER, et al. Isolated ileal loops for ureteral repair. Surg Gynecol Obstet 1956;102:87.

18. Chung BI, Hamawy KJ, Zinman LN, et al. The use of bowel for ureteral replacement for complex ureteral reconstruction: long-term results. J Urol 2006;175: 179–84.

19. Wein AJ, Kavoussi LR, Novick AC, et al. Campbell's urology 10th edition. Chapter 41. Philadelphia: Saunders Elsevier; 2012. p. 1160–2.

20. McDougal WS. Use of intestinal segments and urinary diversion. In: Walsh PC, Retik AB, Vaughan ED, et al, editors. Campbell's urology. 10th edition. Philadelphia: Saunders; 2012. p. 2444–5.

21. Mills RD, Studer UE. Metabolic consequences of continent urinary diversion. J Urol 1999;161(4):1057–66.

22. Stein R, Lotz J, Andreas J, et al. Long-term metabolic effects in patients with urinary diversion. World J Urol 1998;16(4):292–7.

Diagnosis and Surgical Management of Uroenteric Fistula

Harcharan S. Gill, MD, FRCS

KEYWORDS

• Fistula • Urinary • Diverticulitis • Crohn

KEY POINTS

- Uroenteric fistulae can occur between any part of the urinary tract and the small and large bowel. Nomenclature and classification are generally based on the organ of origin in the urinary tract and the termination of the fistula in the segment of the gastrointestinal tract.
- Colovesical fistula secondary to diverticulitis is the commonest fistula that urologist and surgeons treat.
- Enterovesical fistulae are managed either conservatively or surgically.
- Although the principles of management are uniform, surgeons should be familiar with different surgical approaches.

INTRODUCTION

A fistula is an abnormal communication between 2 epithelium-lined cavities. Uroenteric fistulae can occur between any part of the urinary tract and the small and large bowel. Nomenclature and classification are generally based on the organ of origin in the urinary tract and the termination of the fistula in the segment of the gastrointestinal (GI) tract. Fistulae can cause important physiologic, biochemical, and infectious alterations and can often be a source of considerable emotional and psychological distress, thus a methodical and expeditious treatment approach is important for a successful outcome. Although some fistulae heal with conservative management, surgery is often necessary. Constant reassurance in cases in which the fistula will take extended periods to heal is equally important.

Congenital fistulae occur but are rare; most are acquired. Causes of acquired fistulae include trauma, inflammation, radiation, and malignancy, and they can also be iatrogenic. Uroenteric fistulae most frequently occur in a setting of inflammatory bowel disease, and diverticulitis is the commonest cause, accounting for

Disclosure: The author has nothing to disclose.
Department of Urology, Stanford University Hospital, 875 Blake Wilbur Drive, Stanford, CA 94305, USA
E-mail address: Hgill@stanford.edu

Surg Clin N Am 96 (2016) 583–592
http://dx.doi.org/10.1016/j.suc.2016.02.012 **surgical.theclinics.com**

approximately 65% to 79% of cases, and these are mostly colovesical. The second most common cause of fistulae is cancer (10%–20% of cases), followed by Crohn disease (5%-7%). The location and underlying disorder often determine the symptoms. Imaging with contrast in the bowel and intravenous contrast to outline the urinary tract in cross-sectional imaging with a computed tomography (CT) scan or MRI often helps in the diagnosis.

Although every type of fistula has specific methods and procedures necessary for treatment, the basic principles of managing urinary fistulae remain the same and include:

Adequate nutrition

Diversion of the urinary tract

Diversion of the GI tract, or bowel rest

Treat underling inflammatory processes or malignancy

Surgery

Principles of surgery when indicated include the following:

Appropriate timing

Anatomic separation of involved organs, maintaining adequate vascularity

Watertight closure in layers with interposition of omentum

Multiple-layer, tension-free closure with nonoverlapping suture lines

Urinary tract drainage with a stent or catheter

Surgeons should be familiar with a variety of techniques

VESICOENTERIC FISTULAE
Causes

This is the most common uroenteric fistula that surgeons and urologists treat. These fistulae usually occur in the setting of inflammatory bowel diseases such as diverticulitis and Crohn disease. Other causes include colorectal malignancy, radiation, trauma, pelvic abscesses, and iatrogenic surgical procedures. The underlying GI tract disorder determines the anatomic location of the fistula. Ileovesical fistulae are common in Crohn and colovesical fistulae are seen in diverticulitis or malignancies.[1]

Incidence

Diverticulitis is the commonest cause[1-3] and accounts for 65% to 70% of all cases. The peak incidence is between 55 and 65 years of age and it is estimated that 1% to 2% of patients with diverticulitis experience this. The underlying mechanism is a direct extension of ruptured diverticulum or erosion of a peridiverticular abscess into the bladder. The presence of a phlegmon and abscess are the risk factors for fistula formation The second commonest cause is colorectal cancer, which accounts for 10% to 15% of fistulae. Crohn disease accounts for 5% to 6% of vesicoenteric fistulae and the incidence of enterovesical fistulae in patients with Crohn disease is 2% to 4%. The duration of Crohn disease before discovery of the fistula has been reported to be from 6 months to 15 years and in rare cases this can be the initial presentation of this disease. Fistulae from Crohn present earlier in the third decade.[1,4] Regional enteritis, secondary to the transmural inflammation characteristic of Crohn colitis, results in adherence to the bladder with subsequent erosion into the organ and fistula formation. More than 80% of the fistulae are ileovesical, with male predominance presumed to be caused by the protective presence of the uterus in women.[5,6]

Presentation

Although the symptoms may originate from both the urinary tract and the GI tract, urinary symptoms tend to be commoner. The classic presentation syndrome of suprapubic pain, urinary frequency, dysuria, and tenesmus is named after a French physician, R. Gouverneur. Pneumaturia is the commonest symptom noted in 50% to 75% of the cases.[1] Urinary tract symptoms are most common in the early stages of the fistulae and may be nonspecific or dominated by prostatic symptoms, especially in older men. Rarely, patients can present in sepsis when concurrent urinary obstruction exists.[7]

Symptoms of vesicoenteric fistulae include:

Pneumaturia	52%–77%
Fecaluria	42%–51%
Frequency	37%–45%
Fever	12%–41%
Urinary infection	32%–45%
Abdominal pain	25%–33%
Hematuria	8%–22%
Urine per rectum, watery diarrhea	5%–9%

Diagnosis

The diagnosis of enterovesical fistula is primarily clinical, with the symptoms of pneumaturia, fecaluria, and persistent or recurrent urinary tract infections being essentially pathognomonic findings. A high clinical suspicion, detailed history, and selected diagnostic tests are all that are often necessary to establish the diagnosis. The following diagnostic tests are available and each has its potential false-positives and false-negatives:

Cystoscopy
Cross-sectional imaging: CT or MRI
Ultrasonography
Cystography
Upper GI contrast studies with small bowel follow-through
Barium enema
Colonoscopy
Bourne test
Activated charcoal test

Cystoscopy has the highest yield of identifying an abnormality in the bladder but on its own establishes a definitive diagnosis in only 35% to 60% of cases.[3,6,8] Findings on cystoscopy include focal hyperemia, bullous edema, air in the bladder, particulate material, and air extruding from papillary and bullous area in the bladder.

CT with oral contrast is the first test of choice in patients suspected of having fistulae. CT has a dual role of establishing the diagnosis and also identifying the site and segment of bowel involved. The diagnostic accuracy has been reported to be as high as 92% to 100%.[9,10] The classic findings on CT are air in the bladder, bladder wall thickening next to an inflamed or thickened segment of bowel, and presence of colonic diverticula. These finding have the highest yield in diagnosis of colovesical fistulae. Air in the bladder can be a false-positive finding if the patient has had a recent cystoscopy, or has a urinary infection from gas-forming organisms (**Fig. 1**).

Barium enema has a poor yield in the diagnosis of fistulae but may provide valuable information if a malignancy is suspected. Only 14% to 50% of colovesical fistulae were seen or suspected in barium enema.[11] Cystography, similarly, has a poor diagnostic value and is seldom necessary when cystoscopy has been done.

The Bourne test was first described in 1964, and remains an adjuvant test in the evaluations of patients suspected of having colovesical fistulae who have a negative or nondiagnostic barium enema. The first voided urine following a barium enema is collected, spun, and examined radiographically. Presence of radiodense material in the urine is diagnostic. In one report of 28 patients with colovesical fistulae, 7 out of 10 patients who had a negative barium enema had a positive Bourne test as the only positive evidence of the fistula.[10]

Oral activated charcoal test is sometimes indicated in the diagnosis of vesicoenteric fistula. Although it is an inexpensive test it does not localize the site of the fistula. A positive test is when black particles appear in the urine following oral administration of 25 g of activated charcoal. Kavanagh and colleagues[12] reported 5 of 7 patients with vesicoenteric fistulae to have a positive test and advocated the use of this test and cystoscopy as an initial evaluation of patients suspected to have enterovesical fistulae.

Management

The management of enterovesical fistulae can be either operative or nonoperative. The timing of surgical treatment is important and both single and multistage procedures may be necessary. Variables that affect the treatment choice include the underlying disorder, the patient's overall health and nutritional status, location of the fistula, and the presence of bowel obstruction. If a lesion is seen on cystoscopy, a biopsy should be done to rule out malignancy.

Nonsurgical, expectant treatment is an option for a select group of patients. In patients with minimal symptoms, who are not infected and have no underlying malignancy as a cause of the fistula, a trial of conservative therapy should be considered.

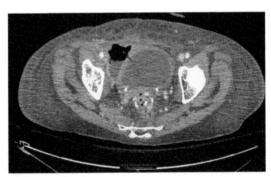

Fig. 1. CT scan in a patient with enterovesical fistula secondary to irradiation for ovarian cancer. Gas in the loop of bowel and fistula tract is seen.

This trial is especially warranted in patients with Crohn disease in whom immediate laparotomy with bowel resection is likely to result in complications. In addition, because of the relapsing nature of Crohn disease, nonoperative management should be tried first. This management includes bowel rest, total parenteral nutrition, antibiotics, and bladder drainage with a catheter.[1,13] Limited success (4 out of 30 patients) has also been reported with nonoperative management in patients with colovesical fistulae secondary to diverticulitis.[14]

The goals of surgical management are to separate the segment of bowel and bladder, close the defects in layers, and interpose healthy tissue like omentum between the 2 suture lines. Repair of the fistula often requires partial cystectomy and resection of involved bowel. The bladder has to remain decompressed with a Foley catheter to facilitate healing, and occasionally the bowel is temporarily diverted with a colostomy or ileostomy. In the presence of pelvic abscesses and severe local inflammation, a staged repair should be performed.

A 1-stage procedure involves removal of the fistula, closure of the involved organs, and primary reanastomosis of the bowel following resection of the involved bowel segment. Patients with an inflammatory cause of the fistula, but without gross contamination or abscess, can be treated with a 1-stage procedure.[14] Most patients with colovesical fistulae present electively with lower urinary tract symptoms, and therefore adequate preoperative support, including nutritional supplementation, and appropriate antibiotics can be used in most cases allowing an elective 1-stage approach.[15]

In Crohn disease, a conservative option with medical therapy including prednisone should be tried before considering surgery. Medical therapy can delay and occasionally obviate surgery. Greenstein and colleagues[16] reported that in 6 of 38 patients, surgery was able to be delayed with medical therapy for a mean of 3 years, and 2 of those patients never required an operation. Gorcey and Katzka[17] prospectively followed 11 patients with enterovesical fistula for up to 21 years with medical therapy. Seven patients ultimately required surgery for indications other than the enterovesical fistula, whereas the other 4 never required surgery. The indications for surgery include acute abdomen in ureteral obstruction, and refractory urinary tract infections, which can be a source of urinary sepsis. When surgery is considered, resection of the affected bowel, primary closure of the bladder, and interposition of an omental patch provides the best results. Occasionally a temporary diverting ileostomy is necessary, which can be taken down within 6 months.[6,18] All patients should have a cystogram at 10 to 14 days before removal of the catheter. In addition, appropriate antibiotics should be used to provide optimal healing of the bladder and bowel.

PROSTATORECTAL AND URETHRORECTAL
Causes

Although congenital rectourethral fistulae (RUF) can occur with imperforate anus, most are acquired. Iatrogenic causes lead this group with surgery, cryotherapy, high-frequency ultrasonography (HIFU), and radiation as the causes. Other causes include trauma, malignancy, and infection.

Incidence

The incidence of rectal injury during radical prostatectomy for prostate cancer ranges from 1% to 2 %.[19–21] The incidence is higher in salvage prostatectomy following irradiation. If the rectal injury is repaired primarily the incidence of prostate urethral fistulae is very small[22]; however, unrecognized injury to the rectum is likely to result in a rectourethral fistula.[20,21,23] The risk factors in the setting of a radical prostatectomy include prior radiation therapy or cryotherapy, rectal surgery, or previous transurethral resection of the prostate.[21] The incidence of fistulae following primary cryotherapy for prostate cancer is also 1% to 2%, but salvage cryotherapy after irradiation has a 3% to 4% rate of fistulae.[22] The reported incidence of prostate-rectal fistulae following brachytherapy is 0.4%, and following HIFU is 2% to 3%.[24] RUF in patients with Crohn disease are often complex and the incidence is less than 1%.

Presentation

Symptoms include urinary infection, fecaluria, hematuria, urinary incontinence, watery diarrhea, and (rarely) sepsis.

Diagnosis

Digital rectal examination often is diagnostic in patients with suspicious history. Definitive diagnosis is made with proctoscopy, urethrogram, barium enema, and a voiding cystourethrogram (**Fig. 2**). Accurate anatomic location is necessary for surgical planning. In complex cases of trauma or malignancy, upper tract imaging should also be done to rule out ureteral involvement.

Management

Conservative management with placement of a catheter with or without temporary bowel diversion is an option for a small and select group of patients, including small

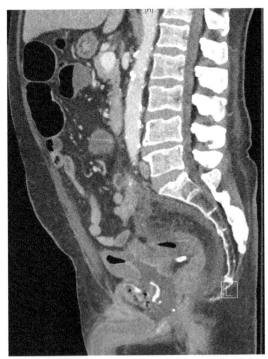

Fig. 2. Patient with fistula between rectum and prostatic urethra following a combination of brachytherapy and external irradiation for prostate cancer. Decompressed bladder with gas and brachytherapy seeds are evident.

postprostatectomy RUF in a nonirradiated patients who are in excellent nutritional status.[25–27] In such cases, fulguration of the fistula tract with application of fibrin glue has also be been reported with limited success.[28]

Surgical treatment is based on the basic principles outlined earlier. The surgical technique and approach are determined by the underlying disorder and the surgeon's experience.[29,30] Although repair of the fistula in 1 or multiple stages is desired, some patients are best managed with permanent urinary and bowel diversion. These patients include those who have a history of extensive irradiation to the pelvis, or have failed multiple attempts at surgical repair. One-stage repair is appropriate for small, surgically induced RUF in the absence of infection or previous irradiation. Staged repair that includes bowel diversion before the repair is best for large fistulae, those with history of irradiation, local infection, and previous failed repairs. Surgical approaches include:

Transanal with division of the anal sphincter

Transanal without division of the anal sphincter

Perineal

Transabdominal

Transrectal, transsphincteric approach, as described in the York Mason procedure, has been reported to have up to 90% success.[31] Meticulous attention to excising the fistula and tension-free closure in layers is critical in obtaining excellent outcome. Transanal approach without division of the sphincter involves dilatation of the anus to provide exposure. Repair technique principles are similar to York Mason with the disadvantage of poor exposure and limited maneuverability.[32] Use of rectal advancement flaps using this approach has also been reported in cases secondary to Crohn disease.[33] A perineal approach is popular with urologists because of familiarity with the local anatomy. This approach gives easy access to interpositional grafts, with the gracilis muscle being the commonest.[34,35] Transabdominal approach provides easy access to omentum for interposition, but has poor success rates compared with other approaches, probably secondary to poor exposure in a deep pelvis.[36,37] Fistulae secondary to radiation therapy and cryotherapy are generally larger, with significant perifistula ischemia. Surgical outcomes for repair are generally poor and therefore these patients often require permanent urinary and fecal diversions.[36,38]

URETEROENTERAL
Causes
Inflammatory bowel disease, such as Crohn disease, remains the commonest cause of ureteroenteric fistula. Other causes include iatrogenic causes, malignancy, radiation, calculus, and infection. Malignancies are either primary urothelial or invasion from surrounding organs.[39] The segment of bowel most likely to be involved is the terminal ileum and thus most cases of ureteroenteric fistula are unilateral, right sided, and usually at the level of the sacral promontory.[40] Rarely, diverticulitis or ulcerative colitis leads to a left-sided ureteroenteric fistula.

Incidence
Ureteroenteric fistulae are uncommon. This condition is a rare complication of Crohn disease[41] but remains the commonest cause. Iatrogenic causes are increasing slightly with the increase in ureteroscopic procedures and interventions.

Presentation

Ureteroenteric fistulae usually present with bowel rather than urinary symptoms. Recurrent urinary infection and flank pain as the presenting symptom have also been reported in some cases.

Diagnosis

Gas in the upper urinary tract collecting system is pathognomonic, but CT IVU (CT intravenous urogram) had the best yield. GI contrast studies are rarely diagnostic.

Management

This involves resection the bowel segment, stenting the ureter, and (rarely) placing a nephrostomy tube. A nephroureterectomy is only indicated in failed cases or if the involved ureter has a nonfunctioning kidney.[41]

RENOENTERAL OR PYELOENTERAL
Causes

Iatrogenic causes secondary to percutaneous renal surgery are increasing slightly compared with the historical cause from chronic infections. Xanthogranulomatous pyelonephritis or other infectious diseases involving the kidney or bowel have in the past been reported as the most common cause of this condition.[42] Other causes include penetrating trauma, complex calculus disease, ingested foreign bodies, and duodenal malignancies.

Presentation

Urinary infection associated with flank pain and fever is the commonest presentation. Patients may also have nonspecific GI symptoms and malaise.[43] It is rarely an incidental finding on imaging. Cloudy and particulate drainage from a nephrostomy tube following a percutaneous procedure should raise the clinical suspicion of a fistula.

Diagnosis

Imaging with CT IVP, nephrostograms (especially in iatrogenic cases), upper GI barium studies, and occasionally barium enema are appropriate.

Management

This is determined by the underlying disorder and renal function. In a poorly or nonfunctioning kidney the optimal treatment is a nephrectomy with repair of the appropriate bowel segment. In patients with normally functioning kidney, conservative treatment with drainage and bowel rest is preferred. A large nephrostomy tube with or without a ureteral stent, in combination with bowel rest, can result in successful closure of the fistula.[43]

REFERENCES

1. Gruner JS, Sehon JK, Johnson LW. Diagnosis and management of enterovesical fistulae in patients with Crohn's disease. Am Surg 2002;68:714–9.
2. Najjar SF, Jamal MK, Savas JF, et al. The spectrum of colovesical fistula and diagnostic paradigm. Am J Surg 2004;188:617–21.
3. McBeath RB, Schiff M, Allen V, et al. A 12-year experience with enterovesical fistulas. Urology 1994;44(5):661–5.

4. Badlani G, Abrams HJ, Levin LEA. Enterovesical fistula in Crohn's disease. Urology 1980;16:599.
5. Chebli JM, Gaburri PD, Pinto JR. Enterovesical fistula in Crohn's disease. Lancet 2004;364(9428):68.
6. Pontari MA, McMillen MA, Garvey RH, et al. Diagnosis and treatment of entero-vesical fistulae. Am Surg 1992;58:258.
7. Mileski WJ, Joehl RJ, Rege RV, et al. One-stage resection and anastomosis in the management of colovesical fistula. Am J Surg 1987;153:75–9.
8. Woods RJ, Lavery IC, Fazio BW, et al. Internal fistulas in diverticular disease. Dis Colon Rectum 1988;31:591–6.
9. Jarrett TW, Vaughan ED. Accuracy of computerized tomography in the diagnosis of colovesical fistula secondary to diverticular disease. J Urol 1995;153:44–6.
10. Amendola MA, Agha FP, Dent TL, et al. Detection of occult colovesical fistula by the Bourne test. AJR Am J Roentgenol 1984;142:715–8.
11. Niebling M, van Nunspeet L, Zwaving H, et al. Management of colovesical fistulae caused by diverticulitis:12 years of experience in one center. Acta Chir Belg 2013;113(1):30–4.
12. Kavanagh DO, Neary P, Bouchier-Hayes DJ, et al. Oral-activated charcoal in the diagnosis of enterovesical fistulae. Ir J Med Sci 2003;172(3):157.
13. Yamamoto T, Keighley MRB. Enterovesical fistulas complicating Crohn's disease: clinicopathological features and management. Int J Colorectal Dis 2000;15(4):211–5.
14. McConnell DB, Sasaki TM, Vetto RM. Experience with colovesical fistula. Am J Surg 1980;140:80–4.
15. Shackley DC, Brew CJ, Bryden AA, et al. The staged management of complex entero-urinary fistulae. BJU Int 2000;86:624–9.
16. Greenstein AJ, Sachar DB, Tzakis A, et al. Course of enterovesical fistulas in Crohn's disease. Am J Surg 1984;147:788–92.
17. Gorcey S, Katzka I. Is operation always necessary for enterovesical fistulas in Crohn's disease? J Clin Gastroenterol 1989;11:396–8.
18. Wade G, Zaslau S, Jansen R. A review of urinary fistulae in Crohn's disease. Can J Urol 2014;21(2):7179–84.
19. Renschler TD, Middleton RG. 30 years of experience with York-Mason repair of recto-urinary fistulae. J Urol 2003;170:1222–5.
20. Guillonneau B, Gupta R, El Fettouh H, et al. Laparoscopic management of rectal injury during laparoscopic radical prostatectomy. J Urol 2003;169:1694–6.
21. McLaren RH, Barrett DM, Zincke H. Rectal injury occurring at radical retropubic prostatectomy for prostate cancer: etiology and treatment. Urology 1993;42:401–5.
22. Chin JL, Pautler SE, Mouraviev V, et al. Results of salvage cryoablation of the prostate after radiation: identifying predictors of treatment failure and complications. J Urol 2001;165:1937–42.
23. Borland RN, Walsh PC. The management of rectal injury during radical retropubic prostatectomy. J Urol 1992;147:905–7.
24. Cordeiro ER, Cathelineau X, Thüroff S, et al. High-intensity focused ultrasound (HIFU) for definitive treatment of prostate cancer. BJU Int 2012;110(9):1228–42.
25. Rassweiler J, Seemann O, Schulze M, et al. Laparoscopic versus open radical prostatectomy: a comparative study at a single institution. J Urol 2003;169:1689–93.
26. Wedmid A, Mendoza P, Sharma S, et al. Rectal injury during robot-assisted radical prostatectomy: incidence and management. J Urol 2011;186(5):1928–33.

27. Noldus J, Fernandez S, Huland H. Rectourinary fistula repair using the Latzko technique. J Urol 1999;161:1518–20.
28. Wilbert DM, Buess G, Bichler KH. Combined endoscopic closure of rectourethral fistula. J Urol 1996;155:256–8.
29. Choi JH, Jeon BG, Choi SG, et al. Rectourethral fistula: systemic review of and experiences with various surgical treatment methods. Ann Coloproctol 2014; 30(1):35–41.
30. Hanna JM, Turley R, Castleberry A, et al. Surgical management of complex rectourethral fistulas in irradiated and nonirradiated patients. Dis Colon Rectum 2014;57(9):1105–12.
31. Rouanne M, Vaessen C, Bitker MO, et al. Outcome of a modified York Mason technique in men with iatrogenic urethrorectal fistula after radical prostatectomy. Dis Colon Rectum 2011;54(8):1008–13.
32. Hata F, Yasoshima T, Kitagawa S, et al. Transanal repair of rectourethral fistula after a radical retropubic prostatectomy: report of a case. Surg Today 2002;32: 170–3.
33. Fazio VW, Jones IT, Jagelman DG, et al. Rectourethral fistulae in Crohn's disease. Surg Gynecol Obstet 1987;164:148–50.
34. Rius J, Nessim A, Nogueras JJ, et al. Gracilis transposition in complicated perianal fistula and unhealed perineal wounds in Crohn's disease. Eur J Surg 2000;166:218–22.
35. Ghoniem G, Elmissiry M, Weiss E, et al. Transperineal repair of complex rectourethral fistula using gracilis muscle flap interposition—can urinary and bowel functions be preserved? J Urol 2008;179:1882–6.
36. Nunoo-Mensah JW, Kaiser AM, Wasserberg N, et al. Management of acquired rectourinary fistulae: how often and when is permanent fecal or urinary diversion necessary? Dis Colon Rectum 2008;51:1049–54.
37. Shin PR, Foley E, Steers WD. Surgical management of rectourinary fistulae. J Am Coll Surg 2000;191:547–53.
38. Marguet C, Raj GV, Brashears JH, et al. Rectourethral fistula after combination radiotherapy for prostate cancer. Urology 2007;69:898–901.
39. Chang JH, Cheng TC, Lin JS. Uretero-enteric fistula. Br J Urol 1998;81(1):162–3.
40. Sigel A, Botticher R, Wilhelm E. Urological complications in chronic inflammatory diseases of the bowel. Eur Urol 1977;3:7–10.
41. Loftus EV Jr, Schoenfeld P, Sandborn WJ. The epidemiology and natural history of Crohn's diseases in population-based patient cohorts from North America: a systematic review. Aliment Pharmacol Ther 2002;16:51–60.
42. Majeed HA, Mohammed KA, Salman HA. Renocolic fistula as a complication to xanthogranulomatous pyelonephritis. Singapore Med J 1997;38:116–9.
43. Desmond JM, Evans SE, Couch A, et al. Pyeloduodenal fistulae. A report of two cases and review of the literature. Clin Radiol 1989;40:267–70.

Diagnosis and Surgical Management of Male Pelvic, Inguinal, and Testicular Pain

Gabriel V. Belanger, MD[a], Graham T. VerLee, MD[b],*

KEYWORDS

- Pelvic pain • Inguinodynia • Orchalgia

KEY POINTS

- Pain in the prostate follows a continuum from acute to chronic, and treatment can be complicated by poor penetration of antibiotics into the reproductive tract.
- Inguinal pain occurs most commonly in the context of a previous herniorrhaphy.
- First-line pharmacotherapy should include gabapentinoids and tricyclic antidepressants, rather than opioids.
- Orchalgia and scrotal pain should prompt an ultrasonography scan to rule out acute disorder.
- Although promising surgical approaches exist to treat chronic scrotal pain, their success depends in part on intervening before central sensitization has occurred.

INTRODUCTION

Pain occurs in the male genitourinary organs, as for any organ system, in response to traumatic, infectious, or irritative stimuli. There are several hypothetical instances in which a knowledge and understanding of chronic genitourinary pain can be of great utility to practicing nonurologists, especially in clinical settings in which urologic consultation services are scarce or not readily available.

Naturally, genitourinary pain should initially be regarded as a symptom of a possible underlying disorder, and every effort should be exerted to identify an organic source, but, when a pertinent causative disorder is effectively excluded from the differential diagnosis, chronic pain then becomes its own diagnosis. Chronic pain in the male genitourinary system is a distressing complaint for the patient, with only subtle objective anatomic and microanatomic findings, if any, and effective treatment options until

Disclosure: The authors have nothing to disclose.
[a] Division of Urology, Maine Medical Center, 22 Bramhall Street, Portland, ME 04102, USA;
[b] Maine Medical Partners Urology, 100 Brickhill Avenue, South Portland, ME 04106, USA
* Corresponding author.
E-mail address: verleg@mmc.org

Surg Clin N Am 96 (2016) 593–613
http://dx.doi.org/10.1016/j.suc.2016.02.014
0039-6109/16/$ – see front matter © 2016 Elsevier Inc. All rights reserved.

recently have been limited.[1] This article demystifies the causes of genital pain and reviews the current approaches to treatment in three regions of the male genital tract commonly affected by chronic pain: the prostate, the inguinal region, and the scrotum.

CHRONIC PAIN PATHOPHYSIOLOGY

Genitourinary pain may be regarded as having either a neuropathic or a nociceptive cause. The term neuropathic pain implies that the peripheral nerves are involved in the primary disorder or have been directly damaged by infection, trauma, or surgery. The resultant pain usually develops in the sensory distribution of the affected peripheral nerve or nerves, and although the original insult has healed, the neurons acquire a pathologic level of activity to autonomously generate impulses in the absence of a stimulus.[2] In contrast, non-neuropathic pain might include that of a persistent somatic nociceptive source, including inflammation of a wound, keloid formation, mass effect from aberrant anatomy such as a recurrent hernia, a foreign body such as a metallic vasectomy clip, or a chronic infection of the prostate or genitalia. There is evidence that additional pathophysiologic processes also contribute to the evolution of chronic pain, including neuroplasticity, afferent hypersensitivity, pain centralization, and deafferentation hypersensitivity, which if present may predispose a patient to treatment failure even if a neuropathic or nociceptive source is identified and corrected.[3]

Several hypotheses exist for the emergence of chronic pain, and these theories are not mutually exclusive. There is evidence that the peripheral and central nervous systems undergo a form of modulation following a long duration of painful stimuli, resulting in sensitization of the pain receptors.[4] Other evidence suggests that, as peripheral nerves regenerate following injury, axons may rejoin erroneously with one another in the dorsal spinal cord such that a depolarization detected by an axon might propagate its signal to an inappropriate neuron proximally, and thus innocent stimuli may be perceived as inordinately noxious.[5]

PROSTATIC PAIN

The term prostatitis refers to a broad array of disease processes. The National Institutes of Health (NIH) developed a classification system for prostatitis in 1995 and proposed universal adoption at the International Prostatitis Collaborative Network workshop in 1998, in Washington, DC[6] (**Table 1**).

CATEGORY I: ACUTE BACTERIAL PROSTATITIS
Clinical Presentation

Prostatitis is a common genitourinary infection, with a lifetime prevalence of up to 16%.[7] A proposed cause of acute bacterial prostatitis (ABP) involves the reflex of

Table 1
NIH prostatitis classification system

Category	Type
I	Acute bacterial prostatitis
II	Chronic bacterial prostatitis
III	Chronic prostatitis/chronic pelvic pain syndrome
IIIA	Inflammatory
IIIB	Noninflammatory
IV	Asymptomatic inflammatory prostatitis

infected urine into the ejaculatory and prostatic ducts of the prostatic urethra. Other possible routes of infection include invasion of rectal bacteria through direct extension or hematogenous spread.[8] Iatrogenic causes include cystoscopic manipulation of the prostate or bacterial seeding via transrectal biopsy.[9] Risk factors for ascending infection include unprotected sexual intercourse, phimosis, indwelling catheter, and instrumentation. Anything leading to urinary stasis, such as distal urethral stricture and benign prostatic hyperplasia, is also a risk factor.[10]

By definition, ABP has a rapid onset. Patients typically present with a combination of pelvic pain and lower urinary tract symptoms (LUTS). The pain is often described as pelvic, perineal, genital, or a combination.[11] In addition to pain, patients may show a wide array of lower urinary tract symptoms. Symptoms may be irritative (urgency, frequency) or obstructive (weakened stream, intermittent stream, acute urinary retention). Patients may also have dysuria. High-grade fever and other signs and symptoms of systemic illness are often present.[11]

In a retrospective analysis of 614 patients diagnosed with ABP by Milan and colleagues,[12] the most common complications in these patients were acute urinary retention (9.7%), prostatic abscess (2.7%), and recurrent infection (12.7%). Patients with ABP secondary to genitourinary tract manipulation also fared much worse overall. Specifically, the investigators noted a higher risk of prostatic abscess, recurrent infections, and infections involving atypical organisms in this group. Patients with ABP are at significant risk of progressing to chronic bacterial prostatitis (CBP).[13]

Diagnosis

Unlike chronic prostatitis, ABP is diagnosed primarily by clinical history, physical examination, and urine culture alone. Given the interconnectivity of the genitourinary tract, a complete urologic physical examination should be performed, including costovertebral angle percussion and palpation of the abdomen, bladder, testicles, and epididymides to rule out associated infectious/inflammatory processes.[11] A gentle palpation of the prostate should be performed as well. The prostate is often described as being tender to palpation and often warm and boggy.[14] Vigorous prostatic massage should be avoided because of the theoretic risk of bacteremia.[14] Therefore, the 2-glass and 4-glass tests used in the diagnosis of chronic prostatitis should be avoided (discussed later).

Urine cultures generally grow out typical uropathogens, with *Escherichia coli* isolated up to 87% of the time. Other organisms include *Pseudomonas*, *Serratia*, *Klebsiella*, and *Enterobacter*.[10] *Chlamydia trachomatis* is rarely isolated.[15] Recent literature has shown an increasing prevalence of fluoroquinolone-resistant and extended-spectrum β-lactamase–producing bacteria in all patients with prostatitis, but especially in those with prostatitis associated with transrectal prostate biopsy.[16,17]

Treatment

Medical

If the patient is febrile or systemically ill, treatment should be with a high-dose, broad-spectrum parenteral antibiotic, such as a broad-spectrum penicillin derivative, third-generation cephalosporin, or a fluoroquinolone until fevers and systemic symptoms have resolved.[11] When clinically stable, the condition can be treated with oral fluoroquinolone or trimethoprim/sulfamethoxazole, if tested susceptible.[18] Treatment duration of 4 weeks is recommended.[19]

Along with treatment of the causative organism, medical management directed at patient symptoms should be considered. Treat concomitantly with nonsteroidal anti-inflammatory medicines for symptomatic pain relief.[18] Treatment with α-blockers has been shown to improve LUTSs in men with prostatic inflammation and should be considered in men in whom LUTSs are an issue.[20,21] Temporary catheterization may be necessary to relieve acute urinary obstruction.

Surgical

Most patients who present with ABP are adequately treated with medical therapy alone; however, a small subset of patients require surgical intervention. In patients who fail to respond rapidly to medical therapy, consider transrectal ultrasonography or computed tomography scan to assess for abscess.[22] Prostatic abscesses smaller than 1 cm can be treated conservatively with antibiotics, whereas larger abscesses benefit from drainage.[23] Percutaneous perineal drainage, transrectal ultrasonography–guided drainage, and transurethral unroofing are all viable methods of treating a prostatic abscess with no clear data recommending one rather than the other.[10] If the abscess is noted to be outside the prostate, consider percutaneous or transrectal drainage.

CATEGORY II CHRONIC BACTERIAL PROSTATITIS
Clinical Presentation

To be chronic, symptoms must be present for more than 3 months.[14] It is the most frequent cause of recurrent urinary tract infection in young to middle-aged men, with 25% to 43% of patients diagnosed with CBP having recurrent urinary tract infection as shown by the 4-glass test.[18] Symptoms are indistinguishable from those of chronic pelvic pain syndrome, which is described in detail later.

Diagnosis

From 4.2% to 7% of men with chronic prostatitis/pelvic pain syndrome have a chronic bacterial infection, as shown by the 4-glass or 2-glass tests.[24] The 4-glass test, the current gold standard, developed in 1968 by Meares and Stamey,[25] is used to distinguish between infections of the urethra, prostate, and bladder (**Fig. 1**).

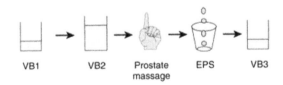

VB1   VB2   Prostate massage   EPS   VB3

4-Glass Test (Meares-Stamey Test)

Classification	Specimen	VB1	VB2	EPS	VB3
CAT II	WBC	−	+/−*	+	+
	Culture	−	+/−*	+	+
CAT IIIA	WBC	−	−	+	+
	Culture	−	−	−	−
CAT IIIB	WBC	−	−	−	−
	Culture	−	−	−	−

Fig. 1. Technique and interpretation of the Meares-Stamey 4-glass lower urinary tract localization test for chronic prostatitis and chronic pelvic pain syndrome. CAT, category; EPS, expressed prostatic secretion; VB, voided bladder; WBC, white blood cell. (*From* Nickel JC. Inflammatory and pain conditions of the male genitourinary tract. In: Wein AJ, editor. Campbell-Walsh urology. 11th edition. Philadelphia: Elsevier; 2016. p. 49, 1104–47.e7; with permission.)

- The first 10 mL of urine represent the urethral specimen (voided bladder 1 [VB1]).[18]
- The second specimen is the midstream urine collection, and assesses the bladder for infection (VB2).
- The third specimen is the prostatic secretions collected at the urethra during vigorous massage (expressed prostatic secretion [EPS]).
- The last specimen contains the first 10 mL of voided urine after a vigorous prostatic massage and further assesses the prostate (VB3).

The 2-glass test assesses for bladder infection versus prostate infection and is much less complicated and costly.[18]

- It involves a midstream urine collection to assess the bladder and the first 10 mL of urine after a vigorous prostatic massage to assess the prostate.
- It has been shown to be a viable alternative to the 4-glass test, and less costly and complicated.[26]

The diagnosis of CBP is made when there is a 10-fold increase in bacteria in the EPS or VB3 specimen compared with the VB1 and VB2 specimens on a 4-glass test. Alternatively a 10- fold increase in bacteria in the post–prostatic massage specimen in the 2-glass test is also diagnostic.[18] In addition, providers should consider obtaining uroflowmetry and postvoid residuals to rule out bladder outlet obstruction as a contributor.[14] Bacterial isolates are similar to those in ABP.[14] In patients with immunodeficiency, consider atypical organisms such as fungus, *Staphylococcus*, *Mycobacterium tuberculosis*, and *Mycobacterium avium*.

Treatment

Fluoroquinolone antibiotics are considered to be the drugs of choice for CBP because prostate concentrations of these drugs have been shown to reach efficacious doses.[14] Bactrim also has proven efficacy.[18] Ultimately, treatment should be tailored appropriately based on culture results. α-Blockers have also been shown to improve symptoms and reduce recurrence in men with CBP.[27] Treatment course should be at least 4 to 6 weeks. If symptoms fail to resolve at 6 weeks, consider prostate imaging to assess for abscess, because this requires drainage, as discussed earlier.[14,18]

CATEGORY III: CHRONIC NONBACTERIAL PROSTATITIS/CHRONIC PELVIC PAIN SYNDROME
Clinical Presentation

Chronic nonbacterial prostatitis (CP)/chronic pelvic pain syndrome (CPPS) is a common disease process affecting around 10% to 16% of men. It is most prevalent in men between 36 and 50 years old and accounts for approximately 8% of visits to urologists and 1% of primary care visits in the United States.[28] The cause is currently unknown and may involve several simultaneous mechanisms. Nickel and colleagues[29] showed no differences in positive cultures in EPS in men with CPPS versus controls. Multiple other studies have failed to show a link between CPPS and sexually transmitted diseases.[28]

Presenting symptoms in patients with IIIA and IIIB disease are essentially indistinguishable. As mentioned previously, they are similar to those with CBP.[14] The most common symptom in these patients is perineal, suprapubic, or penile pain; however, pain can also occur in the testes, groin, or lower back.[30] Pain associated with ejaculation is also common and very concerning to patients and is associated with more severe and refractory symptoms.[31] Other symptoms possibly seen in these patients include obstructive or irritative voiding symptoms, erectile dysfunction, and sexual disturbances.[32–34] The NIH Prostatitis Cohort Study reported that more than half of men had pain related to sexual climax.[30]

Along with physical symptoms, psychological symptoms are common in this patient demographic.[35] Depression, stress, or a history of abuse is common in these patients and their presence may exacerbate primary disease symptoms.[36–38] In addition, a case-control study by Pontari and colleagues[39] showed that patients with chronic prostatitis have a significantly increased lifetime risk of cardiovascular disease, neurologic disease, psychiatric conditions, and infectious disease. Several studies, using standardized quality-of-life measures, have shown similar values to those of patients with myocardial infarction, angina, or Crohn disease.[40,41]

Diagnosis

Symptoms must be present for 3 months to be considered chronic.[24] Physical examination in patients with CP/CPPS is often unremarkable except for pain. Examination and palpation of the external genitalia, groin, perineum, coccyx, external anal sphincter, and internal pelvic floor and sidewalls is essential to look for particular areas of pain because this may facilitate directed treatment.[18]

As with CBP, a 2-glass or 4-glass test is important in diagnosis, mainly ruling out CBP given that the NIH Chronic Prostatitis Cohort Study suggested no significant clinical difference between patients in category IIIA and IIIB.[30]

- Category IIIA CP/CPPS is diagnosed when uropathogenic bacteria are not cultured, but more than 5 to 10 white blood cells (WBCs) per high power field are noted on microscopic analysis of the EPS and/or VB3 specimen.[18]
- Category IIIB CP/CPPS is diagnosed when no uropathogenic bacteria are cultured and fewer than 5 to 10 WBCs per high power field are noted on microscopic analysis.

The NIH Chronic Prostatitis Symptom Index (NIH-CPSI) is a validated patient questionnaire that is invaluable in helping to guide therapy specific to the patient's symptoms.[42,43] It consists of 9 questions that address 3 domains: pain, urinary function, and quality of life. In a complex disease such as CPPS, this tool is invaluable in helping direct treatment. Along with the NIH-CPSI, the NIH Third International Collaborative Network recommends a urinary flow rate and postvoid residual test be performed on every patient with CPPS to help classify symptoms to aid in more directed treatment.[18]

Proposed causes of persistent irritative and obstructive voiding symptoms, often associated with CP/CPPS, include detrusor internal/external sphincter dyssynergia, proximal or distal urethral obstruction, and bladder neck fibrosis/hypertrophy.[44–47] Kaplan and colleagues[48,49] showed that men with a diagnosis of CP/CPPS had symptoms of voiding dysfunction, including 54% with primary bladder neck obstruction, 24% with functional membranous urethral obstruction, 17% with impaired bladder contractility, and 5% with an acontractile bladder. Because of this, videourodynamics may be of some value in selected patients who fail directed therapy, with a component of voiding dysfunction.[48,49]

In patients who fail appropriate antibiotic therapy, transrectal ultrasonography may play a role in diagnosis of medial prostatic cysts, prostatic abscesses, and seminal vesicle obstruction in patients who present with prostatitislike symptoms.[9,50]

Cystoscopy should be performed in all patients presenting with gross hematuria and in those with persistent microscopic hematuria despite appropriate treatment of prostatitis.[51] It should also be considered in patients who fail treatment, to rule out another cause of symptoms, or if the diagnosis is unclear.[18]

Treatment

CP/CPPS encompasses a broad array of patients and symptoms. Because of this, clinicians are often frustrated in choosing the correct treatment modality for these patients. Numerous treatments have shown efficacy in the treatment of this disease spectrum and can be used selectively based on patient symptom domains.

Although patients with CP/CPPS do not grow out bacteria from prostate cultures, by definition, it is thought that bacteria may be the prime cause of patient symptoms in at least a subset of these patients. Nickel and colleagues[52] showed a 45% to 65% NIH-CPSI score in patients with category II, IIIa, and IIIb with treatment of ofloxacin alone, regardless of disease category, suggesting bacteria may play a role even in culture-negative patients. Later studies showed that patients with long-standing symptoms and multiple previous treatments do not benefit from further antibiotic treatment.[53,54] It is reasonable, therefore, to consider antibiotic treatment in a patient newly diagnosed with CP/CPPS, without previous antibiotic treatment.

Given the significant LUTSs experienced in many individuals with CP/CPPS, therapy targeted at this domain is of benefit to patients. Pseudodyssynergia (contraction of the external sphincter during voiding) is one proposed method leading to LUTSs in CP/CPPS patients.[48] This dysfunctional voiding is thought to lead to reflux of urine into the prostatic ducts, leading to inflammation and pain. α-Adrenergic blockade is known to improve outflow obstruction, by causing relaxation of the bladder neck. There are currently 4 randomized controlled trials showing the efficacy of α-adrenergic blockade in treatment of patients with urinary symptoms, as defined by the NIH-CPSI.[55–58]

Category IIIA CP/CPPS involves prostatic inflammation, therefore modulation of prostatic inflammation is another possible treatment modality in these patients. Nonsteroidal antiinflammatory medications have been shown to cause rapid improvement in inflammatory symptoms, such as dysuria, stranguria, and painful ejaculation.[59] High-dose cyclooxygenase-2 inhibitors have also shown efficacy.[60,61] Oral corticosteroid formulations have not shown efficacy in treatment of CP/CPPS at this time.[62]

Some clinicians have proposed pelvic floor dysfunction as a potential cause of CP/CPPS. Clinical data regarding these use of muscle relaxants have been conflicting. One prospective double-blind study showed a significant improvement in patients treated with baclofen compared with placebo,[63] whereas other studies have shown no improvement compared with placebo.[64] At present, data are conflicting. In patients in whom pelvic floor dysfunction is a possible cause for CP/CPPS, use of a striated muscle relaxant is reasonable.

Other possible treatments include hormonal therapy with 5α-reductase inhibitors, phytotherapeutic agents, gabapentinoids, allopurinol, prostatic massage, pudendal nerve entrapment therapy, biofeedback, acupuncture, and psychological support. Each of these modalities has some supporting research, although it is limited and conflicting. More research is needed in these areas.[18]

One recent modality that has shown promise is intraprostatic botulinum toxin injection. It is known that its injection leads to apoptosis and atrophy of the prostate gland. It also results in release of multiple pain mediators, leading to relief of nociceptive pain. One double-blinded randomized controlled trial showed significant NIH-CPSI scores in the treatment group.[65] Although not currently approved in this patient group, it may represent a treatment alternative in refractory and severe disease.

CP/CPPS is a challenging disease with a broad spectrum of symptoms. Pinpointing the correct area to treat can be challenging for any clinician. One new 6-point clinical classification system, called UPOINT (urinary, psychosocial, organ specific, infection, neurologic/systemic, and tenderness of skeletal muscles), classifies patients into 6 domains and was designed to help physicians tailor therapy to these complex patients and has proved efficacious.[66–68]

The treatment of CP/CPPS is often multimodal and complex. The goal of UPOINT is to better characterize the broad array of symptoms with which patients may present in order to develop a better treatment plan that addresses all of the patient's symptoms. Online tools have been developed and validated to assist in classifying patients into UPOINT domains and to assess disease severity.[69] A full discussion of treatment is beyond the scope of this article, but a summary of classification and treatment based on UPOINT is provided in **Table 2**.

Table 2
Phenotypic approach to pelvic pain: UPOINT classification and directed therapy for CP/CPPS

UPOINT Domain	Clinical Criteria	Possible Therapy[a]
Urinary	Bothersome urgency, frequency, and/or nocturia Increased postvoid residual urine Dysuria	Diet modification α-Adrenergic blockers Pyridium Anticholinergic agents
Psychosocial	Depression Maladaptive coping Social dysfunction Stress Anxiety	Cognitive behavior therapy Counseling Antidepressants Antianxiolytics
Organ specific	Specific prostate tenderness Leukocytosis in prostate specimens Hematospermia Extensive prostate calcification Lower urinary tract obstruction	Quercetin α-Adrenergic blockers Prostate massage Surgery
Infection	Exclude patients with clinical category I or II prostatitis[b] Gram-negative bacilli or enterococci in prostate-specific specimens History of previous resolution with antibiotics	Antibiotics
Neurologic/systemic	Pain beyond abdomen and pelvis Associated medical conditions such as irritable bowel syndrome, fibromyalgia	Gabapentinoids Amitriptyline Neuromodulation
Tenderness (of skeletal muscles)	Palpable tenderness, painful spasm or trigger points in pelvis or abdomen	Physiotherapy Muscle relaxants Exercises

[a] Therapies listed are not necessarily evidence based but are suggested on the best available evidence, interpretation of clinical trial data, and clinical experience. Therapies should be targeted against specific symptom or clinical assessment within a particular phenotype. Some treatments are effective only in a subcategory of a specific phenotype and are not effective in others.

[b] This category does not include patients with category II CBP, defined as men with recurrent urinary tract infections (usually same organism) with identical organism identified in prostate-specific specimens between episodes of infection (see text). These patients have the requirements for inclusion in the category III CP/CPPS: genitourinary and/or pelvic pain with no history of recurrent urinary tract infections.

From Nickel JC. Prostatitis and related conditions, orchitis, and epididymitis. In: Wein AJ, Kavoussi LR, Novick AC, et al. Campbell-Walsh Urology. 10th edition. Philadelphia: Elsevier Saunders; 2012. p. 353; with permission.

CATEGORY IV: ASYMPTOMATIC INFLAMMATORY PROSTATITIS

Asymptomatic inflammatory prostatitis is asymptomatic. Patients typically present with another complaint, such as benign prostatic hyperplasia (BPH), prostate cancer, or infertility, and the semen analysis or histologic examination of the prostate shows evidence of inflammation. Because prostatitis is a recognized cause of male infertility, its incidental finding during infertility could necessitate treatment.[70]

INGUINODYNIA

The single most common identifiable predisposing factor in the literature associated with chronic inguinal pain is inguinal herniorrhaphy. By one estimate, up to 27% of all men in the industrialized world may undergo inguinal herniorrhaphy in their lifetimes,[71] and so, even though the procedure might incur an overall low rate of complications, many men might subsequently present annually with persistent postoperative inguinal pain. Although regional practice patterns vary, in North America inguinal hernia repair is most often a procedure performed by general surgeons, and therefore patients who experience postoperative inguinodynia are likely to present to the surgeon who performed their herniorrhaphy. Much of the literature on inguinodynia is likewise written from a general surgical perspective. Inguinodynia of a principally surgical or traumatic cause is discussed later in the article, although other causes might include diabetic neuropathy, herpes zoster infection, and drug-related neuropathy, as can be the case with certain chemotherapy regimens.[72]

DIAGNOSIS

The iliohypogastric, ilioinguinal, and genitofemoral nerves have been collectively dubbed the border nerves by some anatomists,[73] based on their cutaneous innervation of the region between the abdomen and anterior thigh. Surgical incisions in the lower abdomen, even when deliberately made parallel to the Langer lines, risk injury to these nerves, and the resultant neuropathy that follows presents with inguinal pain with possible radiation to the scrotum or medial thigh.[74] Damage to these nerves can occur intraoperatively or postoperatively. Intraoperatively, nerves can be damaged by surgical manipulation but also by stretching; crushing; electrical/thermal damage; partial or complete transection; becoming entrapped in suture during an open repair; or entrapment in tacks, suture, or fixation used during a laparoscopic repair. Postoperatively, nerves can become damaged by envelopment within an inflammatory pseudocapsule surrounding implanted mesh, irritation secondary to an excessive fibrotic reaction, or inflammatory processes such as granuloma or neuroma formation. For the remainder of this article, the term inguinodynia is used to refer to chronic postoperative inguinal pain.

The diagnosis of inguinal pain remains largely based on subjective findings. Efforts to define inguinodynia by quantifying the degree of neuralgia in patients with inguinal pain have shown poor sensitivity. Quantifiable electromyographic abnormalities are present in only 60% of men with proven ilioinguinal or iliohypogastric nerve entrapment, and in fewer than 40% of men with probable entrapment.[75] Diagnosis of inguinal neuralgia is thus made principally on symptoms, although in the absence of an obvious inciting factor, such as herniorrhaphy, other associated disorders, such as zoster infection, should be clinically excluded. Because the initial diagnostic criteria for inguinodynia are so indistinct and lack standardization in the literature, so too are the tools used to measure the success of treatment. Some published studies designed to gauge the effectiveness of one treatment compared with another have done so using various validated quality-of-life questionnaires rather than objective physical findings.

MEDICAL TREATMENT OF POSTOPERATIVE INGUINODYNIA

Commonly prescribed acute pain regimens in the immediate perioperative period following herniorrhaphy typically include acetaminophen and nonsteroidal antiinflammatory drugs followed by low-dose opioids for breakthrough pain. Although this seems to suffice for uncomplicated patients, some patients complain of pain that persists beyond the anticipated convalescence period. The extent of pain at 1 week and 4 weeks postherniorrhaphy correlates with the incidence of ongoing pain after 1 year.[76] Although historically surgeons might have addressed these requests by reordering more prescription narcotics, published consensus guidelines from both the International Association for the Study of Pain and the Neuropathic Pain Special Interest Group have firmly established that opioids do not have a role in first-line treatment of chronic neuropathic pain.[72]

Instead, first-line medications for evolving chronic genitourinary pain include antidepressants and gamma-aminobutyric acid analogues. Secondary amine tricyclic antidepressants (TCAs), including nortriptyline and desipramine, are inexpensive and feature convenient dosing schedules relative to other agents. Their sedative and anticholinergic side effects can limit patient compliance but may become more tolerable with time and are less severe than for tertiary amine TCAs such as amitriptyline. The efficacy of TCAs is optimized by ensuring that an adequate 6-week to 8-week trial is performed.

GABA analogues have been studied for their potential role not only in treatment of postoperative pain but also in the preoperative setting to mitigate the risk of developing chronic neuropathic pain. An elegant meta-analysis confirmed that perioperative administration of a single dose of either pregabalin or gabapentin 1 hour before surgery effectively reduced the risk of chronic postsurgical pain more than placebo in several surgical populations, including inguinal herniorrhaphy. Participants in the treatment arms experienced reduced incidence and severity of chronic pain with 6 months' follow-up.[77] Used over the longer term, these medications can produce dose-related dizziness and sedation that can be ameliorated by starting with low dosages and titrating cautiously.[78]

Guidelines for the treatment of chronic pain describe the use of transdermal medications to assist in regional pain control. However, specific to postoperative inguinodynia, lidocaine patch treatment did not reduce combined resting and dynamic pain ratings compared with placebo in patients with severe, persistent inguinal postherniorrhaphy pain.[79,80]

INTERVENTIONAL TREATMENT OF POSTOPERATIVE INGUINODYNIA

Many regional pain specialists and general surgeons have endeavored to treat postherniorrhaphy pain by targeting the causative peripheral nerve. Although intellectually promising, the results of regional interventions have been mixed.[74] High-level evidence is lacking regarding the interventional and surgical treatment of inguinodynia.[3] Efforts even to inject a temporary local analgesic into the nerves of the groin have had limited results: a double-blinded placebo-controlled study showed no statistical difference between the pain relief of men who received ultrasonography-guided ilioinguinal and iliohypogastric nerve blocks with lidocaine compared with those who received placebo injections.[81] This finding may indicate that peripheral neuropathy has a more complex pathophysiology than can be addressed by a neuroablative approach.

Cryoablation of the ilioinguinal and genitofemoral nerve has been described. In a small series, 9 male patients underwent a mapping procedure using focal low-volume nerve blocks in the distribution of the ilioinguinal and/or genitofemoral nerves to localize the nerve that was most affected, and then the nerve was surgically explored and interrogated with a nerve stimulator to confirm proper identification of the causal nerve. The nerve was then frozen to $-70°C$ for 3 minutes to create a 5-mm ice ball at 3 locations proximal to the suspected neuropathic source. All 9 patients experienced significant relief of pain and diminishment of analgesic use, for a mean follow-up of 8 months.[82] The theoretic advantage of cryoablation compared with other forms of ablation is the selective destruction of axons and myelin with the relative preservation of the epineural and perineural tissues, which theoretically reduces the tendency of the axon termini to form neuromas.[3]

Pulsed radiofrequency ablation (PRFA) has been described for treatment of postsurgical groin pain. One study reported adequate relief in 3 patients after 6 months' follow-up,[83] and another study used PRFA of the T12 to L2 nerve roots with all 5 patients claiming 75% to 100% pain relief with 6 to 9 months' follow-up.[84] However, a larger review concluded that the evidence favoring PRFA for inguinodynia is of marginal quality.[85]

SURGICAL NEURECTOMY FOR TREATMENT OF POSTOPERATIVE INGUINODYNIA

Although pharmacologic therapy is typically well tolerated, its efficacy remains limited for the treatment of chronic neuropathic pain and medical treatment is rarely definitive.[1] In randomized clinical trials assessing efficacious medications for neuropathic pain, often less than half of patients report experiencing satisfactory pain relief with medical treatment alone.[72] Open excision of the ilioinguinal nerve has facilitated improvements in postherniorrhaphy pain.[86] Inguinal exploration with nerve sectioning was offered historically to patients with chronic postherniorrhaphy neuropathic pain, with mixed success.[76] Laparoscopic approaches have likewise been described.[87] An important step is the use of local anesthesia to selectively block the individual nerves in an office setting; failure of an adequate local anesthetic to ameliorate pain has negative predictive value in the efficacy of surgical neurectomy.[74]

A triple neurectomy procedure has been described whereby the ilioinguinal nerve, the iliohypogastric nerve, and the genital branch of the genitofemoral nerve are individually identified and ligated proximal to the site of the previous herniorrhaphy incision. The approach to open neurectomy is via the original open herniorrhaphy incision, if present. Ideally, all 3 pertinent nerves are identified and traced back to their most proximal origins at the abdominal wall, then ligated and divided. The practice of positioning the transected nerve endings into nearby muscle tissue has been suggested as a way to protect the nerve terminus from the inevitable postoperative inflammation within the healing surgical wound, although data are lacking in the efficacy of this principle in the prevention of nociceptive pain following denervation.[88]

Importantly, specific risks of neurectomy procedures include permanent sensory deficits, because the nerves involved all provide cutaneous sensory innervation. In addition, the variable loss of motor innervation of the oblique muscles may result in abdominal wall laxity. Patients who elect to proceed with neurectomy for inguinodynia must make it their goal to feel numbness rather than to feel pain[89]; for this reason, critics of neurectomy have condemned its indiscriminate use.[90]

CHRONIC ORCHALGIA

Pain in the scrotum has presented a long-standing conundrum to urologists and pain experts. Acute pain in the scrotum, although outside the scope of this article, should initially be evaluated to rule out testicular torsion, acute epididymitis and/or orchitis, and scrotal trauma, as well as pain from a referred source such as a ureteral stone. Testis cancer rarely manifests with orchalgia and is more commonly painless, but this too is important to exclude because tumors with internal or external hemorrhage may manifest with pain. Scrotal Doppler ultrasonography is a crucial test in the initial work-up for orchalgia to rule out torsion, neoplasm, and genital trauma. However, scrotal ultrasonography is otherwise an inherently insensitive and nonspecific test: ultrasonic abnormalities such as epididymal cysts or varicoceles may be present in asymptomatic men as well as in those with orchalgia, whereas some men with debilitating orchalgia may manifest with a normal scrotal ultrasonography scan. Furthermore, some patients with orchalgia have some identifiable abnormalities on ultrasonography, but the locus of the pain may be something separate from the appreciable cyst or varicocele, and the ultrasonic anomalies may be incidental and unconnected to the patient's symptoms.

More than 2% to 3% of all outpatient urology office visits are devoted to chronic scrotal and testicular pain,[91] defined as testicular discomfort lasting more than 3 months and of a magnitude sufficient to significantly affect the man's quality of life.[92] Roughly half of these men have no history of trauma or infection to explain the onset of pain, and patients have variable presentations in terms of timing, severity, reproducibility, and radiation.[93]

A unique subset of men who develop chronic orchalgia have a history of vasectomy; patients who undergo vasectomy incur at least a 1% to 2% chance of developing significant chronic scrotal pain after the procedure.[94,95] Because of inconsistencies in the accrual of such data, the likelihood of any chronic discomfort after a vasectomy is not clear but may be as low as 0.1% or as high as 54%.[96,97] Chronic discomfort has been attributed to obstruction and congestion of the epididymal ducts, nerve entrapment by scar tissue, or formation of an inflammatory sperm granuloma following the initial contact between the immune system and sperm cells.[4] Of the men who develop chronic discomfort, some develop the pain instantly after the vasectomy, whereas others heal quickly from the initial procedure and then progress to chronic pain only years later.[98]

Physical examination in patients with orchalgia is geared toward the exclusion of associated disorders, including neoplasm, cysts, varicoceles, and inguinal hernias. Acute intense focal tenderness of the epididymis is suggestive of an active infection, and may merit an empiric 10-day to 20-day course of a fluoroquinolone or trimethoprim-sulfamethoxazole followed by a period of convalescence before arriving at the conclusion that the patient's pain is chronic and does not have an infectious cause. Note that infectious epididymitis cannot occur de novo in a patient after vasectomy, unless the pathogen ascended into the epididymis before or during the procedure.

SPERMATIC CORD BLOCK

A helpful diagnostic step is the option of a spermatic cord block with local anesthesia. Although by definition a local anesthetic provides only temporary analgesia at best, the efficacy of the block may help to localize the patient's complaint to the branches of the genitofemoral and ilioinguinal nerves within the spermatic cord, and may help to prognosticate the efficacy of future surgical efforts to mitigate neuropathic pain in a particular patient.[99] In addition, it provides the patient with a reasonable simulation of the result that can be obtained with surgery to denervate the spermatic cord. It is performed by injection of 10 to 20 mL of 0.25% bupivacaine or 1% lidocaine without epinephrine either at a point just lateral to the pubic tubercle or in the immobilized scrotal portion of the spermatic cord (**Fig. 2**).[100] For patients with clear symptoms of testicular or epididymal hypersensitivity on examination, our practice is to offer a cord block only as an option. In patients who present with a chronic ache in the scrotum that is not reproducible on examination and does not exacerbate with palpation, our practice is to insist on a cord block before considering surgery, because it is less clear in this group of patients whether an operation on the peripheral nerves will alleviate pain.

SURGICAL TREATMENT OF CHRONIC SCROTAL PAIN

Historically, the ultimate definitive surgical treatment of orchalgia is orchiectomy. Surgical removal of the testis carries the risk of inadequate androgen synthesis as well as a non-negligible psychological burden.[101] Not only is orchiectomy an intellectually unsatisfying treatment modality from the physician's perspective, orchiectomy also does not guarantee relief of scrotal pain, with up to 45% of men noting incomplete resolution of pain.[93]

Beginning in the early 1990s, an effort began to maintain the endocrine and reproductive functionality of the testis while effectively nullifying its visceral innervation.[102,103] The goal of such a procedure is to identify and selectively sever the visceral sensory nerve fibers that course through the spermatic cord to the testis and epididymis, thereby rendering it incapable of generating and propagating action potentials to carry a noxious stimulus to the brain. The task was more complicated in practice than in theory, because there proved to be significant variability in the caliber, number, and location of the various branches of the spermatic cord nerves. The variability is such that surgeons could not reliably confirm whether all the relevant

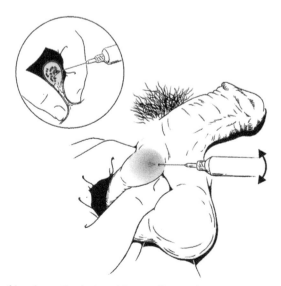

Fig. 2. Injection of local anesthesia to achieve a diagnostic spermatic cord block. (*From* Issa MM, Hsiao K, Bassel YS, et al. Spermatic cord anesthesia block for scrotal procedures in outpatient clinic setting. J Urol 2004;172(6 Pt 1):2359; with permission.)

nerve fibers had been severed.[73] Over time, the procedure was refined to use a converse methodology: rather than attempt to identify and cut selected nerves within the spermatic cord, surgeons endeavored to identify, dissect, retract, and spare the structures vital for the testis to thrive, and then severed all other extraneous spermatic cord structures. At a minimum, the testis requires arterial blood supply and lymphatic drainage to sustain its endocrine function, and a vas deferens to export sperm if desired. All other venous, muscular, and connective tissues could be cut sharply, because it is among this tissue that the many spermatic cord branches of the genitofemoral and ilioinguinal nerves reside. Interestingly, despite ligation of essentially all venous tissue within the spermatic cord, venous congestion of the testis is not common and venous drainage is thought to occur via collaterals in the scrotum.[4]

The procedure is performed with a dual-headed confocal surgical microscope under general anesthesia. A 3-cm to 4-cm subinguinal incision is made roughly 1 to 2 cm lateral to the pubic tubercle, and the spermatic cord is delivered in its entirety. The cord is exposed with a latex Penrose drain through which a sterile tongue depressor is placed to offer additional stiffness. Using microsurgical techniques, the cremasteric muscle fibers are circumferentially divided and the internal spermatic fascia is exposed. A microscopic Doppler probe is used to identify branches of the testicular artery, which is skeletonized bluntly and retracted with a vessel loop. Lymphatic vessels are likewise skeletonized and retracted. Structures to be sacrificed are ligated with 4-0 silk and divided. Smaller vessels can be cauterized with bipolar microforceps. The vas deferens is skeletonized of its richly innervated adventitia, although in some cases it is wise to identify and preserve the vasal artery to ensure adequate collateral perfusion of the testis. Patients who are ambivalent about the preservation of fertility may have the vas divided. The cord is returned to its subinguinal location, and the incision is closed (**Fig. 3**).

In concept, microsurgical denervation in this manner allows the patient to remain reproductively and endocrinologically intact, and unaware of any untoward neuropathic stimuli that might be initiated by his testis or epididymis and halted before the action potential reaches the inguinal ring. Results of a retrospective data series seem to support this hypothesis, because 71% of men noted complete durable relief for a median follow-up of 20 months.[104] Despite these promising early results, even as both the technique and patient selection became more refined, there have continued to be some patients for whom the microdenervation fails, either partially or entirely. Several hypotheses exist to explain the failure of a microdenervation to treat orchalgia (**Fig. 4**). First, the stimulus that activates the brain to perceive pain in the scrotum may reside cephalad to the operative site of the denervation procedure, and thus would not be interrupted by this technique. Second, the branches of the genitofemoral nerve severed by the microdenervation may autostimulate, similar to the pathophysiology of neuroma formation and progression to so-called phantom pain. Third, the arteries, lymphatics, or vas may be entwined so intimately with neural fibers that they must be spared in order to avoid damaging the structures with overzealous microdissection, and noxious action potentials could be transmitted via these fibers. Fourth, the inflammatory response invoked by the microdissection surgical incision may entrap and stimulate the same nerves that it is intended to denervate. In addition, the process of central sensitization of the scrotal pain may have begun before the microdenervation, such that even elimination of the original stimulus fails to temper the hypersensitivity.[4]

Like the study of chronic pain elsewhere in the body, orchalgia is an entity with a rapidly evolving level of understanding. Although optimal treatment methods are yet to be devised, for many patients the recent invention of a microsurgical cure for

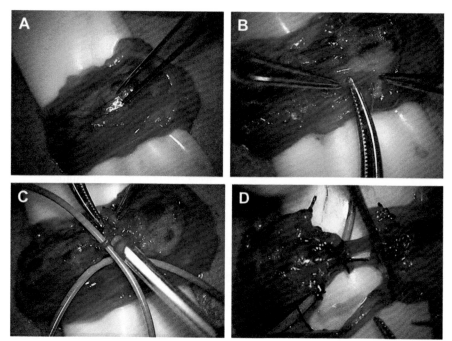

Fig. 3. Microsurgical denervation of the spermatic cord. (*A*) Exposure of the cord via a sub-inguinal approach. (*B*) Identification and dissection of a lymphatic vessel. (*C*) Microscopic Doppler probe used to identify branches of the testicular artery. (*D*) Skeletonized arteries, lymphatics, and vas deferens.

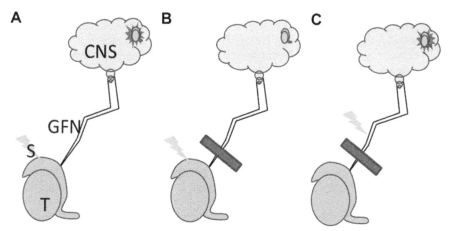

Fig. 4. Chronic neuropathic scrotal pain, spermatic cord denervation, and its possible mechanisms of failure. (*A*) Stimulus (S) causes a depolarization of nociceptive nerves at the testis (T), which propagates its action potential along the genitofemoral nerve to the central nervous system (CNS), where the brain perceives pain in the testis. (*B*) In a denervated testis, the stimulus causes the nerve depolarization but the action potential is not propagated to the CNS, and the brain perceives no pain. (*C*) In a patient who has had unsuccessful treatment with a microdenervation, alternative pathways may exist for the depolarization to propagate to the CNS. Plausible explanations include a more proximal locus of the painful stimulus on the peripheral nerve (as illustrated), persistent intact afferent nerve fibers located too close to the vital lymphovascular structures to safely permit dissection and ligation, formation of a neuroma at the point of nerve ligation, or pain centralization within the brain.

orchalgia has transformed what once was a disorder with poor long-term treatment outcomes into a problem with a potential solution that is not only life-changing for the patient but also gratifying for the surgeon.

REFERENCES

1. Lee CH, Dellon AL. Surgical management of groin pain of neural origin. J Am Coll Surg 2000;191(2):137–42.
2. Kehlet H, Jensen TS, Woolf CJ. Persistent postsurgical pain: risk factors and prevention. Lancet 2006;367(9522):1618–25.
3. Bjurstrom MF, Nicol AL, Amid PK, et al. Pain control following inguinal herniorrhaphy: current perspectives. J Pain Res 2014;7:277–90.
4. Levine L. Chronical scrotal content pain. AUA Update Series 2012;31:367–75.
5. Woolf CJ, Salter MW. Neuronal plasticity: increasing the gain in pain. Science 2000;288(5472):1765–9.
6. Nickel JC, Nyberg LM, Hennenfent M. Research guidelines for chronic prostatitis: consensus report from the First National Institutes of Health International Prostatitis Collaborative Network. Urology 1999;54(2):229–33.
7. Collins MM, Meigs JB, Barry MJ, et al. Prevalence and correlates of prostatitis in the Health Professionals Follow-Up Study cohort. J Urol 2002;167(3):1363–6.
8. Domingue GJ, Hellstrom WJ. Prostatitis. Clin Microbiol Rev 1998;11(4):604–13.
9. Horcajada JP, Vilana R, Moreno-Martínez A, et al. Transrectal prostatic ultrasonography in acute bacterial prostatitis: findings and clinical implications. Scand J Infect Dis 2003;35(2):114–20.
10. Brede CM, Shoskes DA. The etiology and management of acute prostatitis. Nat Rev Urol 2011;8:207–12.
11. Wagenlehner FM, Pilatz A, Bschleipfer T, et al. Bacterial prostatitis. World J Urol 2013;31(4):711–6.
12. Millan-Rodriguez F, Palou J, Bujons-Tur A, et al. Acute bacterial prostatitis: two different sub-categories according to a previous manipulation of the lower urinary tract. World J Urol 2006;24(1):45–50.
13. Ha US, Kim ME, Kim CS, et al. Acute bacterial prostatitis in Korea: clinical outcome, including symptoms, management, microbiology and course of disease. Int J Antimicrob Agents 2008;31(Suppl 1):96–101.
14. Shoskes DA. Chronic prostatitis/chronic pelvic pain syndrome. Totowa (NJ): Humana Press; 2008.
15. Schneider H, Ludwig M, Hossain HM, et al. The 2001 Giessen Cohort Study on patients with prostatitis syndrome – an evaluation of inflammatory status and search for microorganisms 10 years after a first analysis. Andrologia 2003; 35(5):258–62.
16. Tsu JH, Ma WK, Chan WK, et al. Prevalence and predictive factors of harboring fluoroquinolone-resistant and extended-spectrum beta-lactamase-producing rectal flora in Hong Kong Chinese men undergoing transrectal ultrasound-guided prostate biopsy. Urology 2015;85(1):15–21.
17. Kim JW, Oh MM, Bae JH, et al. Clinical and microbiological characteristics of spontaneous acute prostatitis and transrectal prostate biopsy-related acute prostatitis: is transrectal prostate biopsy-related acute prostatitis a distinct acute prostatitis category? J Infect Chemother 2015;21(6):434–7.
18. Nickel JC. Prostatitis and related conditions, orchitis, and epididymitis. In: Wein AJ, Kavoussi LR, Novick AC, et al, editors. Campbell-Walsh Urology. 10th edition. Philadelphia: Elsevier Saunders; 2012. p. 327–56.

19. Naber KG, Bergman B, Bishop MC, et al. EAU guidelines for the management of urinary and male genital tract infections. Urinary Tract Infection (UTI) Working Group of the Health Care Office (HCO) of the European Association of Urology (EAU). Eur Urol 2001;40(5):576–88.

20. Lee HN, Kim TH, Lee SJ, et al. Effects of prostatic inflammation on LUTS and alpha blocker treatment outcomes. Int Braz J Urol 2014;40(3):356–66.

21. Nickel JC. Alpha-blockers for the treatment of prostatitis-like syndromes. Rev Urol 2006;8(Suppl 4):S26–34.

22. Ulleryd P, Zackrisson B, Aus G, et al. Selective urological evaluation in men with febrile urinary tract infection. BJU Int 2001;88(1):15–20.

23. Chou YH, Tiu CM, Liu JY, et al. Prostatic abscess: transrectal color Doppler ultrasonic diagnosis and minimally invasive therapeutic management. Ultrasound Med Biol 2004;30(6):719–24.

24. Weidner W, Schiefer HG, Krauss H, et al. Chronic prostatitis: a thorough search for etiologically involved microorganisms in 1,461 patients. Infection 1991; 19(Suppl 3):S119–25.

25. Meares EM, Stamey TA. Bacteriologic localization patterns in bacterial prostatitis and urethritis. Invest Urol 1968;5(5):492–518.

26. Nickel JC, Shoskes D, Wang Y, et al. How does the pre-massage and post-massage 2-glass test compare to the Meares-Stamey 4-glass test in men with chronic prostatitis/chronic pelvic pain syndrome? J Urol 2006;176(1):119–24.

27. Barbalias GA, Nikiforidis G, Liatsikos EN. Alpha-blockers for the treatment of chronic prostatitis in combination with antibiotics. J Urol 1998;159(3):883–7.

28. Schaeffer AJ. Epidemiology and evaluation of chronic pelvic pain syndrome in men. Int J Antimicrob Agents 2008;31(Suppl 1):108–11.

29. Nickel JC, Alexander RB, Schaeffer AJ, et al. Leukocytes and bacteria in men with chronic prostatitis/chronic pelvic pain syndrome compared to asymptomatic controls. J Urol 2003;170(3):818–22.

30. Schaeffer AJ, Landis JR, Knauss JS, et al. Demographic and clinical characteristics of men with chronic prostatitis: the national institutes of health chronic prostatitis cohort study. J Urol 2002;168(2):593–8.

31. Shoskes DA, Landis JR, Wang Y, et al. Impact of post-ejaculatory pain in men with category III chronic prostatitis/chronic pelvic pain syndrome. J Urol 2004; 172(2):542–7.

32. Liang CZ, Zhang XJ, Hao ZY, et al. Prevalence of sexual dysfunction in Chinese men with chronic prostatitis. BJU Int 2004;93(4):568–70.

33. Clemens JQ, Brown SO, Kozloff L, et al. Predictors of symptom severity in patients with chronic prostatitis and interstitial cystitis. J Urol 2006;175(3 Pt 1): 963–6 [discussion: 967].

34. Marszalek M, Wehrberger C, Hochreiter W, et al. Symptoms suggestive of chronic pelvic pain syndrome in an urban population: prevalence and associations with lower urinary tract symptoms and erectile function. J Urol 2007;177(5): 1815–9.

35. Keltikangas-Jarvinen L, Mueller K, Lehtonen T. Illness behavior and personality changes in patients with chronic prostatitis during a two-year follow-up period. Eur Urol 1989;16(3):181–4.

36. Ullrich PM, Turner JA, Ciol M, et al. Stress is associated with subsequent pain and disability among men with nonbacterial prostatitis/pelvic pain. Ann Behav Med 2005;30(2):112–8.

37. Hu J, Link CL, McNaughton-Collins M, et al. The association of abuse and symptoms suggestive of chronic prostatitis/chronic pelvic pain syndrome: results

from the Boston Area Community Health Survey. J Gen Intern Med 2007;22(11): 1532–7.

38. Koh JS, Ko HJ, Wang SM, et al. Depression and somatic symptoms may influence on chronic prostatitis/chronic pelvic pain syndrome: a preliminary study. Psychiatry Investig 2014;11(4):495–8.

39. Pontari MA, McNaughton-Collins M, O'Leary MP, et al. A case-control study of risk factors in men with chronic pelvic pain syndrome. BJU Int 2005;96(4): 559–65.

40. McNaughton Collins M, Pontari MA, O'Leary MP, et al. Quality of life is impaired in men with chronic prostatitis: the Chronic Prostatitis Collaborative Research Network. J Gen Intern Med 2001;16(10):656–62.

41. Wenninger K, Heiman JR, Rothman I, et al. Sickness impact of chronic nonbacterial prostatitis and its correlates. J Urol 1996;155(3):965–8.

42. Wagenlehner FM, van Till JW, Magri V, et al. National Institutes of Health Chronic Prostatitis Symptom Index (NIH-CPSI) symptom evaluation in multinational cohorts of patients with chronic prostatitis/chronic pelvic pain syndrome. Eur Urol 2013;63(5):953–9.

43. Litwin MS, McNaughton-Collins M, Fowler FJ Jr, et al. The National Institutes of Health Chronic Prostatitis Symptom Index: development and validation of a new outcome measure. Chronic Prostatitis Collaborative Research Network. J Urol 1999;162(2):369–75.

44. Blacklock NJ. Anatomical factors in prostatitis. Br J Urol 1974;46(1):47–54.

45. Bates CP, Arnold EP, Griffiths DJ. The nature of the abnormality in bladder neck obstruction. Br J Urol 1975;47(6):651–6.

46. Orland SM, Hanno PM, Wein AJ. Prostatitis, prostatosis, and prostatodia. Urology 1985;25(5):439–59.

47. Theodorou CH, Konidaris D, Moutzouris G, et al. The urodynamic profile of prostatodynia. BJU Int 1999;84(4):461–3.

48. Kaplan SA, Santarosa RP, D'Alisera PM, et al. Pseudodyssynergia (contraction of the external sphincter during voiding) misdiagnosed as chronic nonbacterial prostatitis and the role of biofeedback as a therapeutic option. J Urol 1997; 157(6):2234–7.

49. Kaplan SA, Ikeguchi EF, Santarosa RP, et al. Etiology of voiding dysfunction in men less than 50 years of age. Urology 1996;47(6):836–9.

50. Dik P, Lock TM, Schrier BP, et al. Transurethral marsupialization of a medial prostatic cyst in patients with prostatitis-like symptoms. J Urol 1996;155(4):1301–4.

51. Davis R, Jones JS, Barocas DA, et al. Diagnosis, evaluation and follow-up of asymptomatic microhematuria (AMH) in adults: AUA guideline. J Urol 2012; 188(6 Suppl):2473–81.

52. Nickel JC, Downey J, Johnston B, et al. Predictors of patient response to antibiotic therapy for the chronic prostatitis/chronic pelvic pain syndrome: a prospective multicenter clinical trial. J Urol 2001;165(5):1539–44.

53. Nickel JC, Downey J, Clark J, et al. Levofloxacin for chronic prostatitis/chronic pelvic pain syndrome in men: a randomized placebo-controlled multicenter trial. Urology 2003;62(4):614–7.

54. Alexander RB, Propert KJ, Schaeffer AJ, et al. Ciprofloxacin or tamsulosin in men with chronic prostatitis/chronic pelvic pain syndrome: a randomized, double-blind trial. Ann Intern Med 2004;141(8):581–9.

55. Cheah PY, Liong ML, Yuen KH, et al. Terazosin therapy for chronic prostatitis/chronic pelvic pain syndrome: a randomized, placebo controlled trial. J Urol 2003;169(2):592–6.

56. Mehik A, Alas P, Nickel JC, et al. Alfuzosin treatment for chronic prostatitis/ chronic pelvic pain syndrome: a prospective, randomized, double-blind, placebo-controlled, pilot study. Urology 2003;62(3):425–9.

57. Nickel JC, Narayan P, McKay J, et al. Treatment of chronic prostatitis/chronic pelvic pain syndrome with tamsulosin: a randomized double blind trial. J Urol 2004;171(4):1594–7.

58. Tuğcu V, Taşçi AI, Fazlioğlu A, et al. A placebo-controlled comparison of the efficiency of triple- and monotherapy in category III B chronic pelvic pain syndrome (CPPS). Eur Urol 2007;51(4):1113–8.

59. Canale D, Scaricabarozzi I, Giorgi P, et al. Use of a novel non-steroidal anti-inflammatory drug, nimesulide, in the treatment of abacterial prostatovesiculitis. Andrologia 1993;25(3):163–6.

60. Nickel JC, Pontari M, Moon T, et al. A randomized, placebo controlled, multicenter study to evaluate the safety and efficacy of rofecoxib in the treatment of chronic nonbacterial prostatitis. J Urol 2003;169(4):1401–5.

61. Zeng X, Ye Z, Yang W, et al. Clinical evaluation of celecoxib in treating type IIIA chronic prostatitis. Zhonghua Nan Ke Xue 2004;10(4):278–81 [in Chinese].

62. Bates SM, Hill VA, Anderson JB, et al. A prospective, randomized, double-blind trial to evaluate the role of a short reducing course of oral corticosteroid therapy in the treatment of chronic prostatitis/chronic pelvic pain syndrome. BJU Int 2007;99(2):355–9.

63. Osborn DE, George NJ, Rao PN, et al. Prostatodynia—physiological characteristics and rational management with muscle relaxants. Br J Urol 1981;53(6): 621–3.

64. Simmons PD, Thin RN. Minocycline in chronic abacterial prostatitis: a double-blind prospective trial. Br J Urol 1985;57(1):43–5.

65. Falahatkar S, Shahab E, Gholamjani Moghaddam K, et al. Transurethral intraprostatic injection of botulinum neurotoxin type A for the treatment of chronic prostatitis/chronic pelvic pain syndrome: results of a prospective pilot double-blind and randomized placebo-controlled study. BJU Int 2015;116(4):641–9.

66. Shoskes DA, Nickel JC, Dolinga R, et al. Clinical phenotyping of patients with chronic prostatitis/chronic pelvic pain syndrome and correlation with symptom severity. Urology 2009;73(3):538–42.

67. Magri V, Marras E, Restelli A, et al. Multimodal therapy for category III chronic prostatitis/chronic pelvic pain syndrome in UPOINTS phenotyped patients. Exp Ther Med 2015;9(3):658–66.

68. Magri V, Wagenlehner F, Perletti G, et al. Use of the UPOINT chronic prostatitis/ chronic pelvic pain syndrome classification in European patient cohorts: sexual function domain improves correlations. J Urol 2010;184(6):2339–45.

69. Tran CN, Li J, Shoskes DA. An online UPOINT tool for phenotyping patients with chronic prostatitis. Can J Urol 2014;21(2):7195–200.

70. Alshahrani S, McGill J, Agarwal A. Prostatitis and male infertility. J Reprod Immunol 2013;100(1):30–6.

71. Primatesta P, Goldacre MJ. Inguinal hernia repair: incidence of elective and emergency surgery, readmission and mortality. Int J Epidemiol 1996;25(4): 835–9.

72. O'Connor AB, Dworkin RH. Treatment of neuropathic pain: an overview of recent guidelines. Am J Med 2009;122(10 Suppl):S22–32.

73. Rab M, Ebmer J, Dellon LA. Anatomic variability of the ilioinguinal and genitofemoral nerve: implications for the treatment of groin pain. Plast Reconstr Surg 2001;108(6):1618–23.

74. Peng PW, Tumber PS. Ultrasound-guided interventional procedures for patients with chronic pelvic pain - a description of techniques and review of literature. Pain Physician 2008;11(2):215–24.
75. Knockaert DC, Boonen AL, Bruyninckx FL, et al. Electromyographic findings in ilioinguinal-iliohypogastric nerve entrapment syndrome. Acta Clin Belg 1996; 51(3):156–60.
76. Callesen T, Bech K, Kehlet H. Prospective study of chronic pain after groin hernia repair. Br J Surg 1999;86(12):1528–31.
77. Clarke H, Bonin RP, Orser BA, et al. The prevention of chronic postsurgical pain using gabapentin and pregabalin: a combined systematic review and meta-analysis. Anesth Analg 2012;115(2):428–42.
78. Moulin DE, Boulanger A, Clark AJ, et al. Pharmacological management of chronic neuropathic pain - consensus statement and guidelines from the Canadian Pain Society. Pain Res Manag 2007;12(1):13–21.
79. Bischoff JM, Petersen M, Uçeyler N, et al. Lidocaine patch (5%) in treatment of persistent inguinal postherniorrhaphy pain: a randomized, double-blind, placebo-controlled, crossover trial. Anesthesiology 2013;119(6):1444–52.
80. Argoff CE. New analgesics for neuropathic pain: the lidocaine patch. Clin J Pain 2000;16(2 Suppl):S62–6.
81. Bischoff JM, Koscielniak-Nielsen ZJ, Kehlet H, et al. Ultrasound-guided ilioinguinal/iliohypogastric nerve blocks for persistent inguinal postherniorrhaphy pain: a randomized, double-blind, placebo-controlled, crossover trial. Anesth Analg 2012;114(6):1323–9.
82. Fanelli RD, DiSiena MR, Lui FY, et al. Cryoanalgesic ablation for the treatment of chronic postherniorrhaphy neuropathic pain. Surg Endosc 2003;17(2):196–200.
83. Cohen SP, Foster A. Pulsed radiofrequency as a treatment for groin pain and orchialgia. Urology 2003;61(3):645.
84. Rozen D, Parvez U. Pulsed radiofrequency of lumbar nerve roots for treatment of chronic inguinal herniorraphy pain. Pain Physician 2006;9(2):153–6.
85. Werner MU, Bischoff JM, Rathmell JP, et al. Pulsed radiofrequency in the treatment of persistent pain after inguinal herniotomy: a systematic review. Reg Anesth Pain Med 2012;37(3):340–3.
86. Malekpour F, Mirhashemi SH, Hajinasrolah E, et al. Ilioinguinal nerve excision in open mesh repair of inguinal hernia–results of a randomized clinical trial: simple solution for a difficult problem? Am J Surg 2008;195(6):735–40.
87. Chen DC, Hiatt JR, Amid PK. Operative management of refractory neuropathic inguinodynia by a laparoscopic retroperitoneal approach. JAMA Surg 2013; 148(10):962–7.
88. Amid PK. Causes, prevention, and surgical treatment of postherniorrhaphy neuropathic inguinodynia: triple neurectomy with proximal end implantation. Hernia 2004;8(4):343–9.
89. Alfieri S, Amid PK, Campanelli G, et al. International guidelines for prevention and management of post-operative chronic pain following inguinal hernia surgery. Hernia 2011;15(3):239–49.
90. Lichtenstein IL, Shulman AG, Amid PK, et al. Cause and prevention of postherniorrhaphy neuralgia: a proposed protocol for treatment. Am J Surg 1988; 155(6):786–90.
91. Strebel RT, Leippold T, Luginbuehl T, et al. Chronic scrotal pain syndrome: management among urologists in Switzerland. Eur Urol 2005;47(6):812–6.
92. Costabile RA, Hahn M, McLeod DG. Chronic orchialgia in the pain prone patient: the clinical perspective. J Urol 1991;146(6):1571–4.

93. Davis BE, Noble MJ, Weigel JW, et al. Analysis and management of chronic testicular pain. J Urol 1990;143(5):936–9.
94. Sharlip ID, Belker AM, Honig S, et al. Vasectomy: AUA guideline. J Urol 2012; 188(6 Suppl):2482–91.
95. Leslie TA, Illing RO, Cranston DW, et al. The incidence of chronic scrotal pain after vasectomy: a prospective audit. BJU Int 2007;100(6):1330–3.
96. Christiansen CG, Sandlow JI. Testicular pain following vasectomy: a review of postvasectomy pain syndrome. J Androl 2003;24(3):293–8.
97. Morris C, Mishra K, Kirkman RJ. A study to assess the prevalence of chronic testicular pain in post-vasectomy men compared to non-vasectomised men. J Fam Plann Reprod Health Care 2002;28(3):142–4.
98. Nangia AK, Myles JL, Thomas AJ. Vasectomy reversal for the post-vasectomy pain syndrome: a clinical and histological evaluation. J Urol 2000;164(6): 1939–42.
99. Levine L. Chronic orchialgia: evaluation and discussion of treatment options. Ther Adv Urol 2010;2(5–06):209–14.
100. Issa MM, Hsiao K, Bassel YS, et al. Spermatic cord anesthesia block for scrotal procedures in outpatient clinic setting. J Urol 2004;172(6 Pt 1):2358–61.
101. Dellon AL, Hashemi SS, Tollstrup TH. Orchialgia after orchiectomy. Plast Reconstr Surg 2014;134(6):998e–9e.
102. Choa RG, Swami KS. Testicular denervation. A new surgical procedure for intractable testicular pain. Br J Urol 1992;70(4):417–9.
103. Levine LA, Matkov TG, Lubenow TR. Microsurgical denervation of the spermatic cord: a surgical alternative in the treatment of chronic orchialgia. J Urol 1996; 155(3):1005–7.
104. Strom KH, Levine LA. Microsurgical denervation of the spermatic cord for chronic orchialgia: long-term results from a single center. J Urol 2008;180(3): 949–53.

Robotic Surgery of the Kidney, Bladder, and Prostate

Arjun Khosla, MD, Andrew A. Wagner, MD*

KEYWORDS

- Robotic • Laparoscopic • Partial nephrectomy • Pyeloplasty • Cystectomy
- Prostatectomy

KEY POINTS

- Minimally invasive surgery offers many advantages over the traditional open approach, including improved cosmesis, reduced blood loss, decreased pain, shorter hospital stays, and improved convalescence.
- Robot-assisted surgery offers the advantages of a minimally invasive approach with greater technical ease and a shorter learning curve than pure laparoscopy.
- Fueled by the success of the robot-assisted laparoscopic prostatectomy, Urologists are increasingly using the robotic platform for other advanced operations involving the kidney, ureters, bladder, and prostate.
- Robotic surgery has been shown to be safe and effective, with good perioperative, functional, and oncologic outcomes.
- Although cost continues to be a major concern regarding the use of robotic technology, improved efficiency and reduced hospital stays associated with the minimally invasive approach are allowing for better cost-effectiveness.

INTRODUCTION

Robot-assisted laparoscopic surgery has been one of the most important recent technological advances in the practice of surgery. In particular, urology has a long-standing history of embracing advances in surgical technology and many urologic procedures have been replaced with more minimally invasive techniques, both endo-scopic and laparoscopic, with the goal of reducing perioperative morbidity (**Table 1**). Advantages of the minimally invasive approach include increased precision, smaller incisions, reduced intraoperative blood loss, decreased postoperative pain, shorter hospital stays, and improved convalescence while preserving functional and

Division of Urology, Department of Surgery, Beth Israel Deaconess Medical Center, Harvard Medical School, Boston, MA, USA
* Corresponding author. Beth Israel Deaconess Medical Center, 330 Brookline Avenue, Rabb 440, Boston, MA 02215.
E-mail address: awagner@bidmc.harvard.edu

Surg Clin N Am 96 (2016) 615–636
http://dx.doi.org/10.1016/j.suc.2016.02.015
0039-6109/16/$ – see front matter © 2016 Elsevier Inc. All rights reserved.
surgical.theclinics.com

Table 1	
History of minimally invasive urologic surgery	
Year	**Description**
1870	Simon: First open partial nephrectomy
1886	Trendelenburg: First reconstruction for ureteropelvic junction obstruction
1887	Bardenheuer: First open cystectomy performed
1900	Freyer: First open simple prostatectomy
1905	Young: First perineal prostatectomy
1947	Millin: First radical retropubic prostatectomy
1949	Marshall and Whitmore: First open radical cystectomy, pelvic lymphadenectomy described in detail
1949	Anderson and Hynes: First open dismembered pyeloplasty
1982	Walsh: First nerve-sparing open radical retropubic prostatectomy
1983	Arthrobot introduced for orthopedic procedures
1985	PUMA 560 introduced for computed tomography–guided brain biopsy
1988	ROBODOC introduced for hip arthroplasty
1988	PROBOT introduced for transurethral prostate surgery
1992	Schuessler: First laparoscopic radical prostatectomy
1992	Parra: First laparoscopic simple cystectomy
1993	Automated Endoscopic System for Optimal Positioning (AESOP) introduced
1993	Winfield: First laparoscopic partial nephrectomy
1993	Sanchez de Badajoz: First laparoscopic radical cystectomy
1993	Kavoussi and Schuessler: First laparoscopic pyeloplasty
1998	ZEUS and da Vinci Surgical Systems introduced
2000	Approval by the Food and Drug Administration of the da Vinci Surgical System for use in laparoscopic surgery
2000	Abbou: First robotic prostatectomy
2002	Mariano: First laparoscopic simple prostatectomy
2002	Gettman: First robotic pyeloplasty
2002	Menon: First robotic cystectomy
2003	Intuitive Surgical, Inc buys Computer Motion, Inc
2004	Gettman: First robotic partial nephrectomy
2008	Sotelo: First robotic simple prostatectomy

oncologic outcomes. Although standard laparoscopy has been shown to improve outcomes for some urologic surgeries, for example, radical nephrectomy, its adoption for reconstructive procedures has been limited due to the technical challenges and steep learning curves. In addition, traditional laparoscopy may be associated with losses of depth perception, intuitive movement, and dexterity. Robotic surgery with the da Vinci Surgical System (Intuitive Surgical, Inc, Sunnyvale, CA) has grown rapidly through its use in operations that benefit from a minimally invasive approach, but are technically challenging to perform with pure laparoscopy. The robotic system overcomes many of the limitations encountered in standard laparoscopy and offers a reduced learning curve. The advantages of robotic assistance were first noted in urology with the robot-assisted laparoscopic prostatectomy,[1,2] whose wide acceptance and popularity has led to other advanced robotic surgeries, in both adults and children, involving the kidney, ureter, bladder, and prostate (**Table 2**).

Table 2
Advantages and disadvantages of the open, laparoscopic, and robotic approach for partial nephrectomy, radical cystectomy, and radical prostatectomy

Procedure	Advantages	Disadvantages
Partial nephrectomy		
Open (OPN)	Gold standard with proven oncologic outcomes Shorter operative time Decreased cost	Larger incisions Increased perioperative morbidity Increased pain Longer hospitalization Longer recovery
Laparoscopic (LPN)	Enhanced visibility Decreased perioperative morbidity Decreased pain Shorter hospitalization Shorter recovery Improved cosmesis Equivalent oncologic outcomes compared with OPN	Increased cost compared with OPN Additional training required Prolonged learning curve/technically challenging Increased operative time
Robotic (RALPN)	(Same benefits seen with LPN) Enhanced visibility, dexterity, ergonomics, and precision Shorter learning curve/technical ease Decreased warm ischemia time Decreased blood loss Shorter hospitalization than LPN	± Cost Additional training required Limited instrumentation No tactile feedback
Cystectomy		
Open (ORC)	Gold standard with proven oncologic outcomes	Increased blood loss Increased transfusion rate Increased time to return of bowel function Longer hospitalization High complication rate (particularly high-grade, Clavien 3–5)
Laparoscopic (LRC)	Enhanced visibility Improved cosmesis Equivalent oncologic/perioperative outcomes compared with ORC	Cost higher than ORC Additional training required Prolonged learning curve/technically challenging Increased operative time
Robotic (RARC)	(Same benefits seen with LRC) Enhanced visibility, dexterity, ergonomics, and precision Shorter learning curve/technical ease Decreased perioperative morbidity Decreased blood loss Decreased rate of transfusion Decreased time to return of bowel function Shorter hospitalization	Cost higher than ORC/LRC Additional training required Need for an experienced robotic team Limited instrumentation No tactile feedback Increased operative time Less long-term oncologic outcome data available

(*continued on next page*)

Table 2
(continued)

Procedure	Advantages	Disadvantages
Prostatectomy		
Open (ORP)	Long-term data with proven oncologic/functional outcomes	Increased blood loss Increased rate of transfusion Longer hospitalization Increased complication rate
Laparoscopic (LRP)	Enhanced visibility Decreased blood loss Shorter hospitalization Shorter recovery Improved cosmesis	Cost higher than ORP Additional training required Prolonged learning curve/technically challenging Increased operative time No clear benefit over ORP
Robotic (RALP)	(Same benefits seen with LRP) Enhanced visibility, dexterity, ergonomics, and precision Shorter learning curve/technical ease Decreased blood loss Decreased rate of transfusion Decreased perioperative morbidity Shorter hospitalization than LRP Equivalent oncologic/functional outcomes Earlier return of urinary continence Higher rate/faster recovery of potency	Cost higher than ORP/LRP Additional training required Limited instrumentation No tactile feedback

A BRIEF HISTORY OF SURGICAL ROBOTICS

The first surgical robot, known as Arthrobot, was developed in Canada in 1983 and designed to assist in orthopedic procedures. In 1985, the PUMA 560 (Unimate Robot Systems, Ewing Township, NJ) was used for computed tomography–guided brain biopsy. In 1988, orthopedic surgeons used a computer enhancement system called ROBODOC (Integrated Surgical Systems, Santa Monica, CA) to more precisely drill the femur during hip arthroplasty. The first surgical robot assistance seen in urology was in 1988 at Guy's and St. Thomas' Hospital in London with the use of PROBOT to perform transurethral prostate surgery. In 1993, the Automated Endoscopic System for Optimal Positioning (AESOP) (Computer Motion, Inc, Santa Barbara, CA) was released, a voice-activated robotic arm that aided in laparoscopic camera holding and positioning, allowing the surgeon to use both hands without the need of an assistant. The most significant advancements came in 1998 with the introduction of the ZEUS Robotic Surgical System by Computer Motion, Inc and the da Vinci Surgical System. The first da Vinci robot-assisted laparoscopic procedure was a cholecystectomy, performed by Drs Cadiere and Himpens in 1997. In July 2000, the da Vinci robot was given approval by the US Food and Drug Administration for use in laparoscopic procedures and the first reported robot-assisted laparoscopic prostatectomy took place in Paris. In 2003, Intuitive Surgical, Inc bought out Computer Motion, Inc and is currently the only company marketing robot-assisted surgical systems.[3,4]

THE DA VINCI SURGICAL SYSTEM

The da Vinci Surgical System has 3 components: a surgeon's console, a patient-side robotic cart with 4 robotic arms manipulated by the surgeon, and a high-definition

3-dimensional (3D) vision system. Articulating surgical instruments are mounted on the robotic arms, which are introduced into the body through cannulas.[5] Advantages of the robotic system include a stable operator-controlled camera, a magnified high-definition view, 3D stereo visualization through a 2-channel endoscope, improved dexterity with articulating EndoWrist instruments with 7° of freedom, motion scaling, and tremor filtration. These features allow for improved precision and fine dissection in a confined space, and allow for easier and more fluid control during reconstructive maneuvers such as intracorporeal suturing. Disadvantages of the robotic system include the lack of tactile feedback, the need to train additional staff, and increased cost associated with the robot, which includes an upfront purchase price of between $1.4 and $2.1 million, annual maintenance contract of $150,000, and additional disposable supply cost of at least $1500 per case. The value of robotic technology lies in balancing these costs with the improvement in patient care and outcomes relative to other surgical approaches.

ROBOTIC SURGERY OF THE KIDNEY AND URETER
Partial Nephrectomy

The incidence of renal tumors has been increasing over the past several decades with an annual incidence of approximately 61,500 cases and 14,000 deaths in the United States.[6] Due to advances in technology and increased use of cross-sectional imaging, most of these tumors are diagnosed at clinical stage T1 and are amenable to nephron-sparing surgery with partial nephrectomy. Nephron-sparing surgery (NSS) with renal preservation for small renal masses has equivalent oncologic outcomes to radical nephrectomy while lowering the risk of severe chronic kidney disease. Many studies have shown that renal insufficiency is associated with increased cardiovascular events, hospitalization, and mortality.[7] The European Organization for Research and Treatment of Cancer provided the first Level I evidence that long-term oncologic outcomes between partial nephrectomy and radical nephrectomy were equivalent, allowing partial nephrectomy to become a standard of care for small renal masses.[8] Open partial nephrectomy (OPN) was the gold standard for NSS, but it involves large abdominal or flank incisions, longer hospital stays, longer periods of convalescence, increased pain, and more perioperative morbidity.

Initially introduced by Winfield and colleagues[9] in 1993 for a patient with a calyceal diverticulum containing stone, laparoscopic partial nephrectomy (LPN) subsequently emerged as a viable alternative in the surgical management of small renal masses. Retrospective reviews and meta-analyses have shown that although OPN is associated with shorter operative time and decreased cost, minimally invasive partial nephrectomy offers decreased blood loss, lower complication rate, and shorter hospital stay.[10,11] However, many studies have discussed the prolonged learning curve associated with purely LPN, which has prevented its widespread adoption and relegated the technique to experienced laparoscopic surgeons. Furthermore, a population-based study by Abouassaly and colleagues[12] revealed that the introduction of laparoscopic renal surgery decreased the uptake and use of partial nephrectomy for renal cell carcinoma at least partially due to technical ease and decreased surgical morbidity with laparoscopic radical nephrectomy. Gettman and colleagues[13] first reported on the safety and feasibility of robot-assisted laparoscopic partial nephrectomy (RALPN) in 2004, offering the benefits of minimally invasive surgery with facilitation of the major surgical steps of the procedure (tumor dissection, renal reconstruction) and a shorter learning curve. The estimated learning curve for LPN with respect to operative time is 100 to 150 cases. On the other hand, RALPN has drastically shortened the learning curve to approximately 16 cases, with respect to operative time, and 26 cases for warm ischemia time.[10] Ellison and colleagues[14] found that ischemia, blood loss, and operative times improved after the first 33 cases. Kaouk and colleagues[15] showed that once the learning curve was overcome, there was a significant decrease in blood loss, transfusion rate, conversion rate, postoperative complication rate, mean operative time, and length of stay. Interestingly, the increased operative time associated with RALPN may pertain to the preparation and docking of the robot, with Masson-Lecomte and colleagues.[16] showing that actual "skin-to-skin" operative times demonstrated no significant difference. Additionally, when comparing pure LPN to RALPN, studies have found that RALPN offers decreased warm ischemia time, decreased blood loss, and shorter hospital stay with similar perioperative outcomes, complication rates, and oncologic control.[11,17–20]

In fact, the indications for RALPN have expanded to include more complex tumors such as lesions that are multifocal, endophytic, posterior, hilar, and bilateral, and masses larger than 7 cm, and within a solitary kidney. Studies have demonstrated the safety and feasibility of treating these challenging masses in select patients, using renal nephrometry scores to classify their complexity.[19,20] Anatomy-based nephrometry scoring systems allow for standardized academic reporting of tumor characteristics, precise patient-specific surgical planning, and can predict partial nephrectomy outcomes. These scores can inform the surgeon regarding the difficulty during partial nephrectomy for a given mass, and have been correlated with ischemia time, operative time, blood loss, complications, length of stay, and the likelihood of conversion to a radical nephrectomy. Furthermore, nephrometry scoring systems can assist in clinical decision-making on performing a radical nephrectomy versus partial nephrectomy or an open procedure versus a minimally invasive approach.[21]

Overall, the 2 surgical principles for optimizing postoperative functional outcomes following a partial nephrectomy are to maximize volume preservation and to minimize ischemia. Historically, a 1-cm rim of healthy parenchyma was recommended to allow for optimal oncologic control[22]; however, further study demonstrated that the width of the margin does not affect local control.[23] Thus, the width of the negative margin can be kept to a thin, uniform rim of normal parenchyma.[21] RALPN has been associated with equivalent oncologic outcomes when compared with the open and laparoscopic approaches.[10,11] Novel surgical approaches have been developed that reduce ischemic time during partial nephrectomy, including early unclamping, segmental clamping, tumor-specific clamping, and unclamped techniques.[19,21] These techniques may positively impact postoperative renal function, which relies on kidney quality, remnant quality, ischemia type, and the duration of ischemia.[21] Thompson and colleagues[24] examined the importance of warm ischemia time on postoperative renal function, reviewing 362 patients with a solitary kidney who underwent partial nephrectomy. They found that longer warm ischemia time was associated with acute renal failure in the postoperative period and with new-onset stage IV chronic kidney disease during follow-up. Furthermore, when evaluating warm ischemia time in 5-minute increments, a cutoff point of 25 minutes provided the best distinction between patients with and without postoperative renal consequences, leading the authors to conclude that "every minute counts when the renal hilum is clamped."[24] One disadvantage of LPN is the prolonged warm ischemia time and subsequent renal dysfunction, secondary to the technical complexity of intracorporeal suturing. Robotic assistance, through improved dexterity and visualization, has significantly decreased the time for tumor resection and intracorporeal suturing, thus reducing warm ischemia time and leading to improved postoperative renal function.[19] Benway and colleagues[17] performed a multi-institutional analysis of perioperative outcomes following RAPN and LPN, finding that the robotic approach was associated with less intraoperative blood loss (155 vs 196 mL, $P = .03$), decreased hospital stay (2.4 vs 2.7 days, $P < .0001$), and shorter warm ischemia times (19.7 vs 28.4 minutes, $P < .0001$). Our single-center experience, with more than 300 RAPN using the early unclamping technique, has demonstrated an average warm ischemia time of 14.7 minutes. The postoperative complication rate has been 18% with only a 1% rate of severe complications. We have had 5 cases of delayed postoperative bleeding, presumably from arteriovenous fistulas, which all occurred after LPN using the standard technique in which early unclamping was not used.

When considering the various approaches to partial nephrectomy, particularly those involving robotic assistance, cost is an important issue. Yu and colleagues[25] analyzed the Nationwide Inpatient Sample and found that, although the costs associated with robotic surgery were higher for all other procedures studied, the median cost of partial nephrectomy did not vary significantly by approach ($15,724 for RALPN, $12401 for LPN, and $11,817 for OPN [$P = .442$]). Ferguson and colleagues[26] performed a direct-cost analysis that showed no difference in total cost between RALPN and LPN ($13,560 vs $13,439, $P = .29$). Laydner and colleagues[27] reported that the increased cost of RALPN due to instrumentation and supplies can be offset by the decreased cost of postoperative hospitalization and more rapid convalescence. However, it is important to note that in addition to the variable cost per case, the cost associated with RALPN is exacerbated when factoring in the acquisition cost of the robotic platform.[10] Alemozoffar and colleagues[28] similarly compared hospital costs of these approaches, factoring in variable costs, fixed costs, and length of hospital stay. The investigators found that the variable costs (operating room [OR] supplies, time, anesthesia, inpatient care) were similar, the OR supplies contributed a greater cost for the minimally invasive approaches, and the inpatient costs were higher for the OPN. They concluded that RALPN and LPN were less costly alternatives to OPN if maintenance costs were not included, the length of stay was ≤ 2 days, and operative time was ≤ 195 and 224 minutes, respectively. As the robotic procedure becomes more efficient and the robotic platform becomes more available and affordable, the differences in cost, previously thought to be a major disadvantage, are becoming more minimal.

Radical Nephrectomy

The advantages of laparoscopic kidney surgery have been apparent for the past 20 years, with numerous centers demonstrating shorter hospital stay, less blood loss, decreased narcotic use, and quicker return to normal activity when compared with open surgery.[29–31] The current recommendation from the European Association of Urology (EAU) for patients with clinical T2 renal tumors, who are not candidates for nephron-sparing surgery, is to undergo a laparoscopic radical nephrectomy, due to the benefits of lower morbidity compared with open nephrectomy.[32] However, because a radical nephrectomy is a purely extirpative procedure, the advantages of robotics (such as the ease of intracorporeal suturing and complex reconstructive maneuvers) are not necessarily beneficial in this setting. Therefore, the general consensus is that robotic assistance is unnecessary when performing a radical nephrectomy.

Gill and colleagues[33] first reported the feasibility of robotic radical nephrectomy (RRN) in the porcine model, followed by Talamini and colleagues[34] reporting the combined human experience of 4 institutions, demonstrating its safety and efficacy. Petros and colleagues[35] described their experience with 101 consecutive cases of RRN and concluded that robotic assistance allowed for consistent outcomes regardless of procedure complexity. However, the main disadvantages to using robotic assistance for radical nephrectomy is the cost of the procedure with no clearly demonstrated improved outcome or extended indications. In 2001, Guillonneau and colleagues[36] evaluated RRN and found the approach failed to demonstrate benefits over the traditional laparoscopic nephrectomy. A literature review by Asimakopoulos and colleagues[37] showed that although RRN is a safe, feasible, and oncologically effective surgical treatment for clinically localized renal cell carcinoma, there was no advantage of the robotic approach over standard laparoscopy and, in fact, the robotic platform added significant expense and operative time to the procedure. According to a study by Yang and colleagues,[38] compared with laparoscopic nephrectomy, RRN conferred $11,267 more in total charges and $4565 in hospital stay charges without improving patient morbidity. On the other hand, a recent application of robotics in the radical nephrectomy setting involves complex cases of renal vein and vena cava tumor thrombus. There have been small series describing complete vena cava control, tumor thrombus removal, and caval reconstruction using robotic assistance.[35,39] It is likely that, in the hands of very experienced robotic surgeons, this approach may become more commonplace. Until clear evidence supporting the superiority of RRN over less expensive extirpative modalities is gathered, laparoscopic nephrectomy will remain the gold standard for uncomplicated renal masses not amenable to NSS.

Pyeloplasty

Ureteropelvic junction obstruction (UPJO) is the most common congenital anomaly of the ureter and long-term success rates greater than 90% have been reported with the open dismembered pyeloplasty. In an effort to reduce the morbidity associated with the open approach, Kavoussi and Peters[40] and Schuessler and colleagues[41] described the first techniques for laparoscopic dismembered pyeloplasty in 1993. Two years later, Peters and colleagues[42] described the first pediatric laparoscopic pyeloplasty. More recently, robotic approaches have been found to be useful for procedures with a considerable amount of intracorporeal suturing and the first robotic pyeloplasty was described by Gettman and colleagues[43] in 2002.

Multiple series and meta-analyses of minimally invasive pyeloplasty, in adults and pediatric populations, demonstrate a low perioperative morbidity and high success rate.[44] Compared with traditional laparoscopy, robotic pyeloplasty offers reduced morbidity, shorter learning curve, enhanced tissue manipulation, and improved visualization.[44,45] The first reported series by Patel[46] emphasized the procedure's minimal morbidity and easy learning process. Furthermore, small series have examined the challenging scenario of secondary redo-robotic pyeloplasty and have shown it to be a feasible operation with good outcomes and acceptable complication rates. Literature comparing adult patients who underwent open pyeloplasty versus laparoscopic pyeloplasty shows that, although associated with a longer operative time, patients undergoing laparoscopic pyeloplasty required less pain medication and had a shorter length of stay. Bansal and colleagues[47] presented a randomized controlled study of patients undergoing open and laparoscopic pyeloplasty. The investigators found that operative time was shorter for the open pyeloplasty group (122 vs 244 minutes, $P<.01$), whereas pain medication requirement and length of hospital stay were decreased in the laparoscopic group (107.14 vs 682.35 mg diclofenac, $P<.01$); (3.1 vs 8.3 days, $P<.01$). When comparing laparoscopic pyeloplasty with robotic pyeloplasty, perioperative complication rates, diuretic scintigraphy-dependent success rates, and length of stay were found to be similar, whereas the operative time in many studies favored the robotic approach.[44,45] Hemal and colleagues[48] reviewed 60 cases of minimally invasive pyeloplasty and found that robotic pyeloplasty was associated with a significantly shorter operative time (98 vs 145 minutes) and equivalent long-term success rates compared with purely laparoscopic pyeloplasty. Overall, the studies suggest that laparoscopic pyeloplasty is a safe and effective minimally invasive approach to UPJO that offers reduced perioperative morbidity. When available, the robotic platform is quickly emerging as a new standard of care in the management of UPJO in adults, offering similar outcomes to the open and laparoscopic approach with increased precision and a shorter learning curve.

ROBOTIC SURGERY OF THE BLADDER
Radical Cystectomy

Bladder cancer is the fourth most commonly diagnosed malignancy in the United States, with an estimated 74,000 cases to be diagnosed in 2015 ultimately leading to 16,000 deaths.[6] Open radical cystectomy (ORC) with urinary diversion is the gold standard for patients with muscle-invasive bladder cancer and for those with high-risk recurrent non–muscle-invasive disease, providing effective long-term oncologic control and disease-free survival.[49] Despite a better understanding of pelvic anatomy and advances in surgical technique, radical cystectomy is still associated with a significant rate of perioperative complications (approximately 60%), with approximately half of these being high-grade complications (Clavien grade 3–5).[50] In an effort to reduce this morbidity, minimally invasive approaches, most notably laparoscopic and robotic, are being increasingly used. Parra and colleagues[51] first described a laparoscopic simple cystectomy in 1992. Using similar techniques, Sanchez de Badajoz and colleagues[52] reported the first laparoscopic radical cystectomy (LRC) the following year and several studies have supported its feasibility. However, this technically challenging procedure was not widely adopted. The first experience with robot-assisted laparoscopic radical cystectomy (RARC) was reported by Menon and colleagues[53] in 2003. More recently, several studies have demonstrated the feasibility of RARC and its use has steadily increased over the past decade.

Generally, ORC is associated with a high risk of complications and outcomes are associated with hospital and surgeon experience. Although randomized controlled trials and meta-analyses examining RARC have demonstrated decreased blood loss, transfusion rate, time to return of bowel function, and length of hospital stay, the mean operative time was increased. When compared with ORC, the postoperative complication rates, positive surgical margins (PSM), lymph node yield, and quality-of-life outcomes have been equivalent or slightly better for patients undergoing RARC. Nix and colleagues[54] compared patients undergoing ORC and RARC in a randomized controlled trial. Although the overall complication rate and mean hospital stay were not significantly different between the 2 groups, and the OR time was increased with RARC (4.2 vs 3.52 hours, $P<.0001$), the investigators found significant differences favoring the robotic group with regard to estimated blood loss (258 vs 575 mL, $P<.0001$), time to flatus (2.3 vs 3.2 days, $P = .0013$), time to bowel movement (3.2 vs 4.3 days, P .0008), and use of in-house morphine equivalent (89 vs 147 mg, $P = .0044$). Additionally, the mean number of lymph nodes removed from the RARC and ORC groups was 19 and 18, respectively, demonstrating the robotic approach to be noninferior to the open cystectomy. Parekh and colleagues[55] performed a pilot prospective randomized clinical trial comparing ORC and RARC. In their analysis, the 2 groups had no significant differences in oncologic outcomes, such as PSM or lymph node yield. The RARC group was noted to have a decreased estimated blood loss when compared with ORC (400 vs 800 mL). They also noted a trend in the RARC patients toward a decreased rate of excessive length of stay (greater than 5 days, 65% vs 90%, $P = .11$) and fewer transfusions (40% vs 50%, $P = .26$). Bochner and colleagues[56] performed the largest randomized prospective trial to date comparing patients undergoing ORC and RARC and found that RARC patients had a lower mean intraoperative blood loss (516 vs 676 mL, $P = .027$), but significantly longer operative time than the ORC group (456 vs 329 minutes, $P<.001$). Postoperative complications, mean hospital stay, quality-of-life outcomes, and pathologic variables, including PSM and lymph node yield, were similar between the groups. Furthermore, when comparing RARC and pure LRC, study has shown decreased transfusion and perioperative complication rates associated with RARC.[49,56–63] This is significant, as perioperative blood transfusion has been linked to perioperative morbidity and predictors of complications following RARC include age, ASA (American Society of Anesthesiologists score) score, Charlson comorbidity index, body mass index, and blood transfusion.[58,64,65] Although these data are encouraging, it is important to note that many studies may suffer from selection bias.

Measures of surgical quality for radical cystectomy include PSM rates and lymph node yields, both of which have implications for oncologic outcomes. A PSM affects local recurrence, increases the risk of metastatic progression, and decreases cancer-specific survival. The literature has demonstrated that rates of PSM between ORC and RARC are equivalent.[49,56,66] In addition, higher lymph node yields are associated with improved cancer-specific and overall survival. Herr and colleagues[67] described a significant increase in mortality in patients with node-positive disease if fewer than 11 lymph nodes were obtained at the time of ORC. Lymphadenectomy not only provides staging information, but is also considered potentially curative in patients with microscopic nodal metastases. Therefore, it is essential that an adequate lymph node dissection be performed at the time of cystectomy. Several studies have supported that an extended lymph node dissection is feasible with robotic assistance and with increasing experience comes improved lymph node yields, as experience is clearly a crucial factor.[49,56,63,66] Long-term study has shown that overall survival, cancer-specific survival, and recurrence-free survival rates following LRC and RARC are similar to that of ORC.[63,68]

An advantage of the robotic platform for many procedures is that it offers the benefits of minimally invasive surgery with the potential for a shortened learning curve. Whereas Pruthi and colleagues[69] failed to demonstrate a difference in perioperative outcomes among the first 50 cases of RARC with extracorporeal diversion, Hayn and colleagues[70] found significant improvements in mean operative time and lymph node yield for their first 164 cases (180 vs 136 minutes, $P<.001$); (16 vs 24 lymph nodes, $P<.001$). In addition, Richards and colleagues[60] demonstrated reduction in overall complication rate from 70% in their first 20 cases to 30% in the second and third 20 cases ($P = .013$). The International Robotic Cystectomy Consortium (IRCC) suggested that 20 operations are needed to reach a plateau operative time and 30 cases are needed to reach a lymph node count greater than 20.

Some have hypothesized that some of the postoperative complications from the procedure result from the significant amount of bowel manipulation during the reconstructive portion of the case, thus advocating for a totally intracorporeal approach. Currently, the vast majority of urinary diversions are performed extracorporeally with approximately 3% of patients undergoing a totally intracorporeal RARC.[71] High-volume centers are just beginning to accumulate data regarding this approach. However, to date, there appears to be no distinct advantage over the standard extracorporeal diversion. Results from the IRCC found similar overall complication rates, however there were significantly fewer gastrointestinal complications in the intracorporeal group (10% vs 23%).[72] Although RARC with intracorporeal diversion is a feasible operation with reasonable outcomes, it is a complex procedure that may be associated with initially increased operative times. Moreover, it really is feasible only when performed by a very experienced robotic team, often requiring multiple attending surgeons experienced in robotics and significant amount of preoperative planning. Thus, its applicability in most clinical settings is debatable. However, some investigators propose that operative time decreases with experience, and a totally intracorporeal approach enhances the benefits seen with minimally invasive techniques, further reducing perioperative morbidity.[59,63,72]

Differences observed in the cost of performing these cases continues to be an issue. Analyses show that for RARC with an ileal conduit, an additional average cost of $1740 was incurred compared with ORC, whereas RARC with an ileal neobladder adds an additional $3920. The additional costs associated with the robot were primarily related to OR costs (eg, robot, supplies, facilities) and physician costs.[56] Additionally, the difference in hospital stay did not appear to offset the additional costs of equipment and longer operative times associated with the robot. Alternatively, Martin and colleagues[73] found that when hospital costs, including length of stay, medications, transfusions, treatment of complications, and related 30-day readmissions were factored in, RARC was 60% less expensive than ORC. To truly identify the cost difference between these approaches, a well-designed randomized controlled trial is necessary comparing experienced robotic surgeons to equally experienced open surgeons.

ROBOTIC SURGERY OF THE PROSTATE
Radical Prostatectomy

Adenocarcinoma of the prostate is the most commonly diagnosed solid organ malignancy and the second-most common cause of cancer death in the United States, with an estimated 220,800 new cases leading to 27,540 deaths in 2015.[6] Because of prostate cancer screening, most prostate cancers are clinically localized at diagnosis. Despite a spectrum of therapeutic options being available, radical prostatectomy has been shown to offer improved overall and disease-specific survival across all D'Amico risk groups.[74] Open radical prostatectomy (ORP) was initially considered the gold standard for the surgical treatment of localized prostate cancer. Hugh Hampton Young performed the first perineal prostatectomy in 1905.[75] Terrence Milin performed the first radical retropubic prostatectomy in 1947.[76] Anatomic studies by Walsh and Donker more clearly established the vasculature, fascial planes, urethral sphincter, and neurovascular bundles and, using this information, Walsh[77] performed the first nerve-sparing radical retropubic prostatectomy in 1982.[77] The establishment of laparoscopy and growing success of less invasive treatment alternatives for prostate cancer led to the first laparoscopic radical prostatectomy (LRP), described by Schuessler and colleagues[78] in 1992. The investigators[78] described their initial series of 9 patients in 1997, stating that although LRP was feasible, it offered no clear advantage over ORP with regard to oncologic control, urinary continence, potency, length of stay, convalescence, and cosmetic result. In addition, operative times were significantly longer, averaging 9.4 hours.[78] Although LRP was thought by many to offer the advantages of minimally invasive surgery, including decreased blood loss and shorter length of stay, it was generally considered a challenging procedure because it involved 2-dimensional visualization, a counterintuitive nature that led to a steep learning curve, and required advanced laparoscopic skills to perform complex tasks such as intracorporeal suturing. These limitations prevented widespread use of the LRP by the average urologist. A dramatic change occurred in the management of prostate cancer, as well as the evolution of robotic surgery, when the first robot-assisted laparoscopic prostatectomy (RALP) was performed in 2000. The improved 3-dimensional visualization and jointed laparoscopic instruments made laparoscopic dissection technically easier, creating widespread surgeon and patient interest in minimally invasive prostatectomy. Binder and Kramer[1] described the first 10 RALP procedures and Menon and colleagues[2] published the first large series in the United States comparing the robotic and open approaches in 2002. These series and subsequent reports led to the widespread rapid acceptance of the RALP as a safe and efficacious treatment option for clinically localized prostate cancer. In fact, it is likely that more than 80% of all radical prostatectomies will be performed robotically by 2020.[79]

Investigators have studied the perioperative outcomes associated with RALP. The goal of minimally invasive surgery is to reduce postoperative morbidity and multiple meta-analyses have demonstrated that laparoscopic, particularly robot-assisted, prostatectomies were associated with significantly less operative blood loss, fewer transfusions, shorter hospital stay, and fewer intraoperative complications.[80–82] In addition to improved visualization and control of the dorsal venous complex, an advantage of the laparoscopic approach is the positive pressure created by the pneumoperitoneum, which results in a tamponade effect, reducing venous and capillary bleeding during the operation and decreased blood loss during the case. Trinh and colleagues[79] found that men who underwent RALP had a lower transfusion rate, were less likely to experience a perioperative complication, and had a decreased rate of prolonged length of stay than patients who underwent ORP. Similarly, an analysis of the Surveillance, Epidemiology, and End Results (SEER) Medicare data comparing RALP to ORP showed a lower rate of transfusion and lesser likelihood of prolonged length of stay.[83] Studies have shown that the postoperative pain experienced by those who undergo ORP and RALP is similar. This is partially because the infraumbilical midline muscle-splitting incision used for an ORP is generally less painful than those in the upper abdomen because of the latter's involvement with respiration.[75] On the other hand, Pierorazio and colleagues[84] evaluated a single-institution experience over a 20-year period and showed that those who underwent RALP were more likely to experience a prolonged length of stay, develop an ileus, have a urine leak, and require a blood transfusion when compared with ORP. This study had some significant biases, most importantly being the comparison of early experiences with minimally invasive surgery to that of seasoned open surgeons from Johns Hopkins. Additionally, Eastham[85] analyzed the SEER Medicare database and showed that postoperative morbidity was lower in patients who underwent their operation by very high-volume surgeons at very high-volume hospitals. These studies illustrate the importance of surgeon experience, hospital experience, and surgical approach in determining outcomes following prostatectomy. In studies from centers that specialize in RALP, significantly less blood loss and lower transfusion rates have been noted, although overall complication rates are similar in many centers.[86,87]

Oncologic control is the most important outcome in the surgical treatment of cancer. In addition to cancer-specific and overall mortality, biochemical recurrence (BCR) and the rate of PSM have been used as surrogate indicators to measure primary cancer control when evaluating different surgical approaches to prostate cancer. Interestingly, there are no randomized controlled trials assessing oncologic control between RALP and ORP. Furthermore, surgeon partiality and patient preference make performing a randomized controlled trial very difficult in the United States. Retrospective reviews from high-volume centers provide us with most of the data on the subject, although these studies may be limited by selection bias, may lack adequate power, and depend on the experience of one or a few skilled surgeons, so their findings may not be generalizable. Numerous centers have compared the rates of PSM and BCR between ORP and RALP and it is important to note that most studies have shown equivalent outcomes.[74,75] This may be partially attributable to adjustments in surgical technique over the years with regard to apical dissection and nerve-sparing, tailoring the dissection to the location and degree of cancer present.

Functional outcomes are also important in evaluating the surgical approach to prostate cancer. Urinary continence and erectile function are the 2 outcomes most affected after prostatectomy. Assessment of these outcomes is often challenging, as there is no consensus for their definition or management. With regard to urinary continence, commonly defined as requiring 0 to 1 pad per day, some studies have shown that robotic assistance has led to an earlier recovery of continence with at least equivalent long-term outcomes.[74,75,86] In their analysis comparing outcomes of patients undergoing ORP, LRP, and RALP, Frota and colleagues[88] reported continence rates of 90% to 92%, 82% to 96%, and 95% to 96%, respectively. In their largest reported ORP series, including 3477 patients, the investigators[88] describe an overall 93% continence rate. Reviewing 1300 patients undergoing LRP, Stolzenburg and colleagues[89] reported a continence rate of 68% at 3 months, 84% at 6 months, and 92% at 12-month follow-up. In their robotic series, Ahlering and colleagues[90] reported a continence rate of 88% at 12-month follow-up of 670 patients. Similarly, in each of their series of more than 1100 patients, Menon and colleagues[91] and Smith and colleagues[92] reported continence rates following RALP of 96% and 97%. Di Pierro and colleagues[93] compared continence rates between those undergoing ORP and RALP. The investigators[93] found improved 3-month continence after RALP compared with ORP (95% vs 83%, $P = .003$), although this difference was not significant at 12 months (89 vs 80%, $P = .092$). Tewari and colleagues[94] also found that patients who underwent RALP recovered urinary continence more quickly than those who underwent ORP (44 vs 160 days, $P<.05$). Geraerts and colleagues[95] examined continence rates in ORP and RALP patients at 1, 3, 6, and 12 months, only noting a significant difference at 1 month. At 12 months, the continence rates were 96% and 97%, respectively, although the time to continence was significantly shorter in the RALP group (16 vs 46 days, $P = .026$). Numerous operative techniques have been developed to improve urinary control by reducing injury to the urinary sphincter mechanism and preserving urinary continence. Ramirez and colleagues[74] reviewed some of these technical adjustments, including bladder neck preservation, periurethral suspension, periurethral reconstruction, preservation of urethral length, preservation of the puboprostatic ligaments and endopelvic fascia, and use of locoregional hypothermia.

In 1983, Walsh and Mostwin[77] described the nerve-sparing technique during ORP to improve erectile function postoperatively. They demonstrated that erectile dysfunction following a prostatectomy was secondary to injury of the neurovascular bundles on the posterolateral aspect of the prostate. The robotic platform, as well as improvement in our understanding of pelvic neuroanatomy, has allowed for many adjustments in prostatic dissection with the goal of improving postoperative potency rates. Robotic nerve-sparing using the Vattikuti Institute technique with preservation of the "veil of Aphrodite" and lateral prostatic fascia was first described by Menon and colleagues[2] in 2002. Tewari and colleagues[96] developed a grading system to assess the degree of nerve-sparing and performed retrospective validation of the technique. Additionally, use of athermal dissection and traction-free techniques avoids destruction of the nerve and nerve sheath, improving recovery and functional outcomes. Maximal nerve-sparing can be achieved by following the plane between the prostatic capsule and the multilayer tissue of the prostatic fascia, which is recommended for sexually active and functional men without comorbidities and limited-risk disease. Partial nerve-sparing, obtained by following the planes within the multilayer tissue of the prostatic fascia, is recommended for preoperatively potent men without comorbidities and localized intermediate or high-risk disease. Finally, those patients with significant erectile dysfunction, no interest in sexual activity, or a high suspicion of extraprostatic disease should undergo a non–nerve-sparing operation.[97] It is important to keep in mind that one must balance improvement in postoperative erectile function with maintaining oncologic control. A review by Ficarra and colleagues[98] showed that for patients undergoing an RALP, the predictors of postoperative potency were age, baseline erectile function, and the presence of comorbidities. Some studies examining erectile function after prostatectomy have found a higher potency rate at 12 months for patients who underwent an RALP when compared with those who underwent ORP. In a cumulative analysis of multiple single-institution studies comparing potency rates following radical prostatectomy, the 12-month potency was 52.2% after ORP and 75.8% after RALP ($P = .02$).[86] Furthermore, Tewari and colleagues[94] found a shorter time to potency recovery after RALP than after ORP (180 vs 440 days, $P<.05$); however, it is important to note that these are retrospective studies at single tertiary institutions, using definitions of potency that are often not agreed on, and evaluated patients who underwent an ideal, bilateral nerve-sparing procedure, making comparison with ORP challenging. Therefore, when comparing the outcomes of RALP experts to ORP experts, the sexual function outcomes are likely comparable and largely dependent on the expertise of the surgeon.[85]

The learning curve for RALP has been studied extensively. Continued experience and technical refinements of the procedure lead to improved operative parameters and outcomes. Menon and colleagues[2] and Ahlering and colleagues[99] demonstrated the successful transfer of open surgical skills to the robotic platform, and were able to accomplish comparable surgical times in 18 cases and 12 cases, respectively. Similarly, Patel and colleagues,[100] with fellowship training in laparoscopy, reported comparable surgical times and a learning curve of approximately 20 to 25 cases. In addition, Badani and colleagues[101] examined their experience with RALP over a 6-year period (2766 cases), comparing their first 200 cases to the most recent 200 cases. The investigators[101] noted that the mean console time decreased by 19% (121 vs 97 minutes, $P<.05$), despite a 100% increase in previous abdominal surgery history that frequently required adhesiolysis and an increase in the proportion of patients with intermediate-risk and high-risk disease. The investigators[101] also showed a decline in the PSM rates in the more recent cohort, attributed to increased experience of the technical aspects of the robotic surgery, growing familiarity of the laparoscopic anatomy, and developments in the pathologic reporting and processing. On the other hand, the learning curve for LRP is significantly longer, requiring 40 to 60 cases for an experienced laparoscopist and 80 to 100 cases for a laparoscopically naïve surgeon, clearly demonstrating that the robotic platform significantly shortens the learning curve for the minimally invasive prostatectomy.[102–104]

Cost is considered one of the main disadvantages to the robot-assisted approach to prostatectomy. Even when considering the possible shorter hospital stay, RALP is still more expensive than ORP. Lotan and colleagues[105] reported that the ORP had a cost advantage of approximately $487 over the LRP, and $1726 over the RALP. However, recent cost-effective analyses of RALP have indicated that cost equivalence may be achieved between ORP and RALP at high-volume centers where 10 or more cases are performed per week.[103]

Simple Prostatectomy

Benign prostatic hyperplasia (BPH) is a highly prevalent condition among older men, affecting nearly 6.5 million white men aged 50 to 79 years in the United States and 1.1 billion men worldwide.[106,107] Although the most common forms of treatment for symptomatic BPH include watchful waiting, oral medications, and minimally invasive endoscopic surgery such as the transurethral resection of prostate (TURP), open simple prostatectomy (OSP) is considered a standard for patients with larger glands (>80 mL). The operation involves surgical enucleation of the BPH adenoma and has demonstrated improved outcomes with respect to International Prostate Symptom Score (IPSS), urinary flow, quality of life, and postvoid residual (PVR).[108] However, although the open operation may be more effective than medical therapy or a TURP, it can be associated with substantial risks of bleeding, transfusion, prolonged hospital stay, and other complications. Over the past decade, studies have shown that a minimally invasive approach to simple prostatectomy, particularly robot-assisted simple prostatectomy (RASP), may be a viable alternative for these patients.[109–111]

In 1900, Peter Freyer described the first open simple transvesical prostatectomy for BPH.[112] Several decades later, Terrence Millin introduced an effective transcapsular technique.[113] Medical therapy has since refined the indications for surgery and advances in surgical technique have reduced the incidence of perioperative complications and improved long-term functional outcomes.[109] Mariano and colleagues[114] reported the first laparoscopic simple prostatectomy in 2002. With advancements in robotic technology and growing experience with the RALP, Sotelo and colleagues[115] reported the first RASP in 2008, demonstrating that it was a feasible and reproducible procedure with an acceptable complication rate.

There have been several published series on RASP, which have shown it to be consistently associated with improved cosmesis, longer operative times, lower rates of complications, fewer transfusions, and decreased hospital stay when compared with OSP.[111,116] Serretta and colleagues[117] examined 1804 patients who underwent OSP and reported severe bleeding in 11.6%, blood transfusions in 8.2%, sepsis in 8.6%, median hospital stay of 7 days, and reintervention within 2 years (mainly from bladder neck stenosis) in 3.6% of patients. Similarly, Varkarakis and colleagues[118] reported a transfusion rate of 6.8% in the 232 cases of OSP they reviewed. Gratzke and colleagues[119] analyzed the perioperative outcomes of 902 patients undergoing OSP, reporting a mean operative time of 80.8 minutes, overall complication rate of 17.3%, bleeding requiring transfusion in 7.5%, urinary tract infection in 5.1%, and surgical revision due to severe bleeding in 3.7% of patients. The same benefits of the robotic platform observed in RALP (improved visualization, ergonomics, dexterity, and learning curve) also apply to the RASP, resulting in improved outcomes. In 2015, Autorino and colleagues[120] reviewed the outcomes of 1330 consecutive minimally invasive simple prostatectomy cases, including 843 laparoscopic simple prostatectomies and 487 RASP cases. For patients undergoing a RASP, the investigators[120] reported a median operative time of 154.5 minutes, median estimated blood loss of 200 mL, transfusion requirement in 3.5%, median length of stay of 2 days, and overall postoperative complication rate of 16.6% (mostly low-grade, Clavien 1–2). In addition, cost analysis by Matei and colleagues[121] revealed that charges incurred for RASP were 30% less than those for OSP, largely owing to the decreased hospital stay. Although long-term comparative studies to alternative treatment modalities have yet to be published, short-term efficacy outcomes, including IPSS, urinary flow, and resolution of urinary retention and infections have been comparable to published series of OSP.[111,116] RASP has been shown to be a safe and effective treatment option, with improved perioperative outcomes and cost, for the management of symptomatic BPH in patients who are otherwise candidates for OSP.

SUMMARY

As robotic technology continues to evolve, there is likely to be a continued shift in the management of urologic diseases. Innovation has led to improved outcomes while maintaining well-established surgical principles. The robotic platform offers the advantages of minimally invasive surgery with a decreased learning curve compared with the purely laparoscopic approach. Because much of the data we have today are based on retrospective reviews and meta-analyses with inherent limitations, there is a need for further prospective, multicenter, long-term randomized controlled trials. With increased surgeon experience and improved cost-effectiveness, the robot will be increasingly used for complex procedures. It is important to note that although the benefits seen with this technology are very encouraging, long-term surgical outcomes result from a combination of surgeon experience, technique, and operative approach.

REFERENCES

1. Binder J, Kramer W. Robotically-assisted laparoscopic radical prostatectomy. BJU Int 2001;87:408–10.
2. Menon M, Shrivastava A, Tewari A, et al. Laparoscopic and robot assisted radical prostatectomy: establishment of a structured program and preliminary analysis of outcomes. J Urol 2002;168:945–9.
3. Ng AT, Tam PC. Current status of robot-assisted surgery. Hong Kong Med J 2014;20:241–50.
4. Jain S, Gautam G. Robotics in urologic oncology. J Minim Access Surg 2015; 11:40–4.
5. Intuitive Surgical. da Vinci Surgical System. Intuitive Surgical, Inc. 2015. Available at: www.intuitivesurgical.com/products/davinci_surgical_system/. Accessed March 22, 2016.
6. Siegel RL, Miller KD, Jemal A. Cancer statistics. CA Cancer J Clin 2015; 2015(65):5–29.
7. Go AS, Chertow GM, Fan D, et al. Chronic kidney disease and the risks of death, cardiovascular events, and hospitalization. N Engl J Med 2004;351:1296–305.
8. Van Poppel H, Becker F, Cadeddu JA, et al. Treatment of localised renal cell carcinoma. Eur Urol 2011;60:662–72.
9. Winfield HN, Donovan JF, Godet AS, et al. Laparoscopic partial nephrectomy: initial case report for benign disease. J Endourol 1993;7:521–6.
10. Laviana AA, Hu JC. Current controversies and challenges in robotic-assisted, laparoscopic, and open partial nephrectomies. World J Urol 2014;32:591–6.
11. Wu Z, Li M, Liu B, et al. Robotic versus open partial nephrectomy: a systematic review and meta-analysis. PLoS One 2014;9:e94878.
12. Abouassaly R, Alibhai SM, Tomlinson G, et al. Unintended consequences of laparoscopic surgery on partial nephrectomy for kidney cancer. J Urol 2010; 183:467–72.
13. Gettman MT, Blute ML, Chow GK, et al. Robotic-assisted laparoscopic partial nephrectomy: technique and initial clinical experience with DaVinci robotic system. Urology 2004;64:914–8.
14. Ellison JS, Montgomery JS, Wolf JS Jr, et al. A matched comparison of perioperative outcomes of a single laparoscopic surgeon versus a multisurgeon robot-assisted cohort for partial nephrectomy. J Urol 2012;188:45–50.

15. Kaouk JH, Hillyer SP, Autorino R, et al. 252 robotic partial nephrectomies: evolving renorrhaphy technique and surgical outcomes at a single institution. Urology 2011;78:1338–44.
16. Masson-Lecomte A, Yates DR, Hupertan V, et al. A prospective comparison of the pathologic and surgical outcomes obtained after elective treatment of renal cell carcinoma by open or robot-assisted partial nephrectomy. Urol Oncol 2013; 31:924–9.
17. Benway BM, Bhayani SB, Rogers CG, et al. Robot assisted partial nephrectomy versus laparoscopic partial nephrectomy for renal tumors: a multi-institutional analysis of perioperative outcomes. J Urol 2009;182:866–72.
18. Wang AJ, Bhayani SB. Robotic partial nephrectomy versus laparoscopic partial nephrectomy for renal cell carcinoma: single-surgeon analysis of >100 consecutive procedures. Urology 2009;73:306–10.
19. Wang L, Lee BR. Robotic partial nephrectomy: current technique and outcomes. Int J Urol 2013;20:848–59.
20. Bi L, Zhang C, Li K, et al. Robotic partial nephrectomy for renal tumors larger than 4 cm: a systematic review and meta-analysis. PLoS One 2013;8:e75050.
21. Klatte T, Ficarra V, Gratzke C, et al. A literature review of renal surgical anatomy and surgical strategies for partial nephrectomy. Eur Urol 2015;68:980–92.
22. Uzzo RG, Novick AC. Nephron sparing surgery for renal tumors: indications, techniques and outcomes. J Urol 2001;166:6–18.
23. Sutherland SE, Resnick MI, Maclennan GT, et al. Does the size of the surgical margin in partial nephrectomy for renal cell cancer really matter? J Urol 2002; 167:61–4.
24. Thompson RH, Lane BR, Lohse CM, et al. Every minute counts when the renal hilum is clamped during partial nephrectomy. Eur Urol 2010;58:340–5.
25. Yu HY, Hevelone ND, Lipsitz SR, et al. Use, costs and comparative effectiveness of robotic assisted, laparoscopic and open urological surgery. J Urol 2012;187: 1392–8.
26. Ferguson JE 3rd, Goyal RK, Raynor MC, et al. Cost analysis of robot-assisted laparoscopic versus hand-assisted laparoscopic partial nephrectomy. J Endourol 2012;26:1030–7.
27. Laydner H, Isac W, Autorino R, et al. Single institutional cost analysis of 325 robotic, laparoscopic, and open partial nephrectomies. Urology 2013;81:533–8.
28. Alemozaffar M, Chang SL, Kacker R, et al. Comparing costs of robotic, laparoscopic, and open partial nephrectomy. J Endourol 2013;27:560–5.
29. Kavoussi LR, Kerbl K, Capelouto CC, et al. Laparoscopic nephrectomy for renal neoplasms. Urology 1993;42:603–9.
30. Clayman RV, Kavoussi LR, Soper NJ, et al. Laparoscopic nephrectomy: initial case report. J Urol 1991;146:278–82.
31. Dunn MD, Portis AJ, Shalhav AL, et al. Laparoscopic versus open radical nephrectomy: a 9-year experience. J Urol 2000;164:1153–9.
32. Ljungberg B, Bensalah K, Canfield S, et al. EAU guidelines on renal cell carcinoma: 2014 update. Eur Urol 2015;67:913–24.
33. Gill IS, Sung GT, Hsu TH, et al. Robotic remote laparoscopic nephrectomy and adrenalectomy: the initial experience. J Urol 2000;164:2082–5.
34. Talamini MA, Chapman S, Horgan S, et al. A prospective analysis of 211 robotic-assisted surgical procedures. Surg Endosc 2003;17:1521–4.
35. Petros FG, Angell JE, Abaza R. Outcomes of robotic nephrectomy including highest-complexity cases: largest series to date and literature review. Urology 2015;85:1352–8.

36. Guillonneau B, Jayet C, Tewari A, et al. Robot assisted laparoscopic nephrectomy. J Urol 2001;166:200–1.

37. Asimakopoulos AD, Miano R, Annino F, et al. Robotic radical nephrectomy for renal cell carcinoma: a systematic review. BMC Urol 2014;14:75.

38. Yang DY, Monn MF, Bahler CD, et al. Does robotic assistance confer an economic benefit during laparoscopic radical nephrectomy? J Urol 2014;192:671–6.

39. Abaza R. Robotic surgery and minimally invasive management of renal tumors with vena caval extension. Curr Opin Urol 2011;21:104–9.

40. Kavoussi LR, Peters CA. Laparoscopic pyeloplasty. J Urol 1993;150:1891–4.

41. Schuessler WW, Grune MT, Tecuanhuey LV, et al. Laparoscopic dismembered pyeloplasty. J Urol 1993;150:1795–9.

42. Peters CA, Schlussel RN, Retik AB. Pediatric laparoscopic dismembered pyeloplasty. J Urol 1995;153:1962–5.

43. Gettman MT, Neururer R, Bartsch G, et al. Anderson-Hynes dismembered pyeloplasty performed using the da Vinci robotic system. Urology 2002;60:509–13.

44. Autorino R, Eden C, El-Ghoneimi A, et al. Robot-assisted and laparoscopic repair of ureteropelvic junction obstruction: a systematic review and meta-analysis. Eur Urol 2014;65:430–52.

45. Ekin RG, Celik O, Ilbey YO. An up-to-date overview of minimally invasive treatment methods in ureteropelvic junction obstruction. Cent European J Urol 2015;68:245–51.

46. Patel V. Robotic-assisted laparoscopic dismembered pyeloplasty. Urology 2005;66:45–9.

47. Bansal P, Gupta A, Mongha R, et al. Laparoscopic versus open pyeloplasty: comparison of two surgical approaches—a single centre experience of three years. Indian J Surg 2011;73:264–7.

48. Hemal AK, Mukherjee S, Singh K. Laparoscopic pyeloplasty versus robotic pyeloplasty for ureteropelvic junction obstruction: a series of 60 cases performed by a single surgeon. Can J Urol 2010;17:5012–6.

49. Tang K, Xia D, Li H, et al. Robotic vs. open radical cystectomy in bladder cancer: a systematic review and meta-analysis. Eur J Surg Oncol 2014;40:1399–411.

50. Shabsigh A, Korets R, Vora KC, et al. Defining early morbidity of radical cystectomy for patients with bladder cancer using a standardized reporting methodology. Eur Urol 2009;55:164–74.

51. Parra RO, Andrus CH, Jones JP, et al. Laparoscopic cystectomy: initial report on a new treatment for the retained bladder. J Urol 1992;148:1140–4.

52. Sanchez de Badajoz E, Gallego Perales JL, Reche Rosado A, et al. Radical cystectomy and laparoscopic ileal conduit. Arch Esp Urol 1993;46:621–4 [in Spanish].

53. Menon M, Hemal AK, Tewari A, et al. Nerve-sparing robot-assisted radical cystoprostatectomy and urinary diversion. BJU Int 2003;92:232–6.

54. Nix J, Smith A, Kurpad R, et al. Prospective randomized controlled trial of robotic versus open radical cystectomy for bladder cancer: perioperative and pathologic results. Eur Urol 2010;57:196–201.

55. Parekh DJ, Messer J, Fitzgerald J, et al. Perioperative outcomes and oncologic efficacy from a pilot prospective randomized clinical trial of open versus robotic assisted radical cystectomy. J Urol 2013;189:474–9.

56. Bochner BH, Dalbagni G, Sjoberg DD, et al. Comparing open radical cystectomy and robot-assisted laparoscopic radical cystectomy: a randomized clinical trial. Eur Urol 2015;67:1042–50.
57. Orvieto MA, DeCastro GJ, Trinh QD, et al. Oncological and functional outcomes after robot-assisted radical cystectomy: critical review of current status. Urology 2011;78:977–84.
58. Novara G, Catto JW, Wilson T, et al. Systematic review and cumulative analysis of perioperative outcomes and complications after robot-assisted radical cystectomy. Eur Urol 2015;67:376–401.
59. Collins JW, Wiklund NP. Totally intracorporeal robot-assisted radical cystectomy: optimizing total outcomes. BJU Int 2014;114:326–33.
60. Richards KA, Kader K, Hemal AK. Robotic radical cystectomy: where are we today, where will we be tomorrow? ScientificWorldJournal 2010;10:2215–27.
61. Aboumohamed AA, Raza SJ, Al-Daghmin A, et al. Health-related quality of life outcomes after robot-assisted and open radical cystectomy using a validated bladder-specific instrument: a multi-institutional study. Urology 2014;83:1300–8.
62. Ishii H, Rai BP, Stolzenburg JU, et al. Robotic or open radical cystectomy, which is safer? A systematic review and meta-analysis of comparative studies. J Endourol 2014;28:1215–23.
63. Patel R, Szymaniak J, Radadia K, et al. Controversies in robotics: open versus robotic radical cystectomy. Clin Genitourin Cancer 2015;13:421–7.
64. Bostrom PJ, Kossi J, Laato M, et al. Risk factors for mortality and morbidity related to radical cystectomy. BJU Int 2009;103:191–6.
65. Lowrance WT, Rumohr JA, Chang SS, et al. Contemporary open radical cystectomy: analysis of perioperative outcomes. J Urol 2008;179:1313–8 [discussion: 1318].
66. Liss MA, Kader AK. Robotic-assisted laparoscopic radical cystectomy: history, techniques and outcomes. World J Urol 2013;31:489–97.
67. Herr HW, Bochner BH, Dalbagni G, et al. Impact of the number of lymph nodes retrieved on outcome in patients with muscle invasive bladder cancer. J Urol 2002;167:1295–8.
68. Snow-Lisy DC, Campbell SC, Gill IS, et al. Robotic and laparoscopic radical cystectomy for bladder cancer: long-term oncologic outcomes. Eur Urol 2014; 65:193–200.
69. Pruthi RS, Smith A, Wallen EM. Evaluating the learning curve for robot-assisted laparoscopic radical cystectomy. J Endourol 2008;22:2469–74.
70. Hayn MH, Hellenthal NJ, Seixas-Mikelus SA, et al. Is patient outcome compromised during the initial experience with robot-assisted radical cystectomy? Results of 164 consecutive cases. BJU Int 2011;108:882–7.
71. Smith AB, Raynor M, Amling CL, et al. Multi-institutional analysis of robotic radical cystectomy for bladder cancer: perioperative outcomes and complications in 227 patients. J Laparoendosc Adv Surg Tech A 2012;22:17–21.
72. Ahmed K, Khan SA, Hayn MH, et al. Analysis of intracorporeal compared with extracorporeal urinary diversion after robot-assisted radical cystectomy: results from the International Robotic Cystectomy Consortium. Eur Urol 2014;65:340–7.
73. Martin AD, Nunez RN, Castle EP. Robot-assisted radical cystectomy versus open radical cystectomy: a complete cost analysis. Urology 2011;77:621–5.
74. Ramirez D, Zargar H, Caputo P, et al. Robotic-assisted laparoscopic prostatectomy: an update on functional and oncologic outcomes, techniques, and advancements in technology. J Surg Oncol 2015;112(7):746–52.

75. Finkelstein J, Eckersberger E, Sadri H, et al. Open versus laparoscopic versus robot-assisted laparoscopic prostatectomy: the European and US experience. Rev Urol 2010;12:35–43.

76. Perrier C. Mes premières prostatectomies rétropubiennes (opération de Millin). Praxis 1947;36:315.

77. Walsh PC, Mostwin JL. Radical prostatectomy and cystoprostatectomy with preservation of potency. Results using a new nerve-sparing technique. Br J Urol 1984;56:694–7.

78. Schuessler WW, Schulam PG, Clayman RV, et al. Laparoscopic radical prostatectomy: initial short-term experience. Urology 1997;50:854–7.

79. Trinh QD, Sammon J, Sun M, et al. Perioperative outcomes of robot-assisted radical prostatectomy compared with open radical prostatectomy: results from the nationwide inpatient sample. Eur Urol 2012;61:679–85.

80. Parsons JK, Bennett JL. Outcomes of retropubic, laparoscopic, and robotic-assisted prostatectomy. Urology 2008;72:412–6.

81. Coelho RF, Rocco B, Patel MB, et al. Retropubic, laparoscopic, and robot-assisted radical prostatectomy: a critical review of outcomes reported by high-volume centers. J Endourol 2010;24:2003–15.

82. Tewari A, Sooriakumaran P, Bloch DA, et al. Positive surgical margin and perioperative complication rates of primary surgical treatments for prostate cancer: a systematic review and meta-analysis comparing retropubic, laparoscopic, and robotic prostatectomy. Eur Urol 2012;62:1–15.

83. Gandaglia G, Sammon JD, Chang SL, et al. Comparative effectiveness of robot-assisted and open radical prostatectomy in the postdissemination era. J Clin Oncol 2014;32:1419–26.

84. Pierorazio PM, Mullins JK, Ross AE, et al. Trends in immediate perioperative morbidity and delay in discharge after open and minimally invasive radical prostatectomy (RP): a 20-year institutional experience. BJU Int 2013;112:45–53.

85. Eastham JA. Do high-volume hospitals and surgeons provide better care in urologic oncology? Urol Oncol 2009;27:417–21.

86. Eifler JB, Cookson MS. Best evidence regarding the superiority or inferiority of robot-assisted radical prostatectomy. Urol Clin North Am 2014;41:493–502.

87. Raynor MC, Pruthi RS. Robot-assisted surgery: applications in urology. Open Access J Urol 2010;2:85–9.

88. Frota R, Turna B, Barros R, et al. Comparison of radical prostatectomy techniques: open, laparoscopic and robotic assisted. Int Braz J Urol 2008;34:259–68 [discussion: 268–9].

89. Stolzenburg JU, Rabenalt R, Do M, et al. Endoscopic extraperitoneal radical prostatectomy: the University of Leipzig experience of 1,300 cases. World J Urol 2007;25:45–51.

90. Ahlering TE, Gordon A, Morales B, et al. Preserving continence during robotic prostatectomy. Curr Urol Rep 2013;14(1):52–8.

91. Menon M, Shrivastava A, Kaul S, et al. Vattikuti Institute prostatectomy: contemporary technique and analysis of results. Eur Urol 2007;51:648–57 [discussion: 657–8].

92. Smith JA Jr, Chan RC, Chang SS, et al. A comparison of the incidence and location of positive surgical margins in robotic assisted laparoscopic radical prostatectomy and open retropubic radical prostatectomy. J Urol 2007;178:2385–9 [discussion: 2389–90].

93. Di Pierro GB, Baumeister P, Stucki P, et al. A prospective trial comparing consecutive series of open retropubic and robot-assisted laparoscopic radical prostatectomy in a centre with a limited caseload. Eur Urol 2011;59:1–6.

94. Tewari A, Srivasatava A, Menon M. Members of the VIPT. A prospective comparison of radical retropubic and robot-assisted prostatectomy: experience in one institution. BJU Int 2003;92:205–10.

95. Geraerts I, Van Poppel H, Devoogdt N, et al. Prospective evaluation of urinary incontinence, voiding symptoms and quality of life after open and robot-assisted radical prostatectomy. BJU Int 2013;112:936–43.

96. Tewari AK, Srivastava A, Huang MW, et al. Anatomical grades of nerve sparing: a risk-stratified approach to neural-hammock sparing during robot-assisted radical prostatectomy (RARP). BJU Int 2011;108:984–92.

97. Montorsi F, Wilson TG, Rosen RC, et al. Best practices in robot-assisted radical prostatectomy: recommendations of the Pasadena Consensus Panel. Eur Urol 2012;62:368–81.

98. Ficarra V, Novara G, Ahlering TE, et al. Systematic review and meta-analysis of studies reporting potency rates after robot-assisted radical prostatectomy. Eur Urol 2012;62:418–30.

99. Ahlering TE, Skarecky D, Lee D, et al. Successful transfer of open surgical skills to a laparoscopic environment using a robotic interface: initial experience with laparoscopic radical prostatectomy. J Urol 2003;170:1738–41.

100. Patel VR, Tully AS, Holmes R, et al. Robotic radical prostatectomy in the community setting–the learning curve and beyond: initial 200 cases. J Urol 2005;174: 269–72.

101. Badani KK, Kaul S, Menon M. Evolution of robotic radical prostatectomy: assessment after 2766 procedures. Cancer 2007;110:1951–8.

102. Ahlering TE. Robotic versus laparoscopic radical prostatectomy. Nat Clin Pract Urol 2004;1:58–9.

103. Patel HR, Linares A, Joseph JV. Robotic and laparoscopic surgery: cost and training. Surg Oncol 2009;18:242–6.

104. Guillonneau B, el-Fettouh H, Baumert H, et al. Laparoscopic radical prostatectomy: oncological evaluation after 1,000 cases at Montsouris Institute. J Urol 2003;169:1261–6.

105. Lotan Y, Cadeddu JA, Gettman MT. The new economics of radical prostatectomy: cost comparison of open, laparoscopic and robot assisted techniques. J Urol 2004;172:1431–5.

106. Wei JT, Calhoun E, Jacobsen SJ. Urologic diseases in America project: benign prostatic hyperplasia. J Urol 2008;179:S75–80.

107. Irwin DE, Kopp ZS, Agatep B, et al. Worldwide prevalence estimates of lower urinary tract symptoms, overactive bladder, urinary incontinence and bladder outlet obstruction. BJU Int 2011;108:1132–8.

108. Ou R, You M, Tang P, et al. A randomized trial of transvesical prostatectomy versus transurethral resection of the prostate for prostate greater than 80 mL. Urology 2010;76:958–61.

109. Lucca I, Shariat SF, Hofbauer SL, et al. Outcomes of minimally invasive simple prostatectomy for benign prostatic hyperplasia: a systematic review and meta-analysis. World J Urol 2015;33:563–70.

110. Banapour P, Patel N, Kane CJ, et al. Robotic-assisted simple prostatectomy: a systematic review and report of a single institution case series. Prostate Cancer Prostatic Dis 2014;17:1–5.

111. Patel ND, Parsons JK. Robotic-assisted simple prostatectomy: is there evidence to go beyond the experimental stage? Curr Urol Rep 2014;15:443.

112. Freyer PJ. A new method of performing perineal prostatectomy. Br Med J 1900; 1:698–9.

113. Millin T. The surgery of prostatic obstructions. Ir J Med Sci 1947;(257):185–9.

114. Mariano MB, Graziottin TM, Tefilli MV. Laparoscopic prostatectomy with vascular control for benign prostatic hyperplasia. J Urol 2002;167:2528–9.

115. Sotelo R, Clavijo R, Carmona O, et al. Robotic simple prostatectomy. J Urol 2008;179:513–5.

116. Sosnowski R, Borkowski T, Chlosta P, et al. Endoscopic simple prostatectomy. Cent European J Urol 2014;67:377–84.

117. Serretta V, Morgia G, Fondacaro L, et al. Open prostatectomy for benign prostatic enlargement in southern Europe in the late 1990s: a contemporary series of 1800 interventions. Urology 2002;60:623–7.

118. Varkarakis I, Kyriakakis Z, Delis A, et al. Long-term results of open transvesical prostatectomy from a contemporary series of patients. Urology 2004;64:306–10.

119. Gratzke C, Schlenker B, Seitz M, et al. Complications and early postoperative outcome after open prostatectomy in patients with benign prostatic enlargement: results of a prospective multicenter study. J Urol 2007;177:1419–22.

120. Autorino R, Zargar H, Mariano MB, et al. Perioperative outcomes of robotic and laparoscopic simple prostatectomy: a European-American multi-institutional analysis. Eur Urol 2015;68:86–94.

121. Matei DV, Brescia A, Mazzoleni F, et al. Robot-assisted simple prostatectomy (RASP): does it make sense? BJU Int 2012;110:E972–9.

Index

Note: Page numbers of article titles are in **boldface** type.

Printed and bound by CPI Group (UK) Ltd, Croydon, CR0 4YY

07/10/2024

01040504-0007